PSYCHOLOGY

for Nurses and Health Professionals

Second edition

RICHARD GROSS
NANCY KINNISON

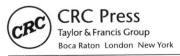 **CRC Press**
Taylor & Francis Group
Boca Raton London New York

CRC Press is an imprint of the
Taylor & Francis Group, an **informa** business

CRC Press
Taylor & Francis Group
6000 Broken Sound Parkway NW, Suite 300
Boca Raton, FL 33487-2742

© 2014 by Taylor & Francis Group, LLC
CRC Press is an imprint of Taylor & Francis Group, an Informa business

No claim to original U.S. Government works

Printed on acid-free paper
Version Date: 20130606

International Standard Book Number-13: 978-1-4441-7992-7 (Paperback)

This book contains information obtained from authentic and highly regarded sources. While all reasonable efforts have been made to publish reliable data and information, neither the author[s] nor the publisher can accept any legal responsibility or liability for any errors or omissions that may be made. The publishers wish to make clear that any views or opinions expressed in this book by individual editors, authors or contributors are personal to them and do not necessarily reflect the views/opinions of the publishers. The information or guidance contained in this book is intended for use by medical, scientific or health-care professionals and is provided strictly as a supplement to the medical or other professional's own judgement, their knowledge of the patient's medical history, relevant manufacturer's instructions and the appropriate best practice guidelines. Because of the rapid advances in medical science, any information or advice on dosages, procedures or diagnoses should be independently verified. The reader is strongly urged to consult the drug companies' printed instructions, and their websites, before administering any of the drugs recommended in this book. This book does not indicate whether a particular treatment is appropriate or suitable for a particular individual. Ultimately it is the sole responsibility of the medical professional to make his or her own professional judgements, so as to advise and treat patients appropriately. The authors and publishers have also attempted to trace the copyright holders of all material reproduced in this publication and apologize to copyright holders if permission to publish in this form has not been obtained. If any copyright material has not been acknowledged please write and let us know so we may rectify in any future reprint.

Library of Congress Cataloging-in-Publication Data

Gross, Richard D., author.
  [Psychology for nurses and allied health professionals]
  Psychology for nurses and health professionals / Richard Gross and Nancy Kinnison. -- Second edition.
    p. ; cm.
  Preceded by: Psychology for nurses and allied health professionals / Richard Gross, Nancy Kinnison. London : Hodder Arnold, 2007.
  Includes bibliographical references and index.
  ISBN 978-1-4441-7992-7 (paperback : alk. paper)
  I. Kinnison, Nancy. II. Title.
  [DNLM: 1. Nursing Care--psychology. 2. Patient Care--psychology. 3. Patients--psychology. WY 87]

RT86
610.73--dc23

2013021554

Visit the Taylor & Francis Web site at
http://www.taylorandfrancis.com

and the CRC Press Web site at
http://www.crcpress.com

To Libbey Starr, granddaughter number five, as adorable and beautiful as the other four. What a fortunate Poppa I am!

Richard Gross

To Theresa and Michael and their families, who light up my life.

Nancy Kinnison

Contents

Contents

Preface

The basic approach that we adopted in the first edition of *Psychology for Nurses and Health Professionals* has been retained: psychological theory and research is interpreted and digested through the eyes of an imaginary student, Surena, whose 'From my diary' extracts (indicated by the pen icon in the margin) provide the scenarios that relate to the chapter. Surena does not make her 'appearance' until Chapter 3, when she begins to use the book to help her understand her experiences in her placements. As in your own practice, these do not follow the sequence of the chapters. To help you find your way around the book, we have provided a 'map' in the form of a grid on page xv that shows how Surena's placements and the chapters are related.

Throughout each chapter, Surena makes notes indicated by the notebook icon in the margin. In keeping with the increased emphasis on reflective practice (RP) in higher education, in this edition Surena refers more to RP theories to help her structure and analyse her own. Sometimes she reflects on her feelings about and behaviour towards her patients or applies the psychological material to the patients' and her own behaviour. As she gains experience, she comments on or evaluates the psychological material itself or reflects on ethical and social issues.

Note that in all chapters the psychology content includes critical evaluation of theory and research, which shows the additional higher level academic skills you are expected to develop during your course. To that end, a recurring feature is the 'Time for Reflection...' breaks. These are designed to encourage you to think about the text that follows and to have questions (if not always answers) in your mind to help you understand and digest the studies and theories that you read about. So, instead of just reading in a rather passive way, you will adopt a more critical approach, equipped with some idea of what to expect and what to look out for.

Sometimes the questions are quite specific, and the answers are given directly in the text that immediately follows. At other times, the questions are more general and abstract, and the answers unfold throughout the next few paragraphs. Another kind of question will require you to reflect on your own experiences and views on a particular issue; in these cases, of course, there is no 'correct answer'.

Occasionally, these 'Time for Reflection...' breaks appear as 'Research Questions...'; here, you are asked to think about methodological issues arising from a particular piece of research described in the text.

Frequent references are made to *Psychology: The Science of Mind and Behaviour* (2010), written by one of us (Richard Gross), pointing you in the direction of more detailed discussion of a particular theory or study or discussion of something that space does not allow in the present text at all.

Other features include 'Key Study' and 'Critical Discussion' boxes. Every chapter opens with an introduction and overview, which tells you what is covered in the chapter and sets the scene, and ends with a comprehensive summary, useful for revision.

Based on reviewers' comments, we have changed the number and order of chapters as they appeared in the first edition. We believe the order is more logical and gives the book greater overall coherence. While dropping three chapters from the first edition, much of the material has been moved into other chapters. In addition, there is a brand new chapter on neuropsychological and genetic aspects of illness and a substantial amount of updating and reordering of material – both within and between chapters.

Finally, Richard Gross has produced an easily accessible Web site. This includes additional material to complement the textbook as well as ways of assessing your knowledge and understanding.

It seems self-evident that to provide holistic care for patients, all health professionals need to have a theoretical knowledge and understanding of psychology. Knowing how to apply it is less obvious, and, of course, there is no one best or correct way to do it. We believe that our approach is supremely relevant to the evolving demands of patient care and hope that you will find it both useful and enjoyable. The 'for' in the title explicitly relates to nurses and allied health professionals in their different roles; implicitly, and as demonstrated throughout the book, it also relates to you as an individual.

Richard Gross and Nancy Kinnison

Free web resources

PowerPoint chapter summaries, MCQs and extension material are available to download from the CRC Press website: http://www.crcpress.com/product/isbn/9781444179927.

Acknowledgements

The authors thank Naomi Wilkinson for commissioning this second edition while still at Hodder Education and for taking the project with her when she moved to Taylor & Francis (United Kingdom). They also thank Ed Curtis, project editor at Taylor & Francis (Florida), for his support and guidance, as well as Dennis Troutman at diacriTech in New Hampshire and Paul Abraham and Dhayanidhi Karunanidhi at diacriTech in Chennai, India.

As with the first edition, Richard thanks Nancy for providing what he could not – the essential ability to 'translate' psychological theory into the language of nursing practice.

Nancy's thanks extend further to Alison and Michael Stuckey for their enduring support, to Laura-Jane Harris for her collaboration on the scenarios and to the care practitioners and patients for sharing so generously with me their thoughts, experiences and feelings on which they are based. For reasons of confidentiality you must remain anonymous – but you know who you are...

Nancy owes a very special debt of gratitude to Richard for his general text-book (an unrivalled reference throughout my teaching career) and for his patient guidance and encouragement during our further work on this edition. Again, it has been a privilege and a pleasure.

Authors

Richard Gross studied psychology and philosophy at Nottingham University, followed by a master's degree in the sociology of education and mass communications at Leicester University School of Education. After completing a postgraduate certificate in education, he taught psychology for more than 25 years on a variety of further and higher education courses, including 'A' level, access to higher education, and nursing diploma and degree courses. He has published a number of psychology textbooks, including *Psychology: The Science of Mind and Behaviour* (1st edition 1987, now in its 6th edition [2010]), *Key Studies in Psychology* (6th edition, 2012), *Themes, Issues and Debates in Psychology* (3rd edition, 2009), and *Being Human: Psychological and Philosophical Perspectives* (2012).

Nancy Kinnison worked as a staff nurse in Cornwall following her general training at the Royal Devon and Exeter Hospital. Her experience included gynaecology, dermatology and children's wards and casualty. During this time, she obtained the diploma in nursing (Part A–theory) and then became a night sister at the Royal Cornwall Hospital (Treliske). Following her divorce, she obtained a degree in sociology and social administration (health care) at Southampton University and then a postgraduate teaching certificate at Garnett College in London. Throughout this time she was an 'agency nurse' working in hospitals in Cornwall, Southampton and Roehampton (London). While teaching in London (where she was fortunate to meet Richard Gross), she taught sociology, psychology and health education and also piloted and managed the new BTEC National Diploma in Health Studies. Later, she moved to Bath College of Further Education to take a position that included teaching psychology on the postgraduate diploma in nursing, run in collaboration with Bath Royal United Hospital.

Table of diary extracts

1

What is psychology?

Introduction and overview

The opening chapter in any textbook is intended to 'set the scene' for what follows, and this normally involves defining the subject or discipline. In most disciplines, this is usually a fairly simple task. With psychology, however, it is far from straightforward. Definitions of psychology have changed frequently during its relatively short history as a separate field of study. This reflects different, and sometimes conflicting, theoretical views regarding the nature of human beings and the most appropriate methods for investigating them. While most psychologists would consider themselves to be scientists, they disagree about exactly what science involves and the appropriateness of using certain scientific methods to study human behaviour.

A brief history

The word 'psychology' is derived from the Greek words *psyche* (mind, soul or spirit) and *logos* (knowledge, discourse or study). Literally, then, psychology is the 'study of the mind'.

The emergence of psychology as a separate discipline is generally dated at 1879, when Wilhelm Wundt opened the first psychological laboratory at the University of Leipzig in Germany. Wundt and his co-workers were attempting to investigate 'the mind' through *introspection* to analyse conscious thought into its basic elements, much as chemists analyse compounds into elements. This attempt to identify the structure of conscious thought is called *structuralism*.

Wundt and his co-workers recorded and measured the results of their introspections under *controlled conditions*, using the same physical surroundings, the same 'stimulus' (such as a clicking metronome), the same verbal instructions to each participant and so on. This emphasis on measurement and control marked the separation of the 'new psychology' from its parent discipline of philosophy.

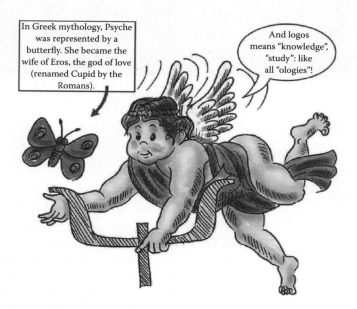

Philosophers had discussed 'the mind' for thousands of years. For the first time, *scientists* (Wundt was a physiologist by training) applied some of scientific investigation's basic methods to the study of mental processes. This was reflected in James's (1890) definition of psychology as

> the Science of Mental Life, both of its phenomena and of their conditions … The Phenomena are such things as we call feelings, desires, cognition, reasoning, decisions and the like.

However, by the early twentieth century, the validity and usefulness of introspection were being seriously questioned, particularly by American psychologist John B. Watson. Watson believed that the results of introspection could never be proved or disproved, since if one person's introspection produced different results from another's, how could we ever decide which was correct? *Objectively*, of course, this is impossible: we cannot 'get behind' an introspective report to check its accuracy. Introspection is *subjective*, and only the individual can observe his/her own mental processes.

Consequently, Watson (1913) proposed that psychologists should confine themselves to studying *behaviour*, since only this is measurable and observable by more than one person. Watson's form of psychology was known as *behaviourism*, which claimed that the only way psychology could make any claim to being scientific was to emulate the natural sciences (physics and chemistry) and adopt its own objective methods. Watson (1919) defined psychology as

> that division of Natural Science which takes human behaviour – the doings and sayings, both learned and unlearned – as its subject matter.

Especially in America, behaviourism (in one form or another) remained the dominant force in psychology up until the late 1950s. The emphasis on the role of *learning* (in the form of *conditioning*) was to make that topic one of the central areas of psychological research as a whole (see Box 2.2).

In the late 1950s, many British and American psychologists began looking to the work of computer scientists to try to understand more complex behaviours that, they felt, had been either neglected altogether or greatly oversimplified by learning theory (conditioning). These complex behaviours were what Wundt, James and other early scientific psychologists had called *mind* or mental processes. They are now called *cognition* or *cognitive processes*, including perception, attention, memory, problem-solving, decision-making, language and thinking in general.

Cognitive psychologists see people as *information-processors*, and cognitive psychology has been heavily influenced by computer science, with human cognitive processes being compared with the operation of computer programs (the *computer analogy*). Cognitive psychology now forms part of *cognitive science*, which emerged in the late 1970s (see Figure 1.1).

Despite the fact that cognitive processes can only be *inferred* from what a person does (they cannot be observed literally or directly), they are now accepted as valid subject matter for psychology, provided they can be made 'public' (as in memory tests or problem-solving tasks). What people say and do

Psychoanalytic theory and Gestalt psychology

- In 1900, Sigmund Freud, a neurologist living in Vienna, first published his *psychoanalytic theory* of personality in which the *unconscious* mind played a crucial role. In parallel with this theory, he developed a form of psychotherapy called *psychoanalysis*. Freud's theory (which forms the basis of the *psychodynamic* approach) represented a challenge and a major alternative to behaviourism (see Chapter 2).
- A reaction against both structuralism and behaviourism came from the *Gestalt* school of psychology, which emerged in the 1920s in Austria and Germany. Gestalt psychologists were mainly interested in perception, which they believed could not be broken down in the way that Wundt proposed, and behaviourists advocated for behaviour. Gestalt psychologists identified several 'laws' or *principles of perceptual organisation* (such as 'the whole is greater than the sum of its parts'), which have made a lasting contribution to our understanding of the perceptual process (see Gross, 2010, for a detailed discussion).

Figure 1.1 The relationship between psychology and other scientific disciplines.

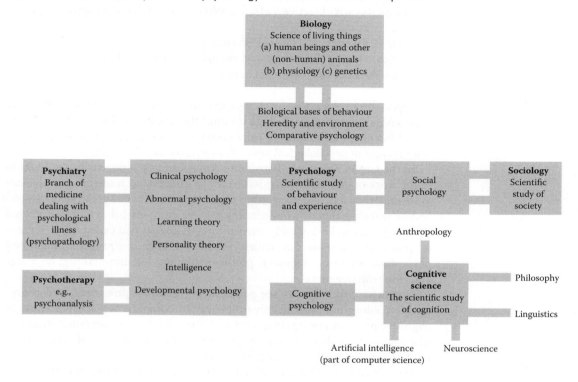

informs us *about* their cognitive processes; however, the processes themselves remain inaccessible to the observer.

The influence of both behaviourism and cognitive psychology is reflected in Clark and Miller's (1970) definition of psychology as

> the scientific study of behaviour. Its subject matter includes behavioural processes that are observable, such as gestures, speech and physiological changes, and processes that can only be inferred, such as thoughts and dreams.

Similarly, Zimbardo (1992) states that 'Psychology is formally defined as the scientific study of the behaviour of individuals and their mental processes'.

Classifying the work that psychologists do

Despite behaviourist and cognitive psychology's influence on psychology's general direction in the past 90 years or so, much more goes on within psychology than has been outlined so far. There are other theoretical approaches or orientations, other aspects of human (and non-human) activity that constitute the special focus of study and different kinds of work that different psychologists do.

A useful, but not hard and fast, distinction can be made between the *academic* and *applied* branches of psychology. Academic psychologists carry out research and are attached to a university or research establishment, where they will also teach undergraduates and supervise the research of postgraduates. Research is both *pure* (done for its own sake and intended, primarily, to increase our knowledge and understanding) and *applied* (aimed at solving a particular problem). Applied research is usually funded by a government institution like the Home Office, National Health Service (NHS) or the Department for Children, Schools and Families or by some commercial or industrial institution. The range of topics that may be investigated is as wide as psychology itself, but they can be classified as focusing either on the processes or *mechanisms* underlying various aspects of behaviour or more directly on the *person* (Legge, 1975).

Process approach

The process approach is divided into three main areas: physiological, cognitive and comparative psychology.

Physiological (or bio)psychology (Chapters 3–5 and 11)

Physiological (or bio)psychologists are interested in the physical basis of behaviour, how the functions of the *nervous system* (in particular the brain) and the *endocrine* (*hormonal*) system are related to and influence behaviour and mental processes. For example, are there parts of the brain specifically concerned with particular behaviours and abilities (*localisation of brain function*)? What role do hormones play in the experience of emotion and how are these linked to brain processes?

A fundamentally important biological process with important implications for psychology is *genetic transmission*. The *heredity and environment* (or *nature–nurture*) issue draws on what geneticists have discovered about the characteristics that can be passed from parents to offspring, how this takes place and how genetic factors interact with environmental ones (see Gross, 2010). Other topics within physiological psychology include motivation and stress (an important topic within *health psychology*).

Cognitive psychology

As seen earlier (page 3), cognitive (or mental) processes include *attention, memory, perception, language, thinking, problem-solving, decision-making, reasoning* and *concept-formation* ('higher-order' mental activities). Social psychology (classified here as belonging to the person approach) is heavily cognitive in flavour: for example, many social psychologists study the mental processes we use when trying to explain people's behaviour (for *social cognition*, see Chapter 10). Also, Piaget's theory (again, belonging to the person approach) is concerned with *cognitive development* (see Chapter 15).

Comparative psychology

Comparative psychology is the study of the behaviour of non-human animals, aimed at identifying similarities and differences between species. It also involves studying non-human animal behaviour to gain a better understanding of human behaviour. The basis of comparative psychology is *evolutionary theory*. Research areas include classical and operant conditioning (see Box 2.2) and evolutionary explanations of human behaviour (see Gross, 2010).

Person approach

Social psychology (Chapters 6–9)

Some psychologists would claim that 'all psychology is social psychology', because all behaviour – public and private – take place within a social context. However, other people usually have a more immediate and direct influence on us when we are actually in their presence (as in *conformity* and *obedience* – see Chapters 8 and 9). Social psychology is also concerned with attitudes and attitude change (see Chapter 6), and prejudice and discrimination (Chapter 7).

Developmental psychology (Chapters 14–19)

Developmental psychologists study the biological, cognitive, social and emotional *changes* that occur in people over time. One significant change within developmental psychology during the past 30 years or so is the recognition that development is not confined to childhood and adolescence, but is a lifelong process (the *lifespan approach*). It is now generally accepted that development continues beyond childhood and adolescence into adulthood and late adulthood (see Figure 1.2).

Figure 1.2 Three generations of the same family.

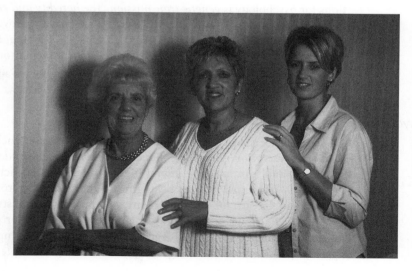

Individual differences

This is concerned with the ways in which people can differ from one another, including *personality* (see Chapter 5), *intelligence* and *psychological abnormality*. Major mental disorders include dementia (see Chapter 11), schizophrenia, depression, anxiety disorders and eating disorders. *Abnormal psychology* is closely linked with *clinical psychology*, one of the major *applied* areas of psychology (see discussion in page 9). Psychologists who study abnormality and clinical psychologists are also concerned with the effectiveness of different forms of treatment and therapy. Each major theoretical approach has contributed to both the explanation and treatment of mental disorders (see Chapter 2).

Comparing the process and person approaches

In practice, it is very difficult to separate the two approaches. However, there are important relative differences between them.

Some important differences between the process and person approaches

- The *process approach* is typically confined to the laboratory (where experiments are the method of choice). It makes far greater experimental use of non-human animals and assumes that psychological processes (particularly learning) are essentially the same in all species and that any differences between species are only *quantitative* (differences of degree).
- The *person approach* makes much greater use of field studies (such as observing behaviour in its natural environment) and of non-experimental methods (e.g. correlational studies, see Chapter 3). Typically, human participants are studied and it is assumed that there are *qualitative* differences (differences in kind) between humans and non-humans.

Areas of applied psychology

Discussion of the person/process approaches has been largely concerned with the *academic* branch of psychology. Since the various areas of applied psychology are all concerned with people, they can be thought of as the *applied* aspects of the person approach.

According to Hartley and Branthwaite (1997), most applied psychologists work in four main areas: *clinical*, *educational* and *occupational psychology* and *government service* (such as *forensic* [or *criminological*] psychologists). In addition, Coolican et al. (2007) identify *counselling*, *sport*, *health* and *environmental psychologists*. Hartley and Branthwaite argue that the work psychologists do in these different areas has much in common: it is the *subject matter* of their jobs that differs, rather than the skills they employ. Consequently, they consider an applied psychologist to be a person who can deploy specialised skills appropriately in different situations (see Box 1.1).

Box 1.1 Seven major skills (or roles) used by applied psychologists.

- *The psychologist as counsellor*: Helping people to talk openly, express their feelings, explore problems more deeply and see these problems from different perspectives. Problems may include school phobia, marriage crises and traumatic experiences (such as being the victim of a hijacking), and the counsellor can adopt a more or less directive approach (see Chapter 2, page 31).
- *The psychologist as colleague*: Working as a member of a team and bringing a particular perspective to a task, namely drawing attention to the human issues, such as the point of view of the individual end user (be it a product or a service of some kind).
- *The psychologist as expert*: Drawing upon psychologists' specialised knowledge, ideas, theories and practical knowledge to advise on issues ranging from incentive schemes in industry to appearing as an 'expert witness' in a court case.
- *The psychologist as toolmaker*: Using and developing appropriate measures and techniques to help in the analysis and assessment of problems. These include questionnaire and interview schedules, computer-based ability and aptitude tests and other *psychometric tests* (mental measurement) (see Chapter 6).
- *The psychologist as detached investigator*: Many applied psychologists carry out evaluation studies to assess the evidence for and against a particular point of view. This reflects the view of psychology as an objective science, which should use controlled experimentation whenever possible (see pages 12–15).
- *The psychologist as theoretician*: Theories try to explain observed phenomena, suggesting possible underlying mechanisms or processes. They can suggest where to look for causes and how to design specific studies that will produce evidence for or against a particular point of view. Results from applied psychology can influence theoretical psychology and vice versa.
- *The psychologist as agent for change*: Applied psychologists are involved in helping people, institutions and organisations, based on the belief that their work will change people and society for the better. However, some changes are much more controversial than others, such as the use of psychometric tests to determine educational and occupational opportunities and the use of behaviour therapy and modification techniques to change abnormal behaviour (see Chapters 2 and 5).

Source: Based on Hartley, J., Branthwaite, A., *The Applied Psychologist*, Open University Press, Buckingham, 2000.

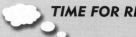

TIME FOR REFLECTION ...

- Which, if any, of the skills identified by Hartley and Branthwaite do you consider to be relevant to nursing (or allied health professions)?
- How do they apply (it might be useful to think in terms of whether they apply *formally* or *informally*, *implicitly* or *explicitly*)?
- Are there any major skills that are used in nursing (or allied health professions) that *are not* included by Hartley and Branthwaite?

The major functions of the clinical psychologist

The functions of a clinical psychologist include the following:

- Assessing people with learning difficulties, administering psychological tests to brain-damaged patients, devising rehabilitation programmes for long-term psychiatric patients and assessing elderly people for their fitness to live independently (see Chapter 11).
- Planning and carrying out programmes of therapy, usually *behaviour therapy/modification* or *psychotherapy* (group or individual) in preference to, or in addition to, behavioural techniques (see Chapter 2).
- Carrying out research into abnormal psychology, including the effectiveness of different treatment methods ('outcome' studies); patients are usually adults, many of whom will be elderly, in psychiatric hospitals, psychiatric wards in general hospitals and psychiatric clinics.
- Involvement in community care, as psychiatric care in general moves out of the large psychiatric hospitals.
- Teaching other groups of professionals, such as nurses, psychiatrists and social workers.

Clinical psychology

Clinical psychologists are the largest single group of psychologists, both in the United Kingdom (Coolican et al., 2007) and in the United States (Atkinson et al., 1990). A related group is 'counselling psychologists', who tend to work with younger clients in colleges and universities rather than in hospitals.

Clinical psychologists work largely in health and social care settings, including hospitals, health centres, community mental health teams, child and adolescent mental health services and social services. They usually work as part of a team with, for example, social workers, medical practitioners and other health professionals. Most work in the NHS, but some work in private practice (see Figure 1.3).

Psychotherapy is usually carried out by psychiatrists (medically qualified doctors specialising in psychological medicine) or psychotherapists (who have

Figure 1.3 Assessing elderly clients in a residential setting.

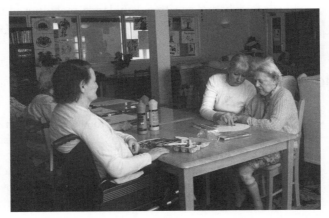

undergone special training, including their own psychotherapy). In all its various forms, psychotherapy is derived from Freud's psychoanalysis (see Chapter 2) and is distinguished both from behavioural treatments and from physical (somatic) treatments (those based on the medical model – see Chapter 3 and Gross, 2010).

Forensic psychology

This is a branch of psychology that attempts to apply psychological principles to the criminal justice system. Areas of research interest include jury selection, the presentation of evidence, eyewitness testimony, improving the recall of child witnesses, false memory syndrome and recovered memory, offender profiling, stalking, crime prevention, devising treatment programmes (such as anger management) and assessing the risk of releasing prisoners.

Educational psychology

Educational psychologists are mostly employed by local education authorities, working in schools, colleges, child and family centre teams (previously called 'child guidance'), the School Psychological Service, hospitals, day nurseries, nursery schools, special schools (day and residential) and residential children's homes. Their functions include the following:

- Administering psychometric tests (particularly intelligence/IQ tests)
- Planning and supervising remedial teaching
- Planning educational programmes for children and adolescents with special educational needs (including the visually impaired and autistic)
- Advising parents and teachers how to deal with children and adolescents with behaviour problems and/or learning difficulties

Occupational (work or organisational) psychology

Occupational psychologists are involved in the selection and training of individuals for jobs and vocational guidance, including administration of aptitude tests and tests of interest. (This overlaps with the work of those trained in *personnel management*.)

Health psychology

This is one of the newer fields of applied psychology.

Health psychologists work in various settings such as hospitals, academic health research units, health authorities and university departments. They may deal with problems identified by health care agencies, including NHS trusts and health authorities, health professionals (such as general practitioners, nurses and rehabilitation therapists) and employers outside the health care system.

The breadth of health psychology

- The use of psychological theories and interventions to prevent damaging behaviours (such as smoking, drug abuse and poor diet) and to change health-related behaviour in community and workplace settings.
- Promoting and protecting health by encouraging behaviours such as exercise, healthy diet and health checks/self-examination.
- Health-related cognitions: Investigating the processes that can explain, predict and change health and illness behaviours (see Chapter 3).
- The nature and effects of communication between health care practitioners and patients, including interventions to facilitate adherence (such as taking medication), preparing patients for stressful medical procedures and so on (see Chapters 3 and 9).
- Psychological aspects of illness: Looking at the psychological impact of acute and chronic illness on individuals, families and carers (see Chapters 3 and 4).

Language of psychology

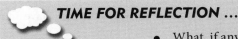

TIME FOR REFLECTION ...

- What, if anything, has come as a surprise to you regarding what goes on in the name of 'psychology'?

As in all sciences, there is a special set of technical terms (jargon) to get used to, and this is generally accepted as an unavoidable feature of studying the subject. But over and above this jargon, psychologists use words that are familiar to us from everyday speech in a *technical way*, and it is in these instances that 'doing psychology' can become a little confusing.

Some examples of this are 'behaviour' and 'personality'. For a parent to tell a child to 'behave yourself' is meaningless to a psychologist's ears: behaving is something we are all doing all the time (even when we are asleep). Similarly, to say that someone 'has no personality' is meaningless because, as personality refers to what makes a person unique and different from others, you cannot help but have one!

Some of the technical terms used throughout the book are defined in the Glossary (pages 439–456).

Formal versus informal psychology

Legge (1975) and others distinguish between *formal* and *informal psychology* (or professional versus amateur, scientific versus non-scientific).

Our common-sense, intuitive or 'natural' understanding is unsystematic and does not constitute a body of knowledge. This makes it very difficult to 'check' an individual's 'theory' about human nature, as does the fact that each individual has to learn from his/her own experience. So part of the aim of formal psychology is to provide such a systematic body of knowledge.

However, rather than negating or invalidating our everyday, common-sense understanding, Legge (1975) believes that most psychological research should be aimed at demonstrating 'what we know already', and then going one step further. Only the methods of science, he believes, can provide us with the public, communicable body of knowledge that we are seeking. According to Allport (1947), the aim of science is 'understanding, prediction and control above the levels achieved by unaided common sense', and this is meant to apply to psychology as much as to the natural sciences.

What do we mean by 'science'?

TIME FOR REFLECTION ...

- What do you understand by the term 'science'?
- What makes a science different from non-science?
- Are there different kinds of science and, if so, what do they have in common?

Asking this question is a necessary first step for considering the appropriateness of attempting to scientifically study human behaviour.

Major features of science

Most psychologists and philosophers of science would probably agree that for a discipline to be called a science, it must possess certain characteristics. These are summarised in Figure 1.4.

What is 'scientific method'?

The account shown in Figure 1.4 of what constitutes a science is non-controversial. However, it fails to tell us how the *scientific process* takes place, the sequence of 'events' involved (such as where the theory comes from in the first place and how it is related to observation of the subject matter) or the exact relationship between theory construction, hypothesis testing and data collection.

Collectively, these 'events' and relationships are referred to as (the) *scientific method*. Table 1.1 summarises some common beliefs about both science and scientific method, together with some alternative views.

Figure 1.4 A summary of the major features of a science.

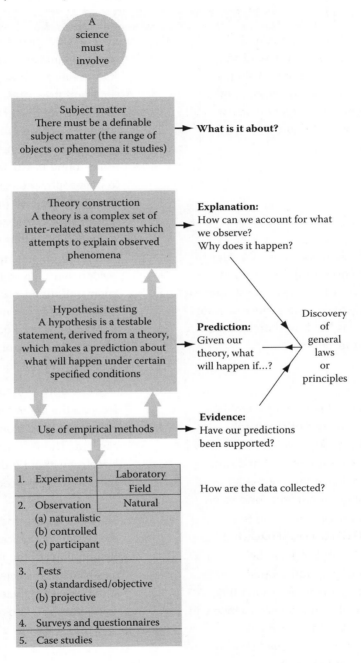

Table 1.1 Some common beliefs and alternative views about 'science' and 'scientific method'.

Common beliefs		Alternative views	
λ	Scientific discovery begins with simple, unbiased, unprejudiced observation: the scientist simply 'samples' the world without any preconceptions, expectations or predetermined theories	λ	There is no such thing as 'unbiased' or 'unprejudiced' observation. Observation is always selective, interpretative, prestructured and directed: we must have at least some idea of what we are looking for, otherwise we cannot know when we have found it. Goldberg (2000) cites a philosophy professor who asserted that what we call 'data' (that which is given) should more accurately be called 'capta' (that which is taken)
ν	From the resulting sensory evidence ('data'/sense data), generalised statements of fact will take shape: we gradually build up a picture of what the world is like based on a number of separate 'samples'	ν	'Data' do not constitute 'facts': evidence usually implies measurements, numbers and recordings, which need to be interpreted in the light of a theory. Facts do not exist objectively and cannot be discovered through 'pure observation'
			'Fact' = data + theory (Deese, 1972)
σ	The essential feature of scientific activity is the use of empirical methods, through which the sensory evidence is gathered: what distinguishes science from non-science is performing experiments and so on	σ	Despite the central role of data collection, data alone do not make a science. Theory is just as crucial, because without it data have no meaning (see preceding point)
τ	The truth about the world (the objective nature of things, what the world is 'really like') can be established through properly controlled experiments and other ways of collecting 'facts': science can tell us about reality as it is independent of the scientist or the activity of observing it	τ	Scientific theory and research reflect the biases, prejudices, values and assumptions of the individual scientist as well as of the scientific community s/he belongs to. Science is not value-free (see Gross, 2010)

Table 1.1 *(Continued)* Some common beliefs and alternative views about 'science' and 'scientific method'.

Common beliefs		Alternative views	
ʋ	Science involves the steady accumulation of knowledge: each generation of scientists adds to the discoveries of previous generations	ʋ	Science involves an endless succession of long, peaceful periods ('normal science') and 'scientific revolutions' (Kuhn, 1962; see Table 2.1)
		ı	Science has a warm, human, exciting, argumentative, creative 'face' (Collins, 1994)

Source: Based on Medawar, P.B., *The Art of the Soluble*, Penguin Books, Harmondsworth, 1963; Popper, K., *Objective Knowledge: An Evolutionary Approach*, Oxford University Press, Oxford, 1972.

Scientific study of human behaviour

Social nature of science: The problem of objectivity

'Doing science' is part of human behaviour. When psychologists study what people do, they are engaging in some of the very same behaviours they are trying to understand (such as thinking, perceiving, problem-solving and explaining). This is what is meant by the statement that psychologists are part of their own subject matter, which makes it even more difficult for them to be objective than other scientists.

According to Richards (1996), it may be impossible for any scientist to achieve complete objectivity. One reason for this relates to the social nature of scientific activity. As Rose (1997) says,

> How biologists, or any scientists, perceive the world is not the result of simply holding a true reflecting mirror up to nature: it is shaped by the history of our subject, by dominant social expectations and by the patterns of research funding.

According to Richardson (1991), science is a very *social* business. Research must be qualified and quantified to enable others to replicate it: in this way, the procedures, instruments and measures become standardised, so that scientists anywhere in the world can check the truth of reported observations and findings. This implies the need for universally agreed conventions for reporting these observations and findings.

However, even if there are widely accepted ways of 'doing science', 'good science' does not necessarily mean 'good psychology'. Is it valid to study human behaviour and experience as part of the natural world, or is a different kind of approach needed altogether? After all, it is not just psychologists who observe, experiment and theorise (Heather, 1976).

The Psychology experiment as a social situation

To regard empirical research in general, and the experiment in particular, as objective involves two related assumptions:

1. Researchers influence the participant's behaviour (the outcome of the experiment) only to the extent that they decide what hypothesis to test, how the variables are to be operationalised (defined in a way that allows them to be measured), what design to use (e.g. randomly allocating each participant to one experimental condition or testing every participant under each condition) and so on.
2. The only factors influencing the participant's performance are the objectively defined variables manipulated by the experimenter.

TIME FOR REFLECTION ...

- Try to formulate some arguments against these two assumptions.
- What do the experimenter and participant bring with them to the experimental situation that is not directly related to the experiment, and how may this (and other factors) influence what goes on in the experimental situation (see Gross, 2010)?

Experimenters are people too: The problem of experimenter bias

Some examples of experimenter bias

- According to Valentine (1992), experimenter bias has been demonstrated in various experiments, including reaction time, animal learning, verbal conditioning, personality assessment, person perception, learning and ability as well as in everyday life situations.
- What these experiments consistently show is that if one group of experimenters has one hypothesis about what it expects to find and another group has the opposite hypothesis, *both* groups will obtain results that support their respective hypotheses. The results *are not* due to the mishandling of data by biased experimenters: the experimenters' bias somehow creates a changed environment, in which participants actually behave differently.
- In a natural classroom situation, children whose teachers were told they would show academic 'promise' during the next academic year showed significantly greater IQ gains than children for whom such predictions were not made (although this latter group also made substantial improvements). In fact, the children were *randomly* allocated to the two conditions. But the teachers' expectations actually produced the predicted improvements in the 'academic promise' group, demonstrating a *self-fulfilling prophecy* (Rosenthal and Jacobson, 1968).

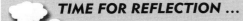

TIME FOR REFLECTION …

- Try to explain the findings from the studies described in Box 'Some examples of experimenter bias'.
- How could experimenter expectations actually bring about the different performances of the two groups of children?

Participants are psychologists too: Demand characteristics

Instead of seeing the person being studied as a passive responder to whom things are done ('subject'), Orne (1962) stresses what the person *does*, implying a far more *active* role. Participants' performance in an experiment could be thought of as a form of *problem-solving behaviour*. At some level, they see the task as working out the true purpose of the experiment and responding in a way that will support the hypothesis being tested.

In this context, the cues that convey the experimental hypothesis to participants represent important influences on their behaviour, and the sum total of those cues are called the *demand characteristics* of the experimental situation. These cues include all explicit and implicit communications during the actual experiment (Orne, 1962). This tendency to identify the demand characteristics is related to the tendency to play the role of a 'good' (or 'bad') experimental participant.

Not only is the experiment a social situation, but science itself is a *culture-related phenomenon*. This represents another respect in which science cannot claim complete objectivity (Moghaddam et al., 1993).

Problem of representativeness

Traditional, mainstream experimental psychology adopts a *nomothetic* ('law-like') approach. This involves generalisation from limited samples of participants to 'people in general', as part of the attempt to establish general 'laws' or principles of behaviour.

TIME FOR REFLECTION …

- The photograph below captures a fairly typical scene as far as participant characteristics in mainstream psychological research are concerned. It depicts one of Asch's famous conformity experiments (see Chapter 8, pages 174–177).
- What are the most apparent characteristics of the experimental participants, and how are they similar to/different from those of Asch (who is pictured furthest right)?

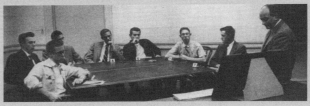

Despite the fact that Asch's experiments were carried out in the early 1950s, very little has changed as far as participant samples are concerned. In American psychology at least, the typical participant is a psychology undergraduate, who is obliged to take part in a certain number of studies as a course requirement and who receives 'course credits' for doing so (Krupat and Garonzik, 1994).

Mainstream British and American psychology has implicitly equated 'human being' with 'member of Western culture'. Despite the fact that the vast majority of research participants are members of Western societies, the resulting findings and theories have been applied to 'human beings', as if culture made no difference (they are 'culture-bound and culture-blind') (Sinha, 1997). This *Anglocentric* or *Eurocentric bias* (a form of *ethnocentrism*) is matched by the *androcentric* or *masculinist bias* (a form of *sexism*), according to which the behaviours and experiences of men are taken as the standard against which women are judged (see Gross, 2009).

In both cases, while the bias remains implicit and goes unrecognised (and is reinforced by psychology's claim to be objective and value-free), research findings are taken as providing us with an objective, scientifically valid account of what 'women/people in general are like'. Once we realise that scientists, like all human beings, have prejudices, biases and values, their research and theories begin to look less objective, reliable and valid than they did before.

Problem of artificiality

Criticisms of traditional empirical methods (especially the laboratory experiment) have focused on their *artificiality*, including the often unusual and bizarre tasks that people are asked to perform in the name of science. Yet, we cannot be sure that the way people behave in the laboratory is an accurate indication of how they are likely to behave outside it (Heather, 1976).

What makes the laboratory experiment such an unnatural and artificial situation is the fact that it is almost totally structured by one 'participant' – the experimenter. This relates to *power differences* between experimenters and their 'subjects', which is as much an *ethical* as a practical issue (see Gross, 2009).

Traditionally, participants have been referred to as 'subjects', implying something less than a person, a dehumanised and depersonalised 'object'. According to Heather (1976), it is a small step from reducing the person to a mere thing or object (or experimental 'subject') to seeing people as machines or machine-like ('mechanism' = 'machine-ism' = mechanistic view of people). This way of thinking about people is reflected in the popular definition of psychology as the study of 'what makes people tick'.

Problem of internal versus external validity

If the experimental setting (and task) is seen as similar or relevant enough to everyday situations to allow us to generalise the results, we say that the study has high *external* or *ecological validity*. But what about *internal validity*? Modelling itself on natural science, psychology attempts to overcome the

> ## Box 1.2 Some difficulties with the notion of experimental control
>
> - While it is relatively easy to control the more obvious *situational variables*, this is more difficult with *participant variables*, either for practical reasons (such as the availability of these groups) or because it is not always obvious exactly what the relevant variables are. Ultimately, it is down to the experimenter's judgement and intuition: what she/he believes it is important (and possible) to control (Deese, 1972).
> - If judgement and intuition are involved, then control and objectivity are matters of degree, whether in psychology or physics (see Table 1.1).
> - It is the *variability/heterogeneity* of human beings that makes them so much more difficult to study than, say, chemicals. Chemists do not usually have to worry about how two samples of a particular chemical might differ from each other, but psychologists need to allow for *individual differences* between participants.
> - We cannot just assume that the IV (or 'stimulus' or 'input') is identical for every participant, definable in some objective way, independent of the participant and exerting a standard effect on everyone.
> - Complete control would mean that the IV alone was responsible for the DV, so that experimenter bias and the effect of demand characteristics were irrelevant. But even if complete control were possible (even if we could guarantee the *internal validity* of the experiment), a fundamental dilemma would remain. The greater the degree of control over the experimental situation, the more different it becomes from real-life situations (the more artificial it gets and the lower its *external validity*).

problem of the complexity of human behaviour by using experimental control. This involves isolating an independent variable (IV) and ensuring that *extraneous variables* (variables other than the IV likely to affect the dependent variable [DV]) do not affect the outcome (see Coolican, 2004). But this begs the crucial question: *how do we know when all the relevant extraneous variables have been controlled?* (See Box 1.2).

To discover the relationships between variables (necessary for understanding human behaviour in natural, real-life situations), psychologists must 'bring' the behaviour into a specially created environment (the laboratory), where the relevant variables can be controlled in a way that is impossible in naturally occurring settings. However, in doing so, they construct an artificial environment and the resulting behaviour is similarly artificial – it is no longer the behaviour they were trying to understand!

Conclusions

During the course of its life as a separate discipline, definitions of psychology have changed quite fundamentally, reflecting the influence of different theoretical approaches. Initially through the influence of behaviourism, psychology has taken the natural sciences as its model (*scientism*). In this chapter, we have highlighted some of the major implications of adopting methods of investigating the natural world and applying them to the study of human behaviour and experience. Ultimately, whatever a particular science may claim to have discovered about the phenomena it studies, scientific activity remains just one more aspect of human behaviour.

CHAPTER SUMMARY

- Early psychologists, such as Wundt, attempted to study the mind through *introspection* under controlled conditions, aiming to analyse conscious thought into its basic elements (*structuralism*).
- Watson rejected introspectionism's *subjectivity* and replaced it with *behaviourism*. Only by using the methods of natural science and studying observable behaviour could psychology become a true science.
- *Gestalt psychologists* criticised both structuralism and behaviourism, advocating that 'the whole is greater than the sum of its parts'. Freud's *psychoanalytic theory* was another major alternative to behaviourism.
- *Cognitive psychologists* see people as *information processors*, based on the *computer analogy*. Cognitive processes, such as perception and memory, are an acceptable part of psychology's subject matter.
- *Academic* psychologists are mainly concerned with conducting *research* (*pure* or *applied*), which may focus on underlying *processes/mechanisms* or on the *person*.
- The process approach consists of physiological, cognitive and comparative psychology, while the person approach covers developmental and social psychology and individual differences.
- Most applied psychologists work in clinical, counselling, forensic, educational or occupational psychology. Newer fields include health and sport psychology.
- A distinction is commonly made between *informal/common-sense* and *formal/scientific psychology*. The latter aims to go beyond common-sense understanding and to provide a public, communicable body of knowledge.
- A science must possess a definable subject matter, involve theory construction and hypothesis testing and use empirical methods for data collection. However, these characteristics fail to describe the scientific process or scientific method.
- Science is a very *social* activity and consensus among the scientific community is paramount. This detracts from psychology's claim (or that of any other science) to *objectivity*.
- Environmental changes are somehow produced by experimenters' expectations (*experimenter bias*), and *demand characteristics* influence participants' behaviours by helping to convey the experimental hypothesis. The experiment is a social situation and science itself is *culture related*.
- The *artificiality* of laboratory experiments is largely due to their being totally structured by experimenters. Also, the higher an experiment's *internal validity*, the lower its *external validity* becomes.

2 Theoretical approaches

Introduction and overview

Different psychologists make different assumptions about what particular aspects of a person are worthy of study, and this helps to determine an underlying model or image of what people are like. In turn, this model or image determines a view of psychological normality, the nature of development, preferred methods of study, the major cause(s) of abnormality and the preferred methods and goals of treatment.

An approach is a perspective that is not as clearly outlined as a theory. As we shall see, all the major approaches include two or more distinguishable theories but, within an approach, they share certain basic principles and assumptions that give them a distinct 'flavour' or identity. The focus here is on the *behaviourist, psychodynamic, humanistic* and *biological* approaches (see Gross, 2010, for a discussion of the cognitive, evolutionary and social constructionist approaches).

Behaviourist approach

Basic principles and assumptions

As we saw in Chapter 1, Watson revolutionised psychology by rejecting the introspectionist approach and advocating the study of observable behaviour. What was revolutionary when he first delivered his 'behaviourist manifesto' (Watson, 1913; see Box 2.1) has become almost taken-for-granted, 'orthodox' psychology. Belief in the importance of empirical methods, especially the experiment, as a way of collecting data about humans (and non-humans) that can be quantified and statistically analysed is a major feature of *mainstream psychology* (see Gross, 2010).

Box 2.1 Watson's (1913) 'behaviourist manifesto'

Watson's article, 'Psychology as the behaviourist views it', is often referred to as the 'behaviourist manifesto', a charter for a truly scientific psychology. Three features of this 'manifesto' deserve special mention.

1. Psychology must be purely *objective*, excluding all subjective data or interpretations in terms of conscious experience. This redefines psychology as the 'science of behaviour' (rather than the 'science of mental life').

2. The goals of psychology should be to *predict* and *control* behaviour (as opposed to describing and explaining conscious mental states), a goal later endorsed by Skinner's *radical behaviourism* (see below).

3. There is no fundamental (*qualitative*) distinction between human and non-human behaviour. If, as Darwin had shown, humans evolved from more simple species, then it follows that human behaviour is simply a more complex form of the behaviour of other species (the difference is merely *quantitative* – one of degree). Consequently, rats, cats, dogs and pigeons became the major source of psychological data. Since 'psychological' now meant 'behaviour' rather than 'consciousness', non-humans that were convenient to study, and whose environments could easily be controlled, could replace people as experimental subjects.

Source: Based on Fancher, R.E., *Pioneers of Psychology*, Norton, New York, 1979; Watson, J.B., *Psychol. Rev.*, 20, 158–177, 1913.

According to Skinner (1987),

> 'Radical' behaviourists ... recognise the role of private events (accessible in varying degrees to self-observation and physiological research), but contend that so-called mental activities are metaphors or explanatory fictions and that behaviour attributed to them can be more effectively explained in other ways.

For Skinner, these more effective explanations of behaviour come in the form of the *principles of reinforcement* derived from his experimental work with rats and pigeons (see Box 2.2). What is 'radical' about Skinner's radical behaviourism is his rejection of thoughts, feelings and other private events as possible explanations (i.e. causes) of behaviour. According to Nye (2000), Skinner's ideas are also radical because he applied the same type of analysis to covert behaviour (thoughts and feelings) occurring 'within the skin' as he did to overt, publicly observable behaviours: in both cases, they can be translated into the language of reinforcement theory. He stressed the importance of identifying *functional relations* (cause-and-effect connections) between environmental conditions and behaviours.

Box 2.2 Basic principles and assumptions made by the behaviourist approach

- Behaviourists emphasise the role of environmental factors in influencing behaviour, to the near exclusion of innate or inherited factors. This amounts essentially to a focus on *learning*. The key form of learning is *conditioning*, either *classical*, which formed the basis of Watson's behaviourism, or *operant*, which is at the centre of Skinner's radical behaviourism (Figure 2.1).

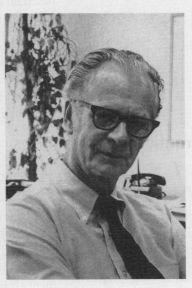

Figure 2.1 B.F. Skinner (1904–1990).

- *Classical conditioning* is also known as *Pavlovian*, after Pavlov, the Russian physiologist, who famously discovered that dogs learn to salivate at anything that has become associated with food. For example, if a bell is rung (the conditioned stimulus) repeatedly just before the dog is given food (the unconditioned stimulus), the dog will eventually salivate when it hears the bell (without food having to be given). Salivating to food is an unconditioned response (i.e. unlearned), but it becomes a conditioned response to the bell. In both cases, salivation is an *automatic* response (hence, this form of learning is also known as *respondent* conditioning). The learner is responding *passively* to environmental events.
- *Operant conditioning* is also known as *instrumental* conditioning. This denotes the fact that the animal's behaviour is instrumental in producing certain *consequences*. In Skinner's experiments with rats, for example, they had to press a lever to receive a *positive reinforcement* (a food pellet) or a *negative reinforcement* (the switching off of an electric shock), or lever pressing would result in an electric shock (*punishment*). Reinforcement (positive or negative) makes the behaviour that produced it *more likely* to be repeated, while punishment makes it *less likely* to be repeated. Here, the learner is *actively* influencing what happens to it by manipulating its environment.
- Behaviourism is often referred to as 'S–R' psychology ('S' standing for 'stimulus' and 'R' for 'response'). However, only in classical conditioning is the stimulus seen as triggering a response in a predictable, automatic way, and this is what is conveyed by 'S–R' psychology.
- Both types of conditioning are forms of *associative learning*, whereby associations or connections are formed between stimuli and responses that did not exist before learning took place.
- The mechanisms proposed by a theory should be as simple as possible. Behaviourists stress the use of *operational definitions* (defining concepts in terms of observable, measurable events).
- The aim of a science of behaviour is to *predict* and *control* behaviour (see Box 2.1).

Theoretical contributions

Behaviourism made a massive contribution to psychology, at least up to the 1950s, and explanations of behaviour in conditioning terms recur throughout the subject (see Gross, 2010). For example, apart from learning and conditioning, imagery as a form of organisation in memory and as a memory aid is based on the principle of association, and the interference theory of forgetting is largely couched in stimulus–response terms. Language, moral and gender development have all been explained in terms of conditioning. The behaviourist approach also offers one of the major models of abnormal behaviour.

Theorists and researchers critical of the original, 'orthodox' theories have modified and built on them, making a huge contribution in the process. One noteworthy example is Bandura's (1971) *social learning theory* (renamed *social cognitive theory* in 1989).

Practical contributions

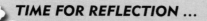

TIME FOR REFLECTION ...

- Try to think of examples of your work (including patients' and colleagues' behaviour, as well as your own) where behaviourist principles (such as reinforcement) and assumptions might help explain what happens.

The emphasis on experimentation, operational definitions and the measurement of observable events has been a major influence on the practice of scientific psychology in general (what Skinner, 1974, called the 'science of behaviour'). This is quite unrelated to any views about the nature and role of mental events. Other, more 'tangible', contributions include the following:

- *Behaviour therapy* and *behaviour modification* (based on classical and operant conditioning, respectively) as major approaches to the treatment of abnormal behaviour and one of the main tools in the clinical psychologist's 'kit bag' (see Box 1.4, page 9).
- *Behavioural neuroscience*, an interdisciplinary field of study, using behavioural techniques to understand brain function and neuroscientific techniques to throw light on behavioural processes.
- *Behavioural pharmacology*, which involves the use of *schedules/contingencies of reinforcement* to assess the behavioural effects of new drugs that modify brain activity (schedules of reinforcement refer to how often and regularly/predictably reinforcements are given following some desired behaviour); most importantly, the research has illustrated how many behavioural effects of drugs are determined as much by the current behaviour and reinforcement contingencies as by the effects of the drug on the brain (Leslie, 2002; see also Chapter 12).
- *Biofeedback* as a non-medical treatment for stress-related symptoms, derived from attempts to change rats' autonomic physiological functions through the use of operant techniques (see Chapter 5).

An evaluation of behaviourism

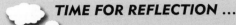

TIME FOR REFLECTION ...

- Do you agree with Skinner's claim that thoughts and other 'covert behaviours' do not *explain* our behaviour (because they cannot *determine* what we do)?

Skinner's claim that human behaviour can be predicted and controlled in the same way as the behaviour of non-humans is usually accepted only by other behaviour analysts. Possessing language allows us to communicate with each other and to think about 'things' that have never been observed (and may not even exist), including rules, laws and principles (Garrett, 1996). While these can only be expressed in or thought about in words, much of our behaviour is governed by them. According to Garrett, when this happens 'behaviour is now shaped by what goes on inside their [people's] heads ... and not simply by what goes on in the external environment'. So, what people *think* is among the important variables determining what they do and say – the very *opposite* of what Skinner's radical behaviourism claims.

Behaviour analysts recognise the limitations of their approach. For example, Leslie (2002) admits that 'operant conditioning cannot provide a complete account of psychology from a behavioural perspective, even in principle'. Similarly, O'Donohue and Ferguson (2001) acknowledge that the science of behaviour cannot account for creativity, as in music, literature and science.

Psychodynamic approach

The term 'psychodynamic' denotes the active forces within the personality that motivate behaviour and the inner causes of behaviour (in particular the *unconscious conflict* between the different structures that compose the whole personality). While Freud's was the original psychodynamic theory, the approach includes all those theories based on his ideas, such as those of Jung (1964), Adler (1927) and Erikson (1950). Freud's *psychoanalytic theory* is psychodynamic, but the psychodynamic theories of Adler, Jung and Erikson are not psychoanalytic. So the two terms *are not* synonymous. However, because of their enormous influence, Freud's ideas will be emphasised in the rest of this section.

Basic principles and assumptions

Freud's concepts are closely interwoven, making it difficult to know where a description of them should begin (Jacobs, 1992). Fortunately, Freud himself stressed the acceptance of certain key theories as essential to the practice of *psychoanalysis*, the form of psychotherapy he pioneered and from which most others are derived (see Box 2.3 and page 28).

Box 2.3 Major principles and assumptions of psychoanalytic theory

- Much of our behaviour is determined by unconscious thoughts, wishes, memories and so on. What we are consciously aware of at any one time represents the tip of an iceberg: most of our thoughts and ideas are either not accessible at that moment (*preconscious*) or are totally inaccessible (*unconscious*). These unconscious thoughts and ideas can become conscious through the use of special techniques, such as *free association*, *dream interpretation* and *transference* – the cornerstones of psychoanalysis.

- Much of what is unconscious has been made so through *repression*, whereby threatening or unpleasant experiences are 'forgotten', locked away from our conscious awareness. This is a major form of *ego defence* (see Chapter 5). Freud (1914) (see Figure 2.2) singled out repression as a special cornerstone 'on which the whole structure of psychoanalysis rests'. Repression is closely related to *resistance*, interpretation of which is another key technique used in psychoanalysis.

- According to the theory of *infantile sexuality*, the sexual instinct or drive is active from birth and develops through a series of five *psychosexual stages*. The most important of these is the *phallic stage* (spanning the ages 3 to 5/6), during which all children experience the *Oedipus complex*. This refers to the 'family romance', which in the case of boys refers to their 'falling in love' with their mother and becoming jealous of their father, whom they also fear will punish them through castration.

- Freud used the German word *trieb*, which translates as 'drive', rather than *instinkt*, which was meant to imply that experience played a crucial role in determining the 'fate' of sexual (and aggressive) energy.

- Related to infantile sexuality is the general *impact of early experience* on later personality (see Chapter 14). According to Freud (1949), '… the child is psychologically father of the man and … the events of its first years are of paramount importance for its whole subsequent life'.

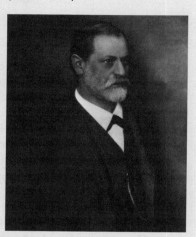

Figure 2.2 Sigmund Freud (1856–1939).

Theoretical contributions

As with behaviourist accounts of conditioning, many of Freud's ideas and concepts (such as 'respression' and 'unconscious') have become part of the vocabulary of mainstream psychology.

Freud's contribution is extremely rich and diverse, offering theories of motivation, dreams and the relationship between sleep and dreams, moral and gender development, aggression, abnormality and forgetting. Psychoanalytic theory also influenced Adorno et al.'s (1950) theory of the authoritarian personality (a major account of prejudice; see Chapter 7).

Finally, Freud's theories have stimulated the development of alternative theories, often resulting from the rejection of some of his fundamental principles and assumptions, but reflecting his influence enough for them to be described as psychodynamic.

Some major alternative psychodynamic theories

TIME FOR REFLECTION …

- Repeat the exercise suggested for the behaviourist approach (see page 23).

- *Ego psychology*, promoted by Freud's daughter, Anna, focused on the mechanisms used by the *ego* (the rational, decision-making part of the personality) to deal with the world, especially the ego defence mechanisms. Freud, by contrast, stressed the influence of the *id*'s innate drives (especially sexuality and aggression) and is often described as an instinct theorist (but see the fourth entry in Box 2.3). (The id represents the infantile, pleasure-seeking part of the personality.) The ego, as well as the id, originates in basic human inheritance and has its own developmental course. It uses neutralised (non-sexual) energy, which makes possible an interest in objects and activities that are not necessarily related to underlying sexual and aggressive drives.
- Erik Erikson, trained by Anna Freud as a child psychoanalyst, also stressed the importance of the ego as well as the influence of social and cultural factors on individual development. He pioneered the *lifespan approach* to development, proposing eight *psychosocial stages*, in contrast with Freud's five psychosexual stages that end with physical maturity (see Chapters 13 and 17 through 19).
- Two of Freud's original 'disciples', Carl Jung and Alfred Adler, broke ranks with Freud and formed their own 'schools' (*analytical psychology* and *individual psychology* respectively). Jung attached relatively little importance to childhood experiences (and the associated personal unconscious) but considerable importance to the *collective* (or *racial*) *unconscious*, which stems from the evolutionary history of human beings as a whole.
- Like Jung, Adler rejected Freud's emphasis on sexuality, stressing instead the *will to power* or *striving for superiority*, which he saw as an attempt to overcome feelings of inferiority faced by all children as they grow up. He also shared Jung's view of the person as an *indivisible unity* or whole and Erikson's emphasis on the *social* nature of human beings.
- The *object relations school* (the 'British school') was greatly influenced by Melanie Klein's (1932) emphasis on the infant's earliest (pre-Oedipal) relationships with its mother. It places far less emphasis on the role of instincts and more on the *relationship with particular love objects* (especially the mother). Fairbairn (1952), for example, saw the aim of the libido as *object-seeking* (as opposed to pleasure-seeking), and this was extended by Bowlby (1969) in his *attachment theory* (see Chapter 14).

Practical contributions

The current psychotherapy scene is highly diverse, with only a minority using Freudian techniques, but as Fancher (1996) points out,

> Most modern therapists use techniques that were developed either by Freud and his followers or by dissidents in explicit reaction against his theories. Freud remains a dominating figure, for or against whom virtually all therapists feel compelled to take a stand.

Both Rogers, the major humanistic therapist (see pages 30 and 31), and Wolpe, who developed *systematic desensitisation* (a major form of behaviour therapy), were originally trained in Freudian techniques. Perls, the founder of *Gestalt therapy*; Ellis, the founder of *rational emotive therapy*; and Berne, who devised *transactional analysis*, were also trained psychoanalysts.

Even Freud's fiercest critics concede his influence, not just within world psychiatry but in philosophy, literary criticism, history, theology, sociology, and art and literature generally. Freudian terminology is commonly used in conversations between therapists well beyond Freudian circles, and his influence is brought daily to therapy sessions as part of the cultural background and experience of nearly every client (Jacobs, 1992).

Many mental health practitioners (including psychotherapists, counsellors and social workers), although not formally trained as psychoanalysts, have incorporated elements of Freudian thought and technique into their approaches to helping their patients (Nye, 2000).

An evaluation of the psychodynamic approach

- A criticism repeatedly made of Freudian (and other psychodynamic) theories is that they are unscientific because they are *unfalsifiable* (incapable of being disproved) (Eysenck, 1985; Popper, 1959).
- According to Kline (1984, 1989), the theory comprises a collection of hypotheses, some of which are more easily tested than others, some of which are more central to the theory than others and some of which have more supporting evidence than others.
- According to Zeldow (1995), the history of science reveals that those theories that are the richest in explanatory power have proved the most difficult to test empirically. For example, Einstein's general theory of relativity is still untestable. Eysenck, Popper and others have criticised psychoanalytic theory for being untestable. But even if this were true,

> ... the same thing could (and should) be said about any psychological hypotheses involving complex phenomena and worthy of being tested ... psychoanalytic

theories have inspired more empirical research in the social and behavioural sciences than any other group of theories .... (Zeldow, 1995)

- Freud's theory provides methods and concepts that enable us to interpret and 'unpack' underlying *meanings* (it has great *hermeneutic strength*); these meanings (both conscious and unconscious) cannot be measured in any precise way. Freud offers a way of understanding that is different from theories that are easily testable, and it may actually be *more* appropriate for capturing the nature of human experience and action (Stevens, 1995; see also Chapter 1). According to Fancher (1996), 'His ideas about repression, the importance of early experience and sexuality, and the inaccessibility of much of human nature to ordinary conscious introspection have become part of the standard Western intellectual currency'.
- Reason (2000) believes it is time to re-acknowledge Freud's greatness as a psychologist. Like James, he had a rare gift for describing and analysing the phenomenology of mental life. Perhaps Freud's greatest contribution was in recognising that apparent trivia we now commonly call 'Freudian slips' are 'windows on the mind'.

Humanistic approach

Basic principles and assumptions

Although the term 'humanistic psychology' was coined by Cohen (1958), a British psychologist, this approach emerged mainly in the United States during the 1950s. Maslow (1968), in particular, gave wide currency to the term 'humanistic' in America, calling it a 'third force' (the other two being behaviourism and Freudianism). However, Maslow did not reject these approaches but hoped to unify them, thus integrating both subjective/private and objective/public aspects of the person.

Theoretical contributions

Maslow's *hierarchy of needs* (see Gross, 2010) distinguishes between motives shared by both humans and non-humans and those that are uniquely human and can be seen as an extension of the psychodynamic approach. Freud's id would represent physiological needs (at the hierarchy's base), Horney (a major critic of the male bias in Freud's theory) focused on the need for safety and love (corresponding to the next two levels) and Adler (see discussion on page 27) stressed esteem needs (at the fourth level). Maslow added self-actualisation to the peak of the hierarchy (Glassman, 1995).

Box 2.4 Some basic principles and assumptions of the humanistic approach

- Both the psychoanalytic and behaviourist approaches are *deterministic*. People are driven by forces beyond their control, either unconscious forces from within (Freud) or reinforcements from without (Skinner). Humanistic psychologists believe in free will and people's ability to choose how they act.

Figure 2.3 Abraham M. Maslow (1908–1970).

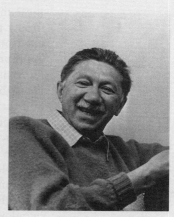

- A truly scientific psychology must treat its subject matter as fully human, which means acknowledging individuals as interpreters of themselves and their world. Behaviour, therefore, must be understood in terms of the individual's *subjective experience*, from the perspective of the actor (a *phenomenological approach*, which explains why this is sometimes called the 'humanistic-phenomenological' approach). This contrasts with the *positivist* approach of the natural sciences, which tries to study people from the position of a detached observer. Only the individual can explain the meaning of a particular behaviour and is the 'expert' – not the investigator or therapist.
- Maslow (Figure 2.3) argued that Freud supplied the 'sick half' of psychology, through his belief in the inevitability of conflict, neurosis, innate self-destructiveness and so on, while he (and Rogers) stressed the 'healthy half'. Maslow saw *self-actualisation* at the peak of a hierarchy of needs, while Rogers talked about the *actualising tendency*, an intrinsic property of life, reflecting the desire to grow, develop and enhance our capacities. A fully functioning person is the ideal of growth. Personality development naturally moves towards healthy growth, unless it is blocked by external factors, and should be considered the norm.
- Maslow's contacts with Wertheimer and other Gestalt psychologists (see Chapter 1) led him to stress the importance of understanding the *whole person*, rather than separate 'bits' of behaviour.

Source: Based on Glassman, W.E., *Approaches to Psychology*, Open University Press, Buckingham, 1995.

According to Rogers (1951), while awareness of being alive is the most basic of human experiences, we each fundamentally live in a world of our own creation and have a unique perception of the world (the *phenomenal field*). It is our *perception* of external reality that shapes our lives (*not* external reality itself). Within our phenomenal field, the most significant element is our sense of *self*, 'an organised consistent gestalt, constantly in the process of forming and reforming' (Rogers, 1959). This view contrasts with those of many other self theorists, who see it as a central, unchanging core of personality (see Chapter 16).

Practical contributions

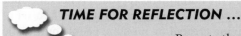

TIME FOR REFLECTION ...

- Repeat the exercise as for the behaviourist and psychodynamic approaches.

By far the most significant practical influence of any humanistic psychologist is Rogers' *client-* (or *person-*)*centred therapy* (see Gross, 2010). Originally (in the 1950s), it was called 'client-centred' therapy (CCT), but since the mid-1970s, it has been known as 'person-centred' therapy (PCT): 'psychotherapy is the releasing of an already existing capacity in a potentially competent individual' (Rogers, 1959).

The change in name was meant to reflect more strongly that the person, in his/her full complexity, is the centre of focus. Also, Rogers wanted to convey that his assumptions were meant to apply broadly to almost all aspects of human behaviour – not just to therapeutic settings. For example, he saw many parallels between therapists and teachers – they are both 'facilitators' of an atmosphere of freedom and support for individual pursuits. According to Nye (2000),

> A wide range of individuals – psychotherapists, counsellors, social workers, clergy and others – have been influenced by Rogers' assumptions that, if one can be a careful and accurate listener, while showing acceptance and honesty, one can be of help to troubled persons.

Nurses can be added to this list, especially in relation to their use of therapeutic conversation (see Chapter 3, Box 3.1).

Rogers helped develop research designs that enable objective measurement of the self-concept and ideal self and their relationship over the course of therapy (see Chapter 16) as well as methodologies for exploring the importance of therapist qualities. These innovations continue to influence therapeutic practice, and many therapists are now concerned that their work should be subjected to research scrutiny.

By emphasising the therapist's personal qualities, Rogers opened up psychotherapy to psychologists and contributed to the development of therapy provided by non-medically qualified therapists (*lay therapy*). This is especially significant in the United States, where (until recently) psychoanalysts had to be psychiatrists (medically qualified). Rogers originally used the term 'counselling' as a strategy for silencing psychiatrists who objected to psychologists practising 'psychotherapy'. In the United Kingdom, the outcome of Rogers' campaign has been the evolution of a counselling profession whose practitioners are drawn from a wide variety of disciplines, with neither psychiatrists nor psychologists dominating. Counselling skills are used in various settings throughout education, the health professions, social work, industry and commerce, the armed services and international organisations (Thorne, 1992).

An evaluation of the humanistic approach

- According to Wilson et al. (1996), the humanistic approach is not an elaborate or comprehensive theory of personality, but should be seen as a set of uniquely personal theories of living created by humane people optimistic about human potential. It has wide appeal to those who seek an alternative to the more mechanistic, deterministic theories.
- Like Freud's theory, many of its concepts are difficult to test empirically (such as self-actualisation) and it cannot account for the origins of personality. Since it describes but does not explain personality, it is subject to the *nominal fallacy* (Carlson and Buskist, 1997) and so cannot really be called a theory.
- Nevertheless, for all its shortcomings, the humanistic approach represents a counterbalance to the psychodynamic (especially Freudian) and the behaviourist approaches and has helped to bring the 'person' back into psychology. Crucially, it recognises that people help determine their own behaviour and are not simply slaves to environmental contingencies or to their past. The self, personal responsibility and agency, choice and free will are now legitimate issues for psychological investigation.

Biological approach

Basic principles and assumptions

Theoretical and practical contributions

We noted in Chapter 1 that biopsychology forms part of the process approach (Legge, 1975) and that a crucially important biological process with important implications for psychology is *genetic transmission* (see Box 2.5). For

Box 2.5 Basic principles and assumptions made by the biopsychological approach

Toates (2001) identifies four strands of the application of biology to understanding behaviour:

1. How things work in the 'here and now', i.e. the immediate *determinants* of behaviour. In some cases, a biological perspective can provide clear insights into what determines people to act in a particular way. For example, when someone treads on a thorn (a cause) and cries out in pain soon afterwards (an effect), we know the pathways of information in the body that mediate between such causes and effects. What this example shows is that behaviour is an integral part of our biological make-up.
2. We inherit *genes* from our parents and these genes play a role in determining the structure of our body; through this structure, and perhaps most obviously through that of our *nervous system* (NS), genes play a role in behaviour.
3. A combination of genes and environment affects the growth and maturation of our body, with the main focus being the NS and behaviour. Development of the *individual* is called *ontogenesis*.

Box 2.5 Basic principles and assumptions made by the biopsychological approach (*Continued*)

4. The assumption that humans have evolved from simpler forms, rooted in Darwin's (1859) theory of *evolution*, relates to both the physical structure of our body and our behaviour: we can gain insight into behaviour by considering how it has been shaped by evolution. Development of *species* is called *phylogenesis* (Figure 2.4).

Figure 2.4 Major subdivisions of the human nervous system (including the main subdivisions of the brain).

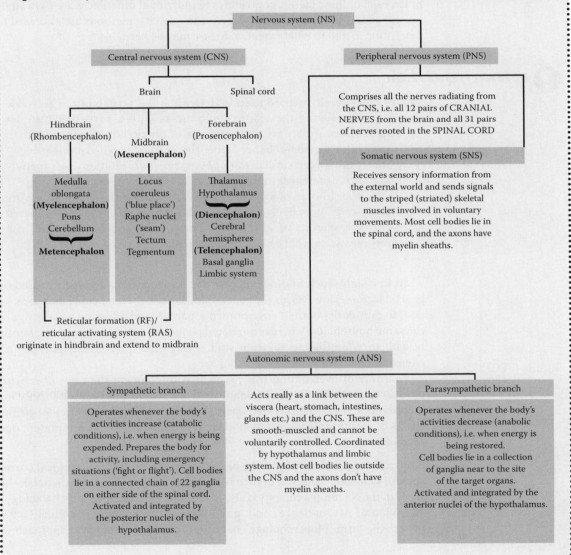

example, *behaviour geneticists* attempt to quantify how much of the variability of any given trait (e.g. intelligence, aggressiveness or schizophrenia) can be attributed to

1. Genetic differences between people (*heritability*)
2. *Shared environments* (i.e. between-family variation, such as socio-economic status)
3. *Non-shared environments* (within-family variations, such as how parents treat each children differently) (Pike and Plomin, 1999)

The two major methods used by behaviour geneticists to determine how much each of these factors contributes to individual differences are twin studies and adoption studies. These same – and related – methods are also used to determine if, and to what extent, a *disease* may be heritable.

 RESEARCH QUESTION ...

- The most basic method used to determine the heritability of a disease involves studying the relatives of patients with a particular disorder to determine if they are at greater risk of developing the disorder than would be expected by chance alone. This method is called *familial aggregation* and is very similar to *family resemblance* studies used to study individual differences in intelligence and schizophrenia.
- If, say, the children of a parent (or both parents) with schizophrenia are significantly more likely to become schizophrenic themselves compared with their cousins or unrelated children, what conclusions could you draw regarding what causes schizophrenia?

At first sight, such findings suggest that schizophrenia is largely caused by genetic factors. However, as the genetic similarity between people increases, so does the similarity of their environments: parents and offspring usually live in the same households, whereas unrelated people do not. In other words, family resemblance/familial aggregation studies *confound* (or confuse) genetic and environmental influences.

One way of overcoming this problem is to compare the rates of schizophrenia among monozygotic (identical) twins reared together with those for monozygotic (MZ) twins reared apart (MZsRA). This helps to *disentangle* the effects of genetic and environmental factors. Studies of MZsRA represent one kind of *adoption study*.

Biopsychology is the study of the biological bases, or the physiological correlates, of behaviour and is a branch of *neuroscience* (or the brain sciences), the study of the NS. Biopsychology is also sometimes referred to as 'psychobiology', 'behavioural neuroscience', and 'physiological psychology'. But Pinel (1993) prefers the term 'biopsychology', because it denotes a biological approach to the study of psychology, where psychology 'commands centre stage': biopsychologists are not interested in biology for its own sake, but for what it can tell them about behaviour and mental (cognitive) processes.

From both an ontogenetic and a phylogenetic perspective, 'the ultimate purpose of the nervous system is to produce and control behaviour' (Pinel, 1993). In general terms,

1. The kind of behaviour an animal is capable of depends very much on the kind of body it possesses; for example, humans can flap their arms as much as they like but they will never fly (unaided) – arms are simply not designed for flying, while wings are. However, we are very skilled at manipulating objects (especially small ones), because that is how our hands and fingers have developed during the course of evolution.
2. The possession of a specialised body is of very little value unless the NS is capable of controlling it: of course, evolution of the one usually mirrors evolution of the other.
3. The kind of NS also determines the extent and nature of the learning a species is capable of. As you move along the phylogenetic (evolutionary) scale, from simple, one-celled amoebae, through insects, birds and mammals, to primates (including ourselves – *Homo sapiens*), the NS gradually becomes more complex. At the same time, behaviour becomes increasingly the product of learning and environmental influence, rather than instinct and other innate, genetically determined factors.

As noted in Chapter 3, the influence of the biological approach can be seen very clearly in the *biomedical model* of illness and disease. The influence of the biological approach is also seen in the concept of addiction, which is based on the *addiction-as-disease model* (see Chapter 12).

According to the biomedical model, disease is something that 'happens to' the individual, originating from either inside or outside the body. While disease may have psychological consequences, there are no psychological causes (i.e. people are just passive victims of forces beyond their control). Similarly, stress is something that inflicts itself on helpless individuals from the outside but that can have very real bodily effects; these include psychophysiological disorders such as hypertension, coronary heart disease and stomach ulcers (see Chapters 4 and 5).

- One major account of how stress makes people ill is Selye's (1956) General Adaptation Syndrome; this describes the interaction between the sympathetic branch of the autonomic nervous system (see Figure 2.4) and the endocrine (hormonal) system.
- Another explanation describes how stressors affect the immune system and is central to *psychoneuroimmunology* (PNI). PNI is defined as the study of psychological factors on the immune system (Ogden, 2004) and so represents a branch of 'mind–body medicine' (but see section on 'Evaluation of the biological approach').

Related to PNI is *psychoneuroendocrinology* (PNE), the study of links between psychological and hormonal processes, and *psychophysiology* (PP), the study of the relationship between psychological manipulations and physiological responses in relation to such diverse behaviours as sleep, problem-solving, reactions to stress, learning, memory, perception and information-processing. The scope of both PNI and PNE is much narrower than that of PP, with specific focus on immune and endocrine responses respectively.

Evaluation of the biological approach

- The biological approach is *reductionist*, that is, it attempts to explain human and non-human psychological processes and behaviour in terms of the operation of physical/physiological structures (such as interactions between neurons/nerve cells and hormones). In turn, these processes are explained in terms of smaller constituent processes, such as synaptic transmission between neurons and nerve cells. Ultimately, reductionism claims that all psychology can be explained in terms of biology, which in turn can be understood in terms of chemistry and physics. Some psychologists believe that this loses sight of the whole person and fails to reflect experience and everyday interaction with other people.

- Reductionism has been effective in scientific research. For example, the greatest insight into the cause and possible cure of Parkinson's disease has been obtained from reducing it to the biological level: we know that Parkinson's disease is caused by the malfunction and death of certain neurons in a particular part of the brain (Toates, 2001). However, while there may be a fairly straightforward causal link between this neuron malfunction and the movement disorder that characterises Parkinson's disease, things are rather more complex when it comes to explaining the associated mood disorder. This, in turn, raises the more general *philosophical* issue regarding the relationship between the brain and the mind (or consciousness) (the 'mind–body' or 'brain–mind' problem; see Gross, 2009).

- As we noted when evaluating PNI, the biological approach tends to remove the person from his/her social context, focusing almost exclusively on physical processes within the body. This is both another form of reductionism and a form of *determinism*. However, outside the laboratory, there is a limit to how far biological manipulation can take place to reveal a simple cause–effect behavioural chain (a major assumption of determinism): biological factors need to be *interpreted* within a context of rather subtle psychological principles (Toates, 2001).

- The Human Genome Project (HGP) was a 13-year research project, aimed at identifying all human genes (the genome), that is, determining the sequences of chemical base pairs that make up human DNA (see Chapter 11). This was duly completed in 2003, the achievement described as a 'landmark event' in the biomedical sciences (Carter, 2004). Hamilton-West (2011) explores the implications of the HGP for identifying disease genes, throwing light on gene–environment interactions, and developing gene-based diagnoses and treatments (see Chapter 11). Several writers discuss the possibility that unethical scientists may abuse this knowledge in the form of genetic manipulation/engineering and selective breeding (eugenics).

- As we have seen, the biological approach does not exclude the role of psychological (i.e. non-physiological) factors, as illustrated by PNI. However, while PNI acknowledges the interaction between stress and the immune system, the source of stress (or stressor) is taken as a given: why the individual experiences something as a stressor in the first place and any attempts at coping with it have no place in PNI-based explanation of how stress makes us ill. By contrast, the *biopsychosocial model* that underlies health psychology (see Box 1.5) takes into account not only individual factors such as personality and coping mechanisms but also the influence of social and cultural factors (such as social norms, the influence of other people and the availability of specific substances and facilities) (see Chapters 3 and 4).

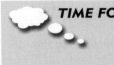

TIME FOR REFLECTION ...

- What is the underlying image of the person associated with each of the major theoretical approaches within psychology?
- Which of these do you consider captures your own experience and your experience of others, most accurately, and why?

Conclusions: can psychology be a science if psychologists cannot agree what psychology is?

As we saw in Chapter 1, definitions of psychology have changed during its lifetime, largely reflecting the influence and contributions of its major theoretical approaches or orientations. In this chapter, we have seen that each approach rests upon a different image of what people are like. Freud's 'tension-reducing person', Skinner's 'environmentally controlled person' and Rogers' 'growth-motivated person' really are quite different from each other (Nye, 2000). The biological approach offers the most tangible image of all – the person as 'flesh-and-blood'.

However, we have also noted some important similarities between different approaches, such as the deterministic nature of Freud's and Skinner's theories. Each approach has something of value to contribute to our understanding of ourselves – even if it is only to reject the particular explanation it offers. The diversity of approaches reflects the complexity of the subject matter, so, usually, there is room for a diversity of explanations.

These different conceptualisations of the person in turn determine what is considered worthy of investigation as well as the methods of study that can and should be used to investigate it. Consequently, different approaches can be seen as self-contained disciplines as well as different facets of the same discipline (Kline, 1988; Kuhn, 1962).

As Table 2.1 shows, Kuhn (and others) believe that psychology is still in a state (or stage) of *prescience*. Whether psychology has, or has ever had, a *paradigm* continues to be hotly debated.

Table 2.1 Stages in the development of a science (σ) and their application to psychology (ν)

σ	*Prescience*: A majority of those working in a particular discipline do not yet share a common or global perspective (*paradigm*), and there are several schools of thought or theoretical orientations
ν	Like Kuhn (1962), Joynson (1980) and Boden (1980) argue that psychology is *preparadigmatic*. Kline (1988) sees its various approaches as involving different paradigms
σ	*Normal science*: A paradigm has emerged, dictating the kind of research that is carried out and providing a framework for interpreting results. The details of the theory are filled in and workers explore its limits. Disagreements can usually be resolved within the limits allowed by the paradigm
ν	According to Valentine (1992), *behaviourism* comes as close as anything could to a paradigm. It provides (1) a clear definition of the subject matter (behaviour as opposed to 'the mind'); (2) fundamental assumptions, in the form of the central role of learning (especially conditioning), and the analysis of behaviour into stimulus–response units, which allow prediction and control; (3) a methodology, with the controlled experiment at its core
σ	*Revolution*: A point is reached in most established sciences where the conflicting evidence becomes so overwhelming that the old paradigm has to be abandoned and is replaced by a new one (*paradigm shift*). When this paradigm shift occurs, there is a return to *normal science*
ν	Palermo (1971) and LeFrancois (1983) argue that psychology has already undergone several paradigm shifts. The first paradigm was *structuralism*, represented by Wundt's introspectionism. This was replaced by Watson's *behaviourism*. Finally, *cognitive psychology* largely replaced behaviourism, based on the computer analogy and the concept of information processing (see Chapter 1). Glassman (1995) disagrees claiming that there is never been a complete reorganisation of the discipline, as has happened in physics

CHAPTER SUMMARY

- Different theoretical *approaches/perspectives* are based on different models/images of the nature of human beings.
- Skinner's *radical behaviourism* regards mental processes as both *inaccessible* and *irrelevant* for explaining behaviour.
- The *behaviourist approach* stresses the role of environmental influences (*learning*), especially *classical* and *operant conditioning*. Psychology's aim is to *predict* and *control* behaviour.
- Bandura's *social learning/social cognitive theory* represents modifications of 'orthodox' learning (conditioning) theory.
- Methodological behaviourism has influenced the practice of scientific psychology in general. Other practical contributions include *behaviour therapy* and *modification*, *behavioural neuroscience* and *pharmacology*, and *biofeedback*.
- The *psychodynamic approach* is based on Freud's *psychoanalytic theory*. Central aspects are the unconscious (especially repression), infantile sexuality and the impact of early experience.
- Freud's ideas have become part of *mainstream psychology*, contributing to our understanding of motivation, sleep and dreams, forgetting, attachment, aggression and abnormality.
- Major modifications/alternatives to Freudian theory include *ego psychology*, Erikson's *psychosocial theory* and the *object relations school*.
- All forms of *psychotherapy* stem directly or indirectly from *psychoanalysis*. Many trained psychoanalysts have been responsible for developing radically different therapeutic approaches, including Rogers, Perls and Wolpe.
- Maslow called the *humanistic approach* the 'third force' in psychology. It believes in free will, adopts a *phenomenological perspective* and stresses the *positive* aspects of human personality.
- Rogers was a prolific researcher into the effectiveness of his *CCT/PCT*, opened up psychotherapy to psychologists and other non-medically qualified practitioners and created a counselling profession that operates within a wide diversity of settings.
- Central to the *biological approach* (a branch of *neuroscience*) is the role of *genes* in determining behaviour through the *NS* (*central NS* and *peripheral NS*). This applies from both a *phylogenetic* and an *ontogenetic* perspective.
- *Behaviour geneticists* attempt to quantify how much of the variability of any given trait can be attributed to *heritability, shared environments* or *non-shared environments*. They do this through the use of *familial aggregation/family resemblance studies*, studies of *separated MZs* and *adoption studies*.

- The influence of the biological approach is clearly seen in the *biomedical model* of illness and disease and the *addiction-as-disease model*.
- Different *theoretical approaches* can be seen as self-contained disciplines, making psychology *pre-paradigmatic* and so still in a stage of *prescience*.
- Only when a discipline possesses a *paradigm* has it reached the stage of *normal science*, after which *paradigm shifts* result in *revolution* (and a return to normal science).

3 Psychological aspects of illness

Introduction and overview

According to Ogden (2004), health psychology (HP) represents one of several challenges that were faced during the twentieth century by the 'biomedical' model (Engel, 1977, 1980). This maintains that disease can be fully explained in terms of deviations from the norm of biological (somatic) factors. More specifically,

- Diseases either come from outside the body and invade it, causing internal physical changes, or originate as internal involuntary physical changes; such diseases can be caused by chemical imbalances, bacteria, viruses or genetic predisposition.
- Individuals are not responsible for their illnesses, which arise from biological changes beyond their control; people who are ill are victims.
- Treatment should consist of vaccination, surgery, chemotherapy or radiotherapy, all of which aim to change the physical state of the body.
- Responsibility for treatment rests with the medical profession.
- Health and illness are qualitatively different, you are either healthy or ill, and there is no continuum between the two.
- Mind and body function independently of each other; the abstract mind relates to feelings and thoughts and is incapable of influencing physical matter.
- Illnesses may have psychological consequences but not psychological causes.

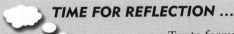 **TIME FOR REFLECTION ...**

- Try to formulate some arguments against the biomedical model.

In opposition to these ideas, HP maintains that human beings should be seen as complex systems. Illness is often caused by a combination of biological (e.g., viruses), psychological (e.g., behaviours and beliefs) and social

Figure 3.1 The biopsychosocial model of health and illness. (Adapted from Ogden, J., *Health Psychology: A Textbook* (2nd edn.), Open University Press, Buckingham, 2000.)

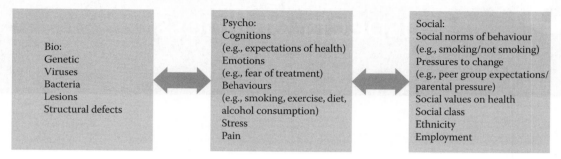

(e.g., employment) factors. These assumptions reflect the 'biopsychosocial' (BPS) model of health and illness (Engel, 1977, 1980), which is summarized in Figure 3.1.

Engel describes illness in terms of interrelated systems with different levels of organisation (such as molecules, cells, person, family or society); these are linked together hierarchically so that change in one system produces change in the others (see Figure 3.2).

According to Stroebe (2000), the BPS model reflects fundamental changes in the nature of illness, causes of death and overall life expectancy during the twentieth century. The influence of non-biological factors (e.g., improvements in medical treatment and significant changes in lifestyle) in major causes of death such as cardiovascular disease and cancer is incompatible with the biomedical model. By conceptualising disease in purely biological terms, the model has little to offer the prevention of chronic diseases through efforts to change people's health beliefs, attitudes and behaviour.

Similarly, the biomedical model, by ignoring the role of psychological and sociocultural factors, is unable to explain the following:

- How pre-operative psychological preparation (including anxiety reduction) can affect wound healing and recovery rate (see Chapter 4)
- The relationship between patients' perception of symptoms and symptom control
- Why patients sometimes do not comply with/adhere to treatment (see Chapter 7)
- How the attitudes towards their illness can affect its course and prognosis in patients with chronic illnesses (such as HIV/AIDS, cancer, obesity and coronary heart disease)
- The enormous diversity in patients' experience/tolerance of pain.

In all these cases, the relationship between the patient and the nurse (or doctor, physiotherapist, etc.) also plays a crucial role. More generally, at each level of the BPS model (see Figure 3.2) the behaviour of people, like that of cells, is shaped by the context in which it takes place.

Figure 3.2 Hierarchy of natural systems. (From Engel, G.L., *Am. J. Psychiatry*, 137, 535–544, 1980.)

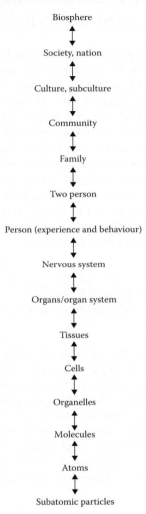

Biosphere

↕

Society, nation

↕

Culture, subculture

↕

Community

↕

Family

↕

Two person

↕

Person (experience and behaviour)

↕

Nervous system

↕

Organs/organ system

↕

Tissues

↕

Cells

↕

Organelles

↕

Molecules

↕

Atoms

↕

Subatomic particles

 From my diary (1): Year 1/Community/District Nurse

My first day in my first placement. Sally, my Community Nurse mentor, started by explaining that seeing patients at home helps us understand 'where they're coming from' (which I now interpret as the biopsychosocial model of health care).

Our first patient was Maisie, a pale, thin woman of 68, who'd had a hysterectomy three weeks previously but whose wound was still oozing. When Sally had dressed it she casually asked her Maisie if she was eating properly as she seemed to have lost weight. Maisie admitted she 'didn't have much of an appetite' and when Sally suggested that might be a factor in her wound being slow to heal, Maisie looked very upset and shook her head; I pretended not to notice, but Sally sat on the bed, took Maisie's hand in hers and asked gently if she was worried about anything. Maisie didn't answer for ages and then, to my embarrassment, began to cry. Sally then asked me if I'd mind waiting in the car, so I said a hasty goodbye to Maisie and left, feeling relieved but also a bit resentful at being dismissed.

Psychoneuroimmunology, behavioural medicine and psychosomatic medicine

The 'systems approach' portrayed in Figure 3.2 is also evident in the relatively new discipline of 'psychoneuroimmunology' (PNI), in which interactions between the brain and the immune system are studied at a neural and biochemical level, together with the resulting implications for health (Hamilton-West, 2011). PNI reflects a holistic view of the person; according to Lorentz (2006), to ensure meeting the needs of the entire individual – mind, body and spirit – holistic nurses promote the concept of the mind–body connection. PNI, therefore, represents one facet of *mind–body medicine* and plays an important role in explaining the link between stress and illness (see Chapter 4).

The BPS model underpins not only HP but also the interdisciplinary field of 'behavioural medicine' (Baum and Posluszny, 1999); it draws on a range of behavioural sciences, including anthropology, epidemiology, sociology and psychology (Schwartz and Weiss, 1977).

TIME FOR REFLECTION ...

- What do you understand by the term 'psychosomatic'?

The BPS model, in acknowledging the role of psychological variables in health, also plays a part in *psychosomatic medicine*. A commonly used term, psychosomatic is often mistakenly taken by the layperson to mean 'imaginary' (or 'all in the mind'), as if the symptoms labelled in this way have no physical (bodily) reality at all. However, as the combination of 'psycho' (mind) and 'somatic' (bodily) suggests, the term refers to physical disorders caused or aggravated by psychological factors, or mental disorders caused or aggravated by physical factors (Lipowski, 1984). Hence, psychosomatic medicine is concerned with the interrelationship between mind and body.

What is health psychology?

Maes and van Elderen (1998) define HP as

> ... a sub-discipline of psychology which addresses the relationship between psychological processes and behaviour on the one hand and health and illness on the other hand ... however ... health psychologists are more interested in 'normal' everyday-life behaviour and 'normal' psychological processes in relation to health and illness than in psycho-pathology or abnormal behaviour ...

However, Turpin and Slade (1998) believe that HP is an extension of clinical psychology (see Chapter 1), focusing specifically on people with physical health problems and their associated psychological needs. They advocate the BPS model (see Figure 3.1).

Either way, HP is firmly grounded in psychological theory and has been defined as

> the aggregate of the specific educational, scientific, and professional contributions of the discipline of psychology to the promotion and maintenance of health, the prevention and treatment of illness, and the identification of aetiologic and diagnostic correlates of health, illness, and related dysfunction, and to the analysis and improvement of the healthcare system and health policy formation (Matarrazo, 1982).

Figure 3.3 shows the connections between HP and related disciplines. In other words, health psychologists

- Conduct research aimed at identifying links between psychological, biological and social variables in the aetiology of illness (reflecting the BPS model)
- Use these research findings to develop, apply and evaluate interventions to improve health.

These interventions may be targeted at any of the following:

Figure 3.3 Health psychology and related disciplines. (From French, D. et al., *Health Psychology* (2nd edn.), BPS Blackwell, Oxford, 2010.)

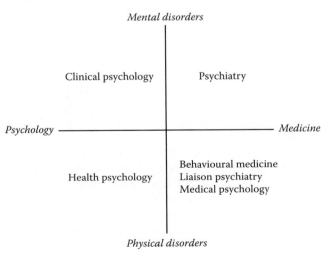

- An 'individual' level (such as psychological interventions to improve pain in patients undergoing surgery; see Chapter 4)
- An 'interpersonal' or 'organisational' level (such as improvements in doctor–patient communication within a hospital or increasing patient adherence with medical advice/instructions; see Chapter 9)
- A 'societal' level (such as public health campaigns to reduce smoking or alcohol consumption; see Chapter 6) (Hamilton-West, 2011)

Interventions can be designed to change psychosocial processes, improve health behaviours and influence neuroendocrine and immune factors and include cognitive behavioural stress management, relaxation, hypnosis, meditation, social support groups, behavioural pain management and biofeedback. These and other interventions are discussed in more detail in pages 67 through 71 and in Chapter 5 in relation to stress and Chapter 10 in relation to applications of models of health behaviour.

Meaning of psychological care

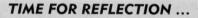

TIME FOR REFLECTION ...

- What do you understand by the term 'psychological care'?
- Why might patients need psychological care as much as they need physical care?

According to Nichols (2005),

> ... Despite 20 years of major expansion and research in psychology – and in particular health psychology – the average-patient test will almost always reveal our failure to develop psychological care as part of the thinking, culture and routines of general hospitals and health centres.

The 'average-patient test' involves visiting your local hospital, picking a ward at random, going with the clinical nurse manager to the third bed on the left or right and asking, 'Who is handling this patient's psychological care and how is it going?'

Despite nursing becoming more psychologically minded during the 1990s via Project 2000, publications encouraging the introduction of psychological approaches into health care and psychologists producing specific local provisions, such as in some stroke, intensive care or cancer units, 'psychological care is still not a common provision in hospitals' (Nichols, 2005). This neglect of psychological care has real – and serious – clinical consequences.

This is my first attempt at reflective writing about my visit to Maisie to explore this idea. I am using Gibbs' model (1988, in Bulman and Shutz, 2008) as it emphasises the importance of feelings, which I think were a significant part of the experience. Maisie was upset but I had no idea why and obviously Sally was concerned for her emotional state. I felt 'in the way' of Maisie talking about it, relieved not to have to deal with it, yet resented being excluded!

TIME FOR REFLECTION …

- List some of the common psychological responses to illness and injury you have noticed in patients.

Nichols includes shock and even post-traumatic stress disorder, confusion and distress, loss of self-worth, lowered personal control and a collapse into dependency. Apart from these responses being highly undesirable in themselves, they can also undermine medical efforts and interfere with rehabilitation. For example, Hemingway and Marmot (1999) found that the probability of cardiac patients suffering a second heart attack increased if they were in 'emotional disarray' and lacked support. Nichols believes this is exactly what psychological care is about – monitoring for signs of such responses and intervening with basic care techniques or referral to psychological treatment. Such a referral represents the link between levels 2 and 3 in a model of psychological care (Nichols, 2003), like that shown in Table 3.1.

Well, at least I achieved the first bit of level 1 this morning, but all I did was recognise Maisie's distress; Sally 'took the relevant action' by sitting down and attending to Maisie.

Nurses, therapists and medical staff (and anyone else involved in the patient's care) can all play a part under the guidance of psychologists (Nichols, 2005).

Table 3.1 The components of psychological care

Level 1 (awareness)	Awareness of psychological issues
	Patient-centred listening
	Patient-centred communication
	Awareness of the patient's psychological state and relevant action
Level 2 (intervention)	Monitoring the patient's psychological state with records kept
	Informational and educational care
	Emotional care
	Counselling care
	Support/advocacy/referral
Level 3 (therapy)	Psychological therapy

Source: Nichols, K., *Psychological Care for Ill and Injured People – A Clinical Guide*, Open University Press, Maidenhead, 2003.

Interestingly, a survey of 354 physiotherapists, chiropractors and osteopaths found that at least 10% continued long-term treatment with patients, even after 3 months or more without demonstrable improvement. Follow-up interviews with a sample of these physical therapy practitioners revealed that many see it as their responsibility to provide psychological support and health advice to patients. Despite international guidelines for the treatment of lower back pain in primary care recommending that patients be referred back to their GP in the absence of any improvement, many of the interviewees were unhappy to discharge patients and were uncertain about what would happen to them once they had left their care (The Psychologist, 2006).

Skilled communication, psychological safety and therapeutic conversation

What Nichols' model calls 'patient-centred listening' and 'patient-centred communication' corresponds with 'skilled communication' (Minardi and Riley, 1988) and 'therapeutic conversation' (Burnard, 1987).

According to Minardi and Riley (1988), the standard of care delivered to patients depends on the quality of the relationships that individual nurses build with them. A prerequisite for the development of such relationships beyond the merely social level is that both participants feel safe enough to openly discuss their feelings. However, most nurses have experienced a patient who consistently under-reports either physical or psychological discomfort. Equally, many nurses hide a variety of feelings under a mask of willing cooperation, in interaction with both patients and colleagues.

This mutual reluctance to express true feelings may reflect perception of the other person as a threat. To reduce this threat, and to ensure a free-flowing discussion, it is necessary to provide a degree of 'psychological safety' for each other.

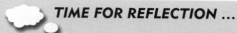

TIME FOR REFLECTION ...

- What do you understand by the term 'psychological safety'?
- With what kinds of communication skills might you show a patient (or colleague) that you understand and support them?

Egan (1977) suggests that the provision of understanding, support and encouragement enables another person to feel secure enough to disclose important emotional concerns. This would involve an individual being listened to, being allowed to speak without interruption and receiving feedback that shows he or she has been understood. It requires recognition of the person's beliefs, values, needs and wishes without judging that person:

It would appear, therefore, that the provision of psychological safety centres around the ability to communicate to an individual that their beliefs, values, needs and wishes are recognised and understood in an open and non-judgemental way (Minardi and Riley, 1988).

Agreeing with Nichols (2005), Minardi and Riley argue that in most nursing situations, the 'recovery of health' involves meeting individuals' emotional needs as much as meeting their physical needs. Such strategies are also a vital part of nurses' relationships with one another: '... the perception of a degree of psychological safety which allows a full and free expression of the concerns and anxieties which may exist in our professional relationships is essential to our work' (Minardi and Riley, 1988).

Later, Sally explained that Maisie wouldn't have said anything while I was there; she knew her well as she'd nursed her husband who'd died of cancer a year ago. I understand now that Sally had established a relationship with her patient that was 'psychologically safe' and which I, a stranger, was compromising.

Psychological safety can be enhanced by what Burnard (1987) calls therapeutic conversations (Box 3.1).

Box 3.1 Five components of the therapeutic conversation

- *Emphasis on the here and now*: Many people find the present painful to live in, whereas the past, however inaccurate our recollection, feels more comfortable. But it is more therapeutic if the nurse stays with the patient's moment-to-moment phenomenology and notes his or her changing verbal and non-verbal cues as they occur. This requires concentration, close awareness of subtle changes and the ability to 'stay awake' and remain focused on the patient.

- *Focus on feelings*: The nurse uses reflection and empathy-building to convey that he or she understands what the patient is feeling. This helps the patient to confront the feelings as they occur, rather than having a theoretical debate about why the patient is feeling this way. This focus on feelings requires training in basic counselling techniques.

- *Empathic understanding*: This involves attempting to enter the other person's frame of reference or way of looking at the world, that is, to see things from their perspective rather than our own. By understanding the patient's belief and value system, we can better appreciate why he or she is experiencing this set of feelings at this time. This too requires training.

- *A non-prescriptive approach*: To be prescriptive is to make suggestions or offer opinions about what the patient should do. It is usually more appropriate in a health-care setting to help the patient to make his or her own decisions and draw his or her own conclusions.

- *The patient should remain the central focus*: Whereas in ordinary social conversation there's a to-and-fro communication between the two speakers, in the therapeutic conversation the patient is 'telling the story' and the nurse is essentially 'listening' (albeit actively listening) (Watts [1986]). This is another skill that can be developed through experiencing what it's like to be heard.

Source: Based on Burnard P., *Nursing Times*, 83(20), 43–45, 1987.

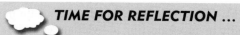 Sally had a good understanding of Maisie's frame of reference, perceived her non-verbal behaviour and focused on her immediate distress. She managed to discover Maisie was getting 'bad indigestion' pain after meals and to avoid it had resorted to not eating. She was convinced she had cancer of the stomach (as her husband had) but was afraid to complain of the pain and have her suspicions confirmed.

TIME FOR REFLECTION …

- Which of the major theoretical approaches discussed in Chapter 2 is most closely related to the various communication skills described in Box 3.1.

KEY STUDY 3.1

Nurses' and students' perceptions of care

The participants were interviewed about their understanding of the phenomenon of care and caring. Transcriptions from the taped interviews were read to develop a 'feeling' for them and to make sense of them. Statements were then categorised according to their perceived meanings and arranged into five main themes, as follows:

1. *Encouraging autonomy*: This relates to 'patient empowerment', wanting to allay patients' fears and anxieties by giving them greater control over their care.
2. *Giving of oneself*: 'Caring, it can be argued, is the essence of giving of oneself' (Bassett, 2002). Nurses give to patients in terms of time, energy and effort. They spend time learning skills and gaining knowledge, both as students and throughout their nursing careers. But to simply provide mechanical care may not be enough in their eyes – providing care without 'genuineness' is not adequate.
3. *Taking risks*: This theme comprises the sub-categories 'taking risks', 'getting a buzz' and 'challenge'. Taking risks in nursing is not about putting patients at risk but refers to testing the boundaries of accepted care, moving from the defined boundaries and developing new and innovative ways of caring for patients. Sometimes, it may be necessary to disobey a doctor's orders if this is in the patient's best interests (see Chapter 8) or to take a stand against colleagues' interpretations of normal nursing procedures or protocols. For students, this means 'standing up' for patients when they feel the care was less than what the patient deserved.
4. *Supporting care*: Certain supporting factors are essential to ensure that care can be delivered effectively. These are managerial, organisational and psychological support systems.
5. *Emotional labour*: This theme was unique to the student participants and seemed to reflect the fact that learning to nurse can constitute an emotional assault. It describes the often difficult things that nurses are expected to do in their daily work, causing them to experience sadness and emotional trauma. If unresolved or buried, these responses may lead nurses to leave nursing or not develop the caring attributes necessary for quality nursing care (see Chapter 4).

Source: Bassett, C., *Nursing Times*, 94(34), 32–34, 2002.

Another answer to the question 'What do we mean by psychological care?' is offered by Bassett (2002) in a study focusing on the lived and expressed experiences of 15 qualified nurses and 6 nursing students (2 from each year of a 3-year advanced diploma in nursing programme).

? RESEARCH QUESTION ...

- What do you consider to be some of the strengths and weaknesses of Bassett's study? (e.g., how confident can we be about the themes applying to nurses in general, was the sample size adequate, and what other methods could be used to explore nurses' perceptions of care?)

This study raises a daunting number of aspects of caring, but it does help me understand the 'emotional labour' bit; my withdrawal at seeing Maisie upset was a way of avoiding emotional involvement. Sally's experience of caring for Maisie's husband until he died must have been demanding.

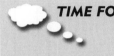

TIME FOR REFLECTION ...

- Draw a diagram summarising the various definitions and components of care discussed in Figure 3.4.
- Try to show the links or connections between them. (See Figure 3.4.)

The final theme in Bassett's study can be seen as related to the concept of 'emotional intelligence': 'a type of social intelligence that involves the ability to monitor one's own and others' emotions, to discriminate among them, and to use the information to guide one's thinking and actions' (Salovey and Mayer, 1990).

People who are able to manage their own feelings well while reading and dealing with other people's emotions are particularly suited to the caring professions. So it is surprising that most nurse education programmes fail to embrace this aspect of training (Evans and Allen, 2002).

According to Evans and Allen,

> Self-awareness is an important part of nursing. The key to self-knowledge lies in intrapersonal intelligence ... If they [students] are able to deal with their own feelings well, they will be able to deal with others confidently, competently and safely.

This explains why we should learn to acknowledge our feelings in the reflective writing we do (Gibbs, 1988, in Jasper, 2003). Recognising my own emotional discomfort is the first step to acknowledging the need to learn how to deal with such situations. Sally's attitude was positive; she explained she had reassured Maisie, but was referring her to the GP for investigations to exclude cancer. This is the support, advocacy and, in this case, medical referral in level 2 of Nichols' model (see Table 3.1).

Figure 3.4 The relationship between different definitions and components of care.

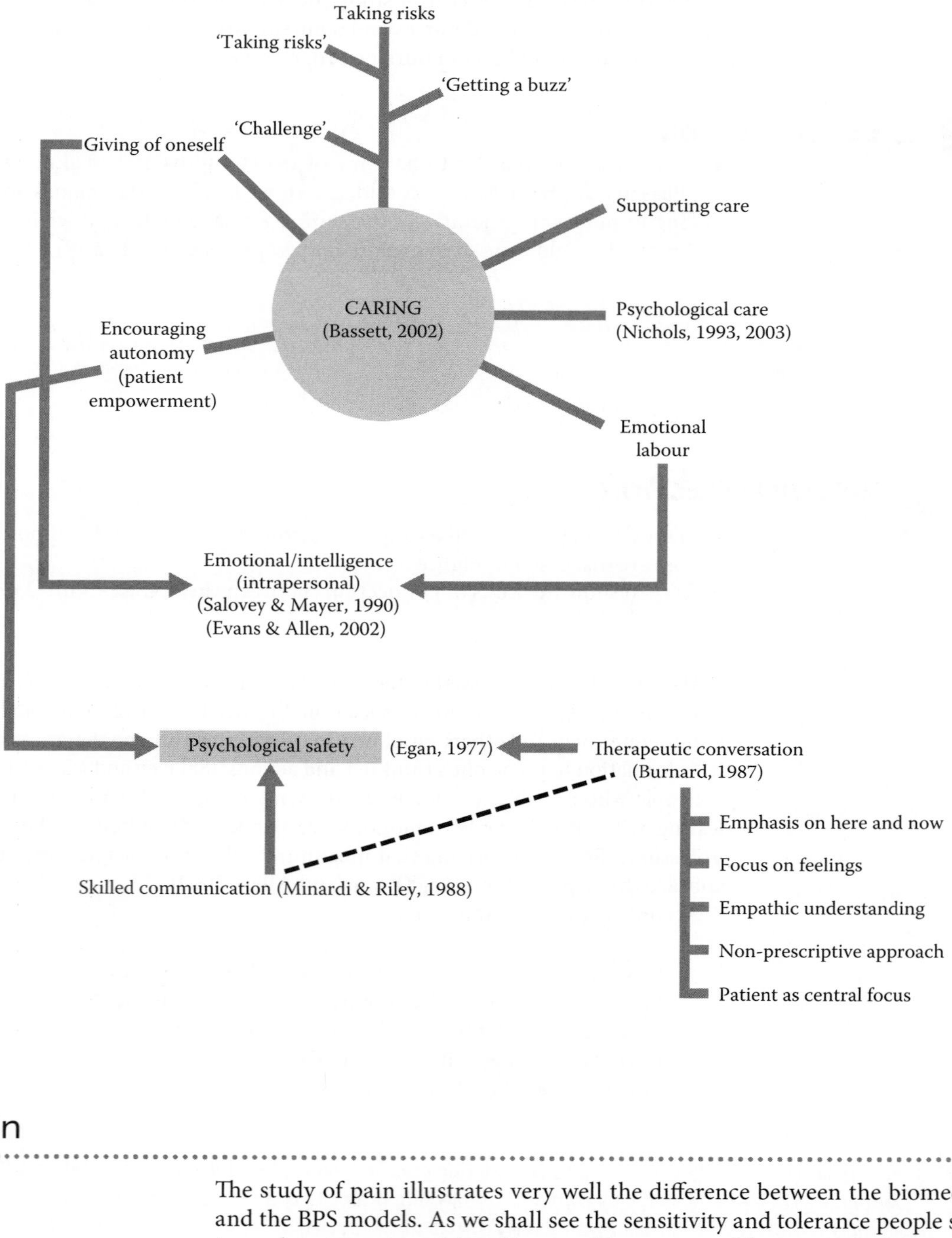

Pain

The study of pain illustrates very well the difference between the biomedical and the BPS models. As we shall see the sensitivity and tolerance people show towards pain varies predictably according to several factors, including gender, ethnicity, personality and culture:

> ... all interacting, overlapping and playing out in the
> tissues and synapses of the body. Indeed, the topic of
> individual differences in pain is like a microcosm of
> science – it's where biology, psychology and sociology
> all meet ... (Jarrett, 2011)

This interaction and overlap between biological, psychological and socio-cultural factors is exactly what a biomedical approach to understanding pain fails to take into account.

According to Eccleston (2011),

> Pain and suffering are fundamental to human being.
> Indeed, we are born into pain, will likely die in pain,
> and we have lives punctuated by painful experience.
> On the brighter side, we are adept at learning how to
> live with pain; we have developed extensive knowledge
> and tools for analgesia and anaesthesia, have created
> social structures that offer respite, succour and prac-
> tical help, and have even developed methods for per-
> sonal growth in our reflection on pain and suffering.

This rather depressing comment on the universality of pain was evident over the next few weeks; it was a recurring problem in our visits. The fact I didn't regard it as significant in itself perhaps reveals an acceptance of its inevitability?

The whole subject of pain obviously requires a good deal of analysis to help me 'make sense of the situation', which is the next stage of Gibbs' Reflective Cycle.

What is pain?

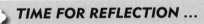

TIME FOR REFLECTION ...

- Can you describe the experience of pain?
- Are there different kinds of pain?
- If so, how do they differ?
- Is pain a purely physical, bodily phenomenon?

According to the International Association for the Study of Pain (IASP, 1986), pain is 'an unpleasant sensory and emotional experience associated with actual or potential tissue damage, or described in terms of such damage'. This definition indicates that pain is a subjective, personal experience involving both sensory (e.g., shooting, burning and aching) and emotional (e.g., frightening, annoying and sickening) qualities. Fear/anxiety can increase the perception of pain, and depression often accompanies chronic pain (Bradley, 1995).

While pain is a physiological 'protective mechanism' for the body (Collins, 1994), this doesn't explain the pain experience, which includes both the pain sensation and certain autonomic responses and 'associated feeling states'

(Zborowski, 1952). For example, understanding the physiology of pain cannot explain the acceptance of intense pain in torture or the strong emotional reactions of certain individuals to the slight sting of a hypodermic needle.

'Pure' pain is never detected as an isolated sensation: it is always accompanied by emotion and meaning, so that each pain is unique to the individual (O'Connell, 2000). Ultimately, the subjective nature of pain makes it difficult to find a satisfactory scientific definition. Box 3.2 describes different types of pain.

Maisie likened her pain to indigestion (a biological explanation), but, as O'Connell (2000) observes above, it had emotional elements to it – her anxiety in case she had cancer (psychological pain) and the effects of her husband's illness and death (spiritual pain). Her progress improved rapidly when her investigations, happily, proved negative!

Communicating the pain experience

According to McCaffrey and Beebe (1994), pain is 'whatever the experiencing person says it is, existing whenever the experiencing person says it does'. However, according to Schott (2004), 'pain is intrinsically impossible to convey to others and therefore language will always prove inadequate'; this difficulty with putting painful experiences into words also applies to other unpleasant sensory and emotional experiences. Pain is especially difficult to convey to

---

Box 3.2 Different types of pain

- *'Acute pain'* serves as a warning to tell people that something is wrong and to seek help. The problems causing the pain can usually be diagnosed and, if treated, will usually get rid of the pain.
- *'Chronic non-malignant pain'* (CNMP) 'persists beyond the point at which healing would be expected to be complete or ... occurs in disease processes in which healing does not take place' (Clinical Standards Advisory Group, 2000). Unlike acute pain, it often serves no purpose. A diagnosis cannot always be given, which can be difficult for the patient to accept. The approach is to manage it, not to cure or remove it. Back pain constitutes a significant proportion of CNMP, but it can be caused by whiplash injuries, arthritis, diabetic neuropathy and trigeminal neuralgia. It can also be secondary to other chronic conditions, such as multiple sclerosis and stroke.
- *'Psychological pain'* is a multifaceted experience that includes feelings of hopelessness, guilt, unresolved anger and fear of the unknown. It is often expressed in body language and physical symptoms (see Chapter 13).
- *'Spiritual pain'*: 'The realisation that life is likely to end soon may well give rise to feelings of the unfairness of what is happening, and at much of what has gone before, and above all a desolate feeling of meaninglessness' (Saunders, 1988). Spiritual pain is often now considered in relation to the care of the bereaved, but it is just as relevant to terminally ill patients (again, see Chapter 13).

Source: Based on Howarth, A., *Nursing Times*, 98(32), 52–53, 2002; Morrison, R., *Nursing Standard*, 6(25), 36–38, 1992; Sheahan, P., *Nursing Times*, 92(17), 63–67, 1996.

those who have not experienced it themselves (or, more accurately, who have not experienced a comparable pain-inducing situation, such as childbirth). Schott (2004) also claims that the meaning of the terms used to describe pain may vary for different patients and different pain experiences; in other words, the same words can convey different things to different people at different times.

Hamilton-West (2011) observes that a number of researchers have suggested that chronic pain patients should receive skills training or therapy aimed at enhancing communication with caregivers and improving caregivers' responses to pain behaviours. Researchers have also recommended that health-care providers are trained to recognise non-verbal signs of pain (either chronic or acute) in patients.

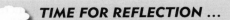 I'm fortunate that childbirth is the worst pain I've experienced in my life and was of comparatively short duration. Thinking about it, although very unpleasant at the time, I didn't have negative feelings about it, then or now.

TIME FOR REFLECTION …

- List some examples of non-verbal expressions of pain.
- What factors do you think might influence patients' experience and expression of pain and nurses' perception of their pain?

Pain assessment

Consistent with this discussion of the difficulties involved in describing one's pain to another person, Daniel and Williams (2010) state that 'any assessment tool is a compromise between the richness of patients' own descriptions and the need for economical and standardized measurement'. How pain is assessed depends on the purpose of the assessment: diagnosis, decision about treatment, evaluation of treatment effects or predicting response to treatment (Turk and Okifuji, 2003). Assessment of persistent pain should consider pain experience, its psychological content and process, its function and use of health-care resources (McDowell and Newell, 1996; Turk and Melzack, 2001; Williams, 2007a).

In the last few weeks, I've met two patients with painful chronic conditions: Sarah is a diabetic who also has rheumatoid arthritis, Alan has osteoarthritis and a leg ulcer and so has both chronic pain and acute pain when his dressing is done. I'm discovering that many patients, especially the older ones, have complicated case histories.

Pain scales

A number of measures have been developed and validated for use in different contexts with different populations:

- 'Visual analogue scales' (VASs) remain one of the most popular forms of measurement (Daniel and Williams, 2010). These are commonly used in clinical settings and require the patient to indicate his or her level of pain by

Figure 3.5 Examples of visual analogue scales.

- Visual analogue scales may be continuous or intermittent:

10 cm unmarked line   No pain _____ Worst possible pain

Coloured analogue scale

Facial anchors

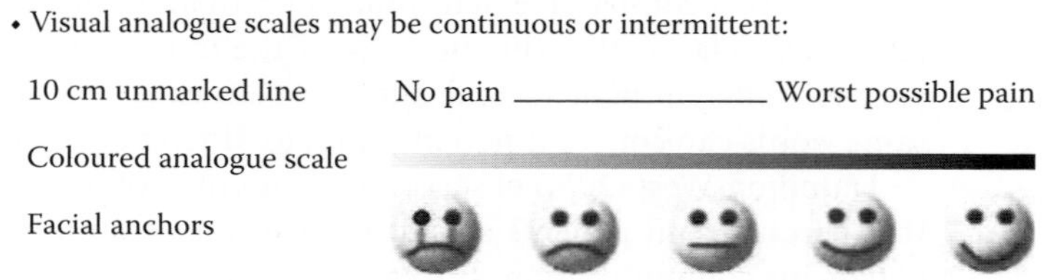

placing a mark on a 10-cm line with anchors at each end (e.g., 'no pain' and 'worst pain imaginable'/'worst possible pain'). Surprisingly, there is almost no research on the effect of verbal anchors for the highest pain levels on these scales. Pain relief is usually measured as a percentage: 50% pain relief is a common, if arbitrary, criterion for successful treatment (Daniel and Williams, 2010). (See Figure 3.5.)

- 'Numerical rating scales' (NRSs) ask the patient to rate his or her pain intensity from 0 to 10 (with '0' being the lowest and '10' the highest).
- 'Verbal rating scales' (VRSs) use pain descriptors representing increasing pain intensity (e.g., 'mild', 'discomforting', 'distressing', 'horrible', and 'excruciating'). While entirely verbal scales are easy to administer and have high face validity (i.e., they appear to be measuring pain, as they are intended to), they can present problems for scaling and scoring (Jensen and Karoly, 2001).
- For use with children and patients with cognitive impairment/learning difficulties, pain can be assessed through the use of visual depictions of faces that represent increasing levels of pain (as shown in Figure 3.5). Pain assessment in neonates and infants is discussed further in Critical Discussion 3.1.
- The scales described in the aforementioned list items are all 'unidimensional', that is, there is no differentiation between different dimensions of pain, such as sensory/intensity, emotional/motivational, cognitive and interference with everyday life. This is a problem because patients find it difficult to distinguish between, say, the intensity of their pain and the distress it causes. So, although these scales claim to measure pain intensity, scores more likely reflect a combination of sensory, emotional and other pain qualities (Knotkova et al., 2004).
- Multidimensional measures designed to address these problems include the McGill pain questionnaire (MPQ) (Melzack, 1975; short form, Melzack, 1987); this includes a pain drawing, a numerical intensity scale and a list of 20 pain descriptors, which tap the sensory, affective and evaluative dimensions of pain.

One day Sally asked Sarah how she was and she said she was 'good' as she was having a 'below five' few days. Apparently, when she sees the consultant he asks her to rate the severity of her pain on a 0–10 scale and she now uses the numerical scale to monitor herself; if it's below five in the morning, it's a good day! So for her, I presume the number is a symbolic summary of all the different aspects of her pain.

CRITICAL DISCUSSION 3.1

Do neonates and young children feel pain?

- Of all patient populations, neonates are the most compromised in terms of their ability to communicate their pain experience. According to Hamilton-West (2011), research into pain in neonates has highlighted problems with how pain is defined, conceptualised, assessed and treated. For example, Anand and Craig (1996) highlighted several problems with the widely accepted IASP definition of pain (see page 53) when applied to neonates: the reliance on self-reporting may have led to the failure to acknowledge and treat pain in infants and young children.

- Consequently, the IASP has amended the definition, stating that 'the inability to communicate verbally does not negate the possibility that an individual is experiencing pain and is in need of appropriate pain-relieving treatment'. However, recent reports conclude that pain-relieving treatments are still underused, particularly in relation to the numerous minor procedures that are part of routine care for neonates (American Academy of Pediatrics, 2006).

- According to Hodges (1998), another widely held myth maintains that narcotic analgesia should not be administered to young children because they will become addicted. This fear of addiction is also relevant to pain management in adults. However, less than 1% of all patients become addicted to opiates and children are no more at risk than adults. Also, addiction is not the same as dependence (see Chapter 12).

- Nurses play a central role in assessing when and how much analgesia is required. Hodges (1998) cites a number of studies that show that nurses often wrongly perceive and underestimate a child's pain compared with the child's own rating.

- McCaffery and Beebe (1994) argue that children are not more tolerant of pain; they just use distraction techniques more effectively than adults. A Royal College of Surgeons report (1990) also concluded that children's pain, although different, is no less severe than adults'.

- Measures of pain in neonates tend to rely on the identification of facial expressions and behaviours associated with pain. For example, a neonatal facial coding system (NFCS) (Grunau and Craig, 1987; Grunau et al., 1990) has been used to study pain in full-term, preterm and older infants. Facial expressions coded using the NFCS have been shown to be more specific to tissue damage than heart rate (Grunau et al., 1998).

- Also, the CRIES (Bildner and Krechel, 1996) instrument was developed to measure post-operative pain in infants up to 6 months of age. A score is provided for each of crying, oxygen requirement, increased vital signs, expression and sleeplessness.

- Another barrier to adequate pain relief is the reluctance of medical and nursing staff to use painful intramuscular injections to deliver analgesics. A major alternative is *patient-controlled analgesia* (PCA), which is suitable for children over the age of 4 or 5 years (Hodges, 1998).

According to King and McCool (2004), even in adults behavioural responses to pain may be more critical indicators than VAS scores, especially in the case of acute, intense pain. Even where VAS scores are used, it's important that behavioural responses are also taken into account; these may be evaluated via unstructured observation or using formal scoring systems, such as the pain behaviour checklist (Kerns et al., 1991).

Sally always finds time to discuss pain management with the patients. Most are stabilized on analgesic regimes and Alan takes extra painkillers an hour before she arrives to do his dressing as his ulcer is so deep. Last time she offered him some gas and air which he stoically refused, but afterwards she said she's going to recommend he has Fentanyl patches; she thinks he's not admitting how much pain he has.

Although pain is reliably expressed in the face, culture and context influence expressiveness (Craig et al., 2001; Williams, 2002). However, facial expression may be the only unique indicator of pain in people with compromised or underdeveloped communication capacities (Hadjistavropoulos et al., 2001). Other motor behaviours, such as guarding, are important and can be assessed by observation (Keefe et al., 2001); this is preferable to self-reporting of these behaviours (Daniel and Williams, 2010).

Daniel and Williams (2010) observe that pain can be operationalised in terms of function, which can be assessed in terms of the following:

- Measures of physical performance
- Impact or interference of pain
- Quality-of-life measures
- Work (or equivalent) status
- Health-care use

Cognitive aspects of pain

Expectancy and acceptance are as much cognitive as emotional dimensions of pain. Trusting the doctor's ability to ease your suffering (whether this takes the form of a cure or merely the relief of pain and suffering) represents part of the 'cognitive appraisal' aspect of pain, that is, the belief that the illness/symptoms are controllable. If we attribute our symptoms to something that's controllable, this should make us feel more optimistic (see Chapter 4). The meaning of our illness may be a crucial factor in how we react to it, including any associated pain.

This applies to Sarah – she understands her illness can't be cured but she's optimistic there will be newer drugs which will control it or improve it. At present she's on Isobrufen for pain and Leflunomide, which has caused her hair to thin; this distresses her.

If patients are allowed to perform necessary painful procedures on themselves (such as debridement of dead skin in severe burn cases), they tend to find the pain is reduced compared with the same procedure performed by a nurse (Melzack and Wall, 1991). This suggests the role of control in influencing the patient's level of anxiety, which, in turn, affects subjective pain (see Chapter 4).

Expectations and the modulatory pathway

Since the 1970s, researchers have been uncovering, piece by piece, a circuit in the brain and spinal cord that functions as a kind of volume control for pain, adjusting the amount a person perceives depending on the circumstances (Fields, 2009). For example, patients with severe chronic pain obtain significant, though temporary, relief from electrical stimulation of a site in the midbrain called the 'periaqueductal grey'. The body's pain-control circuit stretches from the cerebral cortex in the frontal lobes through underlying brain structures (including the periaqueductal grey) to the spinal cord, where pain-sensitive nerve fibres connect to neurons that transmit pain signals from the rest of the body. Neurons in this pathway synthesise endorphins – the body's natural painkillers – that have pharmacological properties identical to the powerful opioid morphine. Endorphins and opioids (which also include opium and heroin: see Chapter 12) attach themselves to the same 'μ-opioid' receptors along this pain modulatory pathway to produce their analgesic effects (see Figure 3.6).

Neuroscientists are finding that cognitive influences on pain operate through this modulatory pathway: the pathway acts as the conduit for a variety of expectation effects, including the prospect of pain relief (i.e., expectation of analgesia) from a 'placebo' (Fields, 2009).

Figure 3.6 Pain modulatory pathway.

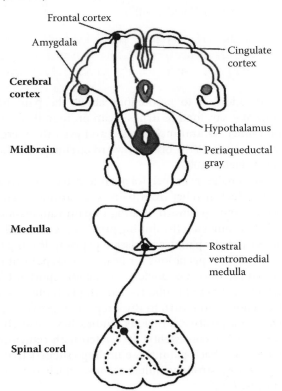

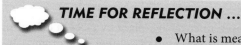

TIME FOR REFLECTION ...

- What is meant by a placebo?
- What is meant by a 'placebo effect'?
- Describe what the placebo condition in a drug trial might be.

A *placebo* denotes an inactive/inert substance, designed to take account of the psychological (as opposed to pharmacological) influences on physiological change (such as the expectation of improvement). A *placebo effect* refers to the positive psychological or physiological changes associated with the administration of a placebo. In drug trials, the placebo condition is the *control condition* and usually involves a sugar pill or some other inactive/inert substance.

However, rather than dismissing the effect of a placebo as a 'mere' placebo effect, implying that it is purely psychological (as a supporter of the biomedical approach would do), Zubieta et al. (2005) found that the placebo effect is a very real, demonstrable biological effect: their data show that cognitive factors (such as expecting pain relief) are capable of influencing physical and emotional states through activation of μ-opioid receptor signalling in the human brain (i.e., the activation of endorphins). Blocking μ-opioid receptors using the drug naloxone removes the placebo effect in patients experiencing pain from recent surgery (Fields, 2009).

Sarah tried acupuncture in the early part of her illness and said it did give relief for a short while, but it didn't last; I must admit I dismissed acupuncture as 'all in the mind'. But could it have been due to stimulation of neurons synthesising endorphins – or the more psychologically influenced effect of expectation?

In addition to predictions about the pain itself, the expectation of a reward – say, food or drugs – can profoundly affect pain intensity. Food, sex and other natural incentives – and even the mere anticipation of such pleasures – activate the brain's reward circuitry, which, in turn, can produce pain relief (Fields, 2009).

The analgesic properties of anticipated rewards are consistent with the placebo effect: if relief from pain is rewarding, then a placebo pill is a sign of a forthcoming reward, leading to pain suppression. Thus, the expectation of relief becomes a self-fulfilling prophecy. Conversely, predicting pain amplifies activity in the pain transmission pathway, leading to greater pain perception.

Positive expectations for healing from painful injuries can result in faster actual recovery. Ozegovic et al. (2009) reported that among 2335 Canadians who had suffered traffic-related whiplash injuries, those who expected to get well enough to return to work reported recovering 42% faster that those who were less positive. Previous studies have also shown that expectations for recovery are consistently associated with returning to work among patients with lower back pain; these findings suggest that a person's outlook on the future can strongly influence how much pain impacts on his or her life (Fields, 2009).

📄   As this seems to be true for both acute and more chronic conditions, perhaps Sarah's optimism is helping her cope with her pain?

Individual differences

People's pain thresholds (the lowest stimulus value reported as painful) clearly differ (although the reasons are much less clear – Starr [1995]). Post-operative pain is influenced by anxiety, neuroticism and extroversion (Taenzer et al., 1986). How pain is communicated may be affected by gender, socialisation and self-efficacy (see Chapter 10) (Miller and Newton, 2006).

Fields (2009) describes a 2007 study of 131,500 Canadians, which showed that among chronic pain patients 11.3% had major depressive disorder; this compared with just 5.3% of individuals without chronic pain. Although we cannot conclude from these data that depression increases the experience of pain, and being in pain may be depressing, depression itself is thought to affect pain perception. Neurochemical changes associated with depression (such as the depletion of the neurotransmitters serotonin and noradrenaline; see Gross [2010]) may reduce normal inhibition or increase facilitation within the descending pain pathway.

Box 3.3 describes the extremes of pain experience that have been reported between individuals.

📄   This describes Maisie's situation perfectly; she was sure she had cancer and stopped eating, which may have adversely affected her recovery. (See page 50.)

According to Tyrer (2010), psychological disorders are more often manifest in patients with chronic pain than in the standard population; the fear of pain in relation to catastrophisation is one of several mechanisms by which pain may be experienced in the absence of sufficient sensory stimuli to account for the intensity of the feelings. However, catastrophising pain is not necessarily a symptom of mental disorder. Patients who score high on catastrophising on a standard questionnaire tend to experience more severe post-operative pain and show more sensitivity to experimentally induced pain compared with those who score

Box 3.3 Extremes of pain experience

Some individuals perceive pain in a malign way through the process of 'catastrophisation' (Asmundson et al., 2004): the cause of the pain is viewed in a horrific light and the individual worries about the effects of this on the body. This process may occur because of previous life experiences, particularly episodes of situations involving pain, anxiety and perceived threats to physical integrity. The symptoms of distress persuade the individual to avoid activities and situations that might give rise to further pain; this reduction in mobility prevents the re-establishment of physical routines that are essential in promoting recovery from injury. In this way, the painful state is reinforced (Peters et al., 2005).

low on the questionnaire (Fields, 2009). Catastrophising may worsen pain by focusing the individual's attention to it and attaching additional emotion to it.

At the opposite end of the responding-to-pain scale are individuals with a chronic indifference to pain (CIP) (or *congenital analgesia*); this is an extremely rare, genetically determined inability to perceive pain (thought to be caused by a mutation in a single gene). Wickelgren (2009) cites the study of a group of such patients living in Pakistan. Although they can sense touch, heat, vibration and their body's position in space, pain has no place in their experience. One boy entertained others by sticking knives in his arms and leaping out of trees; he died jumping off a roof. Those who survive are often deformed and disabled by self-mutilation or broken bones that they failed to notice or for which they refused to rest.

While pain may be difficult to describe in and of itself, the problem is even more evident in relation to patients with cognitive impairments/learning difficulties; they may be unable to communicate their pain experience in the same way as other people (Hamilton-West, 2011). MENCAP (2007) highlighted the cases of six cognitively impaired adults who, they believe, died because health-care professionals failed to recognise their pain and distress and to consult with or involve the families who could have provided vital information relevant to appropriate treatment. As Hamilton-West (2011) observes, the MENCAP report 'highlights the crucial importance of listening to patients and their families and conducting thorough pain assessments in order to inform diagnosis and treatment'.

Apparently older people (like Alan?) are often reluctant to acknowledge and report pain but it should be part of every assessment and should be multidimensional: sensory (the type, location and severity), affective (the emotional effect), and impact (the effect on function).
(Clinical skills in Adult Nursing, ed. Randle, Coffey and Bradbury, 2009).

I don't understand why it should be assumed children's pain isn't as bad as adults' or why they should be able to tolerate it more. And the difficulty in assessment must also apply to anyone unable to communicate their pain, so recognising behavioural signs is important in every branch of nursing.

Pain and gender

The research points overwhelmingly in one direction: whether in the laboratory or the clinic, men demonstrate greater tolerance of, and less sensitivity to, pain than women (Jarrett, 2011). Women are also 10 times more likely to be diagnosed with chronic pain conditions such as fibromyalgia, which is typically associated with all-over body pain, increased pain sensitivity and tenderness when specific parts of the body (the nine paired 'tender points' on either side of the body) are touched ('allodynia'). Women are also at greater risk than men for rheumatoid arthritis and lupus.

Paulson et al. (1998) scanned the brains of 10 women and 10 men while they experienced a heat stimulus applied to their forearm. The participants were told the experiment was testing their ability to discriminate temperatures using a scale from 0 (no heat sensation) to 10 (just barely tolerable pain). Not only did the female participants consistently rate the higher 50°C stimulus as more painful than the males but also their brains showed a greater activity change; this change occurred in both the anterior cingulate cortex (known to be associated with the evaluation of painful stimuli) and posterior insula (which regulates internal bodily states).

Sex hormones may contribute to this gender difference. For example, oestrogen can often increase pain, partly by acting at receptors that sit on pain nerves. During their menstrual cycle, women perceive more pain after ovulation when progesterone – and to a lesser extent oestrogen – levels are high. Hormone replacement therapy (HRT) also increases pain sensitivity, whereas drugs that block oestrogen provide long-term pain relief in certain situations (Wickelgren, 2009).

Further evidence for a biological male–female difference relates to the body's endogenous opioids. Zubieta et al. (2002) gave 14 men and 14 women an excruciatingly painful injection of saline into their cheeks while scanning their brains using positron emission tomography (PET). The researchers found less μ-opioid system activation in the brains of female participants compared with male participants.

Other evidence also points to weaker pain inhibition in women. Intense or long-lasting pain applied to one part of the body, say, an arm, can suppress pain at another site, such as a tooth. The initial pain is thought to invoke the body's descending pain suppression system (Wickelgren, 2009). Cognitive factors believed to help explain gender differences in pain response include catastrophising (see Box 3.3, page 61).

However, men are less likely to want to *admit* they have found a stimulus painful. Several studies have shown that men report lower pain intensity ratings and show greater pain tolerance when the experimenter is female, and at least one study has found that women also report higher pain tolerance when tested by a male experimenter (Jarrett, 2011).

So it seems unfair that it's the women who have the babies! More seriously, I wonder if Alan's refusal of the gas and air had anything to do with it being offered by an attractive, female nurse.

Pain and personality

Since the 1980s, a vast amount of research has been done to discover a small but comprehensive number of basic trait dimensions that can account for the structure of personality and individual differences. There is a growing consensus that personality can adequately be described by five broad constructs or factors, commonly referred to as the 'big five' (see Table 3.2) (Costa and McCrae, 1992; Digman, 1990; Goldberg, 1993; McCrae and Costa, 1989).

A consistent research finding is that people who score higher on neuroticism (or a neuroticism-like factor) tend to show greater sensitivity to pain and reduced tolerance. Vossen et al. (2006) showed that this sensitivity is also reflected in an exaggerated cortical response to pain as measured by an electroencephalogram (EEG) (see Chapter 2).

Table 3.2 The big five personality factors

	Desirable traits	Undesirable traits
1. Extroversion (corresponds to Eysenck's construct)	Outgoing, sociable, assertive	Introverted, reserved, passive
2. Agreeableness	Kind, trusting, warm	Hostile, selfish, cold
3. Conscientiousness	Organised, thorough, tidy	Careless, unreliable, sloppy
4. Emotional stability (or neuroticism) (corresponds to Eysenck's construct)	Calm, even-tempered, imperturbable	Moody, temperamental, narrow
5. Intellect/openness to experience	Imaginative, intelligent, creative	Shallow, unsophisticated, imperceptive

Aspects of personality also seem to predict how people respond to pain relief. According to Pud et al. (2006), both men and women who scored more highly on 'harm avoidance' (a trait resembling neuroticism) showed a larger response to morphine as indicated by their later tolerance of pain. (This was measured by the *cold pressor test*, i.e., immersing the arm into iced water until the pain becomes intolerable.)

People with a chronic pain condition tend to display a characteristic personality profile. For example, Applegate et al. (2005) followed up more than 2000 university students after a 30-year gap and found that those who had scored highly in their youth on measures of femininity (male participants only), paranoia (females only), hypochondriasis or hysteria were also more likely to have a chronic pain condition in middle age.

Conrad et al. (2007) compared 207 patients with 105 pain-free controls. The patients scored higher on harm avoidance and lower on self-directedness (a mix of the big five factors of conscientiousness and extroversion and cooperativeness [similar to agreeableness]). The patients also tended to score higher on depression and state anxiety. People with high harm avoidance who suffer a painful injury will continue to rest, relax and generally be careful even after the injury has healed. Conrad et al. also found that low *self-efficacy* (the belief that we can act effectively and control events that influence our life) (Bandura, 1977, 1986) is associated with chronic pain (see Chapter 9).

However, not everyone agrees with the conclusions of this and other related research. For example, Eccleston (2011) argues that the idea of there being a 'pain personality' is accepted now as popular myth: no evidence exists for any stable personality traits that put one at risk of chronic pain, or for any underlying psychological vulnerability.

Making sense of contradictory research is difficult! And how would we, as nurses, assess the personality of our patients? It seems the best approach, while being aware of the many factors which can affect the perception of pain and its alleviation, is to treat each patient on a highly individual basis.

Cutural and ethnic dimensions pf pain

A patient's cultural background is one of the factors influencing the inferences a nurse makes about his or her physical pain and psychological distress (Davitz et al., 1977). But, equally, nurses' own cultural background can affect the kind of judgments they make about patients' suffering. For example, if nurses from Anglo-Saxon or Germanic backgrounds (the majority of the American sample in Davitz et al.'s study) tend to minimise physical pain and psychological distress, how do these beliefs affect relationships with patients from another culture? They conclude by saying that recognising cultural differences regarding beliefs about suffering can prevent a great deal of misunderstanding and misperceptions and lead to more effective, sensitive patient care.

I didn't even consider an epidural when I had my baby; perhaps my Asian grandmother's influence was still powerful within the family? Both control and meaning influenced my decision; I wanted a natural childbirth, so I anticipated and prepared for the pain and was confident I could manage it (I didn't recognise this as a 'cognitive perspective' at the time!). I also saw the pain as purposeful, unlike Maisie, who would see hers as having a sinister outcome, or Sarah, for whom there is little expectation of reward.

Not only are women more prone to pain, so are certain ethnic groups. African Americans (and others of African or Asian descent) display greater sensitivity to painful stimuli compared with white Caucasian people, at least under laboratory conditions (Jarrett, 2011; Wickelgren, 2009).

Cultural factors related to ethnic identity (such as religion, education and social expressiveness) might give specific meanings to pain or suggest coping strategies. Such shared beliefs and practices may not only influence people's outward expressions of pain but also shape the biological infrastructure underlying the pain experience. One example of this is the endogenous pain control mechanism called 'diffuse noxious inhibitory controls'. This mechanism was demonstrated by Campbell et al. (2008), who induced ischaemic pain by tightening an arm tourniquet; during this procedure, they electrically shocked the participant's ankle. Compared with the African American participants, white participants showed greater reductions in electrical pain ratings; this suggests that African Americans are less effective in controlling pain than white people.

Palmer et al. (2007) found that reports of all-over body pain were four times higher on average among a sample of South Asian participants in the United Kingdom compared with white Europeans. Crucially, such reports were negatively correlated with participants' degree of assimilation into British culture; in other words, the lesser the degree of assimilation, the greater the reported all-over body pain. One possible explanation for these findings is that ethnic differences in pain experience are largely cultural: people who identify with their ethnic group are more likely to be susceptible to these cultural influences. Cultural influences are, in turn, likely to be mediated via neurobiological factors and processes (Jarrett, 2011).

Pain and injury

Pain without injury

The IASP definition recognises that an individual need not suffer actual tissue damage at a specific body site to perceive pain at that site, as in the 'phantom limb' phenomenon (see Gross [2010]). In describing treatment of phantom limb pain, Ramachandran and Blakeslee (1998) maintain that 'pain is an opinion on the organism's state of health rather than a mere reflexive response to an injury. There is no direct hotline from pain receptors to "pain centres" in the brain'.

Two-thirds of amputees suffer pain in their phantom limb. Paraplegics sometimes complain that their legs make continuous cycling movements, which produces painful fatigue, despite the fact that their actual legs are lying immobile on the bed (Curtiss, 1999).

Phantom limb pain is one of several examples of how it is possible to experience pain in the absence of any physical damage/injury. Others include *neuralgia* (nerve pain) and *caucalgia* (a burning pain that often follows a severe wound, such as stabbing), both of which develop after the wound/injury has healed. Tension headaches/migraines are surprisingly difficult to explain: the widely held account in terms of dilation of blood vessels has been discredited in the light of research showing that dilation is more likely to be the *result* than the cause (Melzack and Wall, 1988).

According to Munro (2000), 4.7% of the U.K. population suffers from fibromyalgia/chronic widespread pain (or chronic musculoskeletal pain of no identifiable origin). This often 'overlaps' with other syndromes, such as irritable bowel, temperomandibular disorder and tension headache and is definitely associated with psychiatric disturbance and hypochondriacal anxieties about health. As yet, there is no convincing medical explanation for them.

Objective indicators of tissue damage often correspond poorly with perceived pain. Wickelgren (2009) cites a study that showed that the amount of inflammation in rheumatoid arthritis patients did not parallel the degree of suffering they reported. In people with osteoarthritis, the tissue damage revealed by x-rays often bears little relationship to how much discomfort the patient feels.

So there is a remarkable discrepancy between the biological evidence and the perception of pain! This means that we had better ensure the 'evidence base' that guides nursing practice is not based only on the medical model.

Injury without pain

As we noted earlier in page 62, people with CIP are incapable of feeling pain (a potentially life-threatening disorder), whereas those with *episodic analgesia* experience pain only minutes or even hours after the injury has occurred.

This can sometimes be life-saving, as when soldiers suffer horrific injuries but suffer little/no pain while waiting for medical attention (e.g., Beecher, 1956). Similarly, Curtiss, (1999) cites a study which found that of 138 accident patients in accidents and emergency departments, 37% reported not feeling any pain at the time of the injury (embarrassment seemed to be the most relevant emotion). Most reported pain within an hour of the injury, but in some cases this was delayed by up to 9 hours.

Treating pain

According to the *misdirected problem-solving model* of chronic pain (Eccleston and Crombez, 2007), chronic pain is an active process of searching for solutions: people are seen as actively pursuing pain management. Figure 3.7 represents the psychological processes involved in making sense of pain.

Eccleston (2011) points out how the model helps to guide different approaches to psychological treatment:

- For those who are anxiously hypervigilant for signals of possible pain, with a heightened fear of possible consequences of pain, a behavioural therapeutic treatment focusing on fear exposure is best. (This refers to 'behaviour therapy', based on classical conditioning; see Chapter 2.)
- Where the focus of treatment is on reducing the rigidity of belief in pain as requiring biomedical intervention, and in changing the problem frame from one of needing a cure to one of managing a chronic problem, a variety of methods from *cognitive behavioural therapy* (CBT) are indicated. (Related to CBT is *self-management*; this refers to multiple treatments, such

Figure 3.7 A misdirected problem-solving model of chronic pain.

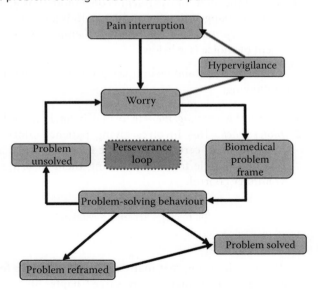

KEY STUDY 3.2

Giving birth the electromyograph way

- Duchene used electromyograph biofeedback to reduce the acute pain associated with childbirth among 40 first-time mothers. This measures muscle tension.
- They were randomly assigned to the experimental or control group; the former attended six weekly training sessions and were provided with biofeedback machines for practice at home. The feedback was provided through both sound and a visual monitor based on the tension of the abdominal muscles, which the women focused on relaxing when they felt a pain or contraction.
- All the women were monitored for pain perception, starting at admission and then at various points during labour, then again at delivery and once more 24 hours after delivery (to recall the overall pain intensity).
- Whereas 14 of the 20 control group women requested and had epidurals for pain relief, only 8 of the experimental group did so (a significant difference). The experimental group's labours were also significantly shorter.

Source: Duchene, P., *Nursing Times*, 86(25), 56, 1990.

as learning coping skills, progressive muscle relaxation training, practice in communicating effectively with family and health-care providers, and providing positive reinforcement for displaying coping behaviour.) Patients are encouraged to take responsibility for managing their pain and to attribute their success to their own efforts.

- Where the focus of treatment is on a more thoroughgoing accommodation of a life changed to one in which pain is a feature – but not a central one – then *acceptance and commitment therapy* (ACT) is emerging as the treatment of choice (see below).

Other methods and techniques used to treat (mainly chronic) pain include the following:

1. *Contingency management* (a form of behaviour modification; see Chapter 2).
2. *Biofeedback*: This involves giving patients information (via monitors or buzzers) about certain autonomic functions (such as blood pressure, heart rate and muscle tension), enabling them to bring these functions under voluntary control.

This helps explain my experience of childbirth. I attended relaxation classes regularly, although not with biofeedback, and became good at relaxing at will which I am convinced helped me cope.

It is worth noting that many of these techniques for treating pain are also used in the management of stress (see Chapter 5).

Acceptance and commitment therapy

Although it may be hard to imagine, life can be lived well with chronic pain. Data from children's and adults' pain management programmes show that large reductions in disability and distress can be achieved even where the reductions in pain are modest or non-existent (Eccleston et al., 2003; Vowles and McCraken, 2009). Also, after appropriate treatment individuals with pain can come to use medical services much less, becoming more confident and reliant on their own ability to cope (Gauntlett-Gilbert and Connell, 2011). How can psychology help to support this?

Psychologists have traditionally distinguished between two kinds of coping (see Chapter 5):

1. *Active coping* includes proactive problem-solving and seeking support.
2. *Passive coping* includes withdrawal or avoidance of activities.

Active coping is complex and contemporary pain researchers split it into two forms:

1. *Assimilative coping* tries to change or solve the problem at hand, such as curing or reducing the pain through medical or non-medical methods;
2. *Accommodative coping* tries to adjust to the difficulty rather than change the problem itself and is quite different from passive acquiescence. This might involve reducing one's ambitions, accepting disability or reminding oneself that others are worse off. It often promotes better adjustment than other forms of active coping in chronic pain.

Although it is entirely natural to resist pain and suffering, it also seems that struggling to change an experience that is uncontrollable and intractable (such as pain) does more harm than good. Preliminary data suggest that assimilative coping is associated with increased distress and disability (Crombez et al., 2008). There is a growing consensus that treating chronic pain as a problem to be solved, or an experience to be avoided, may constitute a problem in itself (Crombez et al., 2008; McCracken and Eccleston, 2003).

This is disturbing as I have always seen it as just that – a problem to be solved! I think Alan is coping passively – he doesn't like doing the exercises he's supposed to do and seems resigned to his fate. Sarah's coping is more active, but it's assimilative; she hasn't really accepted her condition is for life and is still hoping some miracle drug will cure her.

There is a current trend in psychological therapies to help patients to be open, non-defensive and focused on the present moment. One example of this is *mindfulness-based stress reduction* (Kabat-Zinn, 1990); another is ACT (Hayes et al., 1999; Ruiz, 2010). ACT assumes that all suffering is partially uncontrollable. Human beings are hard-wired with a pain system, which is essential in evolutionary terms (as are fear and anxiety) but which, like other systems, may sometimes malfunction. Rigid attempts to control and eliminate suffering (1) are only partially successful and (2) have clear disadvantages, as they attempt to control experiences that are inevitable (Ruiz, 2010). ACT uses methods to help people to be open and focused on the present moment without struggling to eliminate distress.

Perhaps ACT's greatest innovation is to carefully specify the goals of therapy, seeing symptomatic control (such as an improvement in mood) as a secondary aim; the role of therapy is entirely to help individuals identify what they value in their lives and to help them pursue this effectively. Although therapists in all traditions have endorsed similar goals (see Chapter 2), ACT specifically assumes that there's no need to change the presence or frequency of unpleasant thoughts, feelings or sensations to achieve this (Gauntlett-Gilbert and Connell, 2011).

Although ACT has been most extensively developed for treating adult mental health problems, it is highly suited for use in treating paediatric pain. Parents sometimes respond catastrophically to their child's pain; rather than rationalize, restructure or distract them from these thoughts, parents are encouraged to let them be present, observe them as mental phenomena and keep some of their attention connected to the lived present moment. Children are helped to stop struggling with their pain and to allow nasty emotions to be present without being overwhelmed by them. ACT is well suited for children, as most of its therapeutic interventions are metaphorical and experiential (rather than talk based or didactic; see Chapter 2). An example is given in Box 3.4.

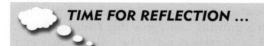

TIME FOR REFLECTION …

Box 3.4 'Walking in the rain'

'Imagine you're walking in the rain – it is really chucking down and you are getting wet. You've got a long way to go and you've got no umbrella. It's cold! You are really fed up and miserable about the situation. What kind of physical posture would you be in? Try doing it. Really feel what this posture is like, sense it in your body.

Now imagine you are in the same rainstorm, just as wet, but this time your attitude is, "OK, I'm getting wet. Nothing to be done about it. Oh well! Wish I'd brought my brolly … yep, I'm still getting wet." What posture would you be in? Again, pay attention to what this feels like.'

Source: Data from Gauntlett-Gilbert, J. and Connell, H. *The Psycholgist, 25*, 198–201, 2011.

This sample clinical technique can provide a vivid physical metaphor of how individuals can react in different ways to discomfort. For the first scenario, people often adopt a hunched forward posture, shoulders up, frowning. With the second, they usually adopt a more relaxed posture. This evokes reflection about which of the two postures involves more effort, which involves more suffering and which is more 'open' to noticing what is going on in the present moment. The second time, the person is not exactly pleased about getting wet – he or she is just fighting it less, using less energy and resistance. It does not have to involve resignation or 'giving in'; rather, it can just involve a degree of acceptance.

It is also useful to ask which time (first or second) the person would get wetter (probably equal). Adopting a more accepting posture does not change the primary source of suffering (the rain, or pain/anxiety in a clinical setting). This is quite different from, for example, promoting relaxation in the hope that it will reduce anxiety.

In adults with chronic pain, acceptance is associated with better functioning and less distress in most areas. Parental acceptance is also associated with better child functioning (McCracken and Gauntlett-Gilbert, 2011).

Multidisciplinary pain management clinics

These are found in most large teaching hospitals and district general hospitals. The clinics comprise a variety of health-care professionals (doctors, nurses, clinical psychologists/psychiatrists, physiotherapists, pharmacists and occupational therapists) who will assess patients and offer expert help in pain management.

Treatment is wide-ranging and may include improving physical and life-style functioning by, for example, improving muscle tone, self-esteem and self-efficacy (see Chapter 10); or reducing boredom and inappropriate pain behaviours (such as being 'rewarded' for 'being in pain'). These are all designed to reduce reliance on drugs.

The subject of pain encompasses most of the psychological approaches described in Chapter 2, biological, cognitive, humanistic and behaviourist. It is therefore, a very complex issue and this analysis shows the inadequacy of the medical model in addressing it.

The tiny incident of a wound dressing taught me the importance of the 'psychological aspect' of care and I should have been more aware of Maisie's non-verbal cues and more sensitive to her need for privacy with Sally. I also discovered that a feeling of incompetency makes me defensive and resentful; therefore I'm pleased I now have a more comprehensive theoretical understanding of pain, which, given its universality, I will certainly need in future.

Gibbs' final stage in the cycle is to ask what I would do again. I hope to be more sensitive to non-verbal cues in general, to concentrate on the patients' feelings and to develop the skills I need to make them feel psychologically safe with me. And I will try to respect a patient's own perception of pain, with all its psychological and social complexity, as the valid one.

CHAPTER SUMMARY

....

- Underlying health psychology (HP) is the biopsychosocial (BPS) model, which is the major alternative to the biomedical model. Only the former is compatible with the influence of non-biological factors as major causes of death and can aid the prevention of chronic diseases.

- Like the BPS model, psychoneuroimmunology (PNI) adopts a systems approach, reflecting a holistic view of the person. The BPS model underpins *behavioural medicine* and also plays a part in *psychosomatic medicine*.

- HP uses research findings regarding the aetiology of illnesses to develop and apply interventions to improve health, at an individual, interpersonal or organisational or societal level.

- Poor *psychological care* can have detrimental effects on patients' physical health. Common psychological responses to illness and injury (including shock, distress and loss of self-worth) can undermine medical treatment and interfere with rehabilitation.

- A major aspect of psychological care is providing *psychological safety*. This can be achieved through *therapeutic conversations* that comprise focus on the here and now, emphasis on feelings, empathic understanding and a non-prescriptive approach, and focus on the patient.

- Care and caring can also be defined in terms of encouraging autonomy, giving of oneself, taking risks, supporting care and *emotional labour*. The last of these is similar to the concept of *emotional (intrapersonal) intelligence*.

- *Pain* is a subjective experience involving both sensory and emotional qualities. This makes it difficult to define pain objectively. It can take many forms, including *acute, chronic non-malignant, psychological* and *spiritual*.

- There are several forms of pain assessment, including visual analogue scales (VASs), numerical rating scales (NRSs) and verbol rating scales (VRSs). These are all unidimensional. Multidimensional measures include the McGill pain questionnaire (MPQ).

- *Cognitive* influences on pain, including cognitive appraisal and expectations, seem to operate through a *modulatory pathway* in the brain and spinal cord; a crucial part of this pathway is the *periaqueductal grey*. The pathway acts as a conduit for the expectation of analgesia from a *placebo*.

- The expectation of reward (e.g., food or sex) can also profoundly affect pain intensity. The *nucleus accumbens* plays a critical role in both signalling reward and controlling pain. This is consistent with the *placebo effect*.

- Individual differences in pain experience include *catastrophisation* at one extreme and *congenital analgesia* (CIP) at the other. Other individual differences include gender, personality and culture.

- Both neuroticism and harm avoidance have been shown to be key personality traits influencing sensitivity to pain and response to analgesia.
- Both women and people of African or Asian descent have been shown to display greater sensitivity to painful stimuli.
- Research into pain in neonates and young children has highlighted problems with how pain in general is defined, conceptualised, assessed and treated.
- Pain can occur in the absence of actual tissue damage, as demonstrated in *phantom limb pain*, *neuralgia* and *caucalgia*. Conversely, injury can occur without pain, as in CIP, *episodic analgesia*, and many trauma patients.
- Treatment of pain can be conducted through behaviour therapy, *cognitive behaviour therapy* (CBT), self-management, *acceptance and commitment therapy* (ACT), *contingency management* (a form of behaviour modification), *biofeedback* and *multidisciplinary pain management clinics*.
- Like mindfulness-based stress reduction, ACT aims to help patients be open, non-defensive and focused on the present moment; it assumes that all suffering is partially uncontrollable. Both approaches advocate *accommodative* (as opposed to *assimilative*) *coping*.

4 Stress: Definitions and causes

Introduction and overview

According to Bartlett (1998),

> … the notion that stress is bad for you and can make you ill has become a modern cultural truism. However, there is also a significant body of research evidence which lends support to this idea … The study of stress must … be central to … health psychology, which concerns, at its most basic level, the role of psychosocial processes in health and disease.

Definitions of stress fall into three categories (Bartlett, 1998; Goetsch and Fuller, 1995):

1. Stress as a *stimulus*
2. Stress as a *response*
3. Stress as an *interaction* between an organism and its environment.

In turn, this classification corresponds very closely to the three models of stress identified by Cox (1978):

1. The *engineering model*, which is mainly concerned with the question 'what causes stress?'
2. The *physiological model*, which is concerned with 'what are the effects of stress?'
3. The *transactional model*, which is concerned with both the aforementioned questions plus 'how do we cope with stress?'

Although stressors are faced by everyone (especially, perhaps, those living in constantly changing Western cultures), some face greater demands than others. As a group, patients (both in and out of hospital) face sources of stress that they did not have to deal with before becoming ill. Similarly, while all occupations are stressful, some are more stressful than others. Several studies have suggested that health workers experience more stress than comparable groups of non-health workers (Jones, 1995). In terms of Warr's (1987) vitamin model, which identifies several environmental factors that affect mental health, nurses and other health professionals are likely to suffer from organisational stressors that are common to many other occupations (such as lack of clarity, conflicting roles, work overload and lack of control). However, nurses often suffer additional stressors that are intrinsic to their job, such as providing terminal care, counselling bereaved parents and dealing with disturbed and violent patients.

 From my diary (11): Year 3/Medical Ward

This incident happened when I was on night duty with Adam (my mentor) on internal rotation from the ward. After changeover, I went to speak to Pauline, who had called in briefly to see her husband (Tom Hendon) who's in for investigations into anaemia. I was just leaving them when, without warning, Tom had a massive haematemesis. It was very frightening – there was blood everywhere, but luckily Adam saw what happened and came quickly to the bed. He was very calm and reassuring to Tom, gave him high flow oxygen and told me quietly to go and fast bleep the F1 on call which I ran to do. When I got back he asked me to take Pauline, who was obviously shocked and distressed, to the visitor's room. I felt a bit panicky myself but tried to appear calm like Adam, got her a coffee and said I'd ask the doctor to see her as soon as possible. When I returned to the ward, Ruth (the F1) had set up an IV and taken blood for the lab, which Adam sent me to deliver and then gave me a list of things to do – prepare a catheter tray, organise the paperwork for observations and fluid balance, check the suction etc . . . . I was too busy to feel upset.

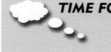 **TIME FOR REFLECTION ...**

- What do you understand by the term 'stress'?
- What makes you feel stressed, and how does it feel?

Stress: Definitions and models

According to the *engineering model* (Cox, 1978), external stresses (stressors) give rise to a stress reaction, or strain, in the individual. Stress is what happens to a person (not what happens within a person). Up to a point, stress is inevitable and can be tolerated, and moderate levels may even be beneficial (*eustress*) (Selye, 1956).

The *physiological model* is primarily concerned with what happens within the person as a result of stress (the response aspects of the engineering model), in particular the physiological changes.

The impetus for this view was Selye's (1956) definition of stress as 'the individual's psychophysiological response, mediated largely by the autonomic nervous system (ANS) and the endocrine system, to any demands made on the individual'. While a medical student, Selye noticed a general malaise or syndrome associated with 'being ill', regardless of the particular illness. The syndrome was characterised by (1) a loss of appetite, (2) an associated loss of weight and strength, (3) loss of ambition, and (4) a typical facial expression associated with illness.

Further examination of extreme cases revealed major physiological changes (confirmed by Cox [1978]). This non-specific response to illness reflected a distinct phenomenon, which Selye called the *'general adaptation syndrome'* (GAS) (see Chapter 5).

The *transactional model* represents a blend of the first two models. It sees stress as arising from an interaction between people and their environment, in particular when there's an imbalance between the person's perception of the demands being made of them by the situation and their ability to meet those demands. Because it is the person's *perception* of this mismatch between demand and ability that causes stress, the model allows for important individual differences in what produces stress and how much stress is experienced. There are also wide differences in how people attempt to cope with stress, psychologically and behaviourally.

For Mr Hendon and his wife, the engineering model would locate stress in his illness; for the nurses, in the demands of their job. The physiological model would be concerned with the changes happening in our bodies in response to external pressures and the transactional one with how we individually perceived and coped with them.

What causes stress?

Consistent with the transactional model, the causes of stress do not exist objectively, and individuals differ in what they see as a stressor in the first place (Lazarus, 1966). So, in this section, we are really identifying *potential* stressors, the kinds of events or experiences that most people are likely to find exceed their capacity to handle the demands that are involved.

Lazarus (1966) is saying stress is what each individual perceives it to be. So although Adam and I shared the same experience, Adam may not have perceived it as a stressor because he knew how to cope with the situation.

Disruption of circadian rhythms

The word *'circadian'* ('about 1 day') describes a particular periodicity or rhythm of a number of physiological and behavioural functions, which can be seen in almost all living creatures. Many studies have shown that these rhythms persist if we suddenly reverse our activity pattern and sleep during the day and are active during the night. This indicates that these rhythms are internally controlled (*endogenous*).

However, our circadian rhythms are kept on their once-every-24-hours schedule by regular daily environmental (*exogenous*) cues called *zeitgebers* (German for 'time givers'). The most important zeitgeber is the daily cycle of light and dark. If we persist with our reversal of sleep and activity, the body's circadian rhythms will reverse (after a period of acclimatisation) and become synchronised to the new set of exogenous cues.

TIME FOR REFLECTION ...

- What is it about the disruption of circadian rhythms that could account for the effects of shift work?

Individual differences and the effects of shift work

Some people take 5–7 days to adjust, others take up to 14, and some may never achieve a complete reversal. But not all physiological functions reverse at the same time: body temperature usually reverses inside a week for most people, whereas the rhythms of the adrenocortical hormone take much longer. During the changeover period, the body is in a state of *internal desynchronisation* (Aschoff, 1979). This is very stressful, and shift workers often report experiencing insomnia, digestive problems, irritability, fatigue and even depression when changing work shifts. In shift work, the zeitgebers stay the same, but workers are forced to adjust their natural sleep–wake cycles to meet the demands of changing work schedules (Pinel, 1993) (Key Study 4.1).

Body temperature is endogenously controlled, which explains why I felt shivery (when it naturally dropped) in the early hours of the morning.

This explains why some nurses are less disturbed by night duty, although, as night duty rarely exceeds seven nights, others could be in a permanent state of internal desynchronisation. Or perhaps regular night nurses have learned to ignore external cues, like the patients who slept in spite of lights on all round them. A case of endogenous cues overcoming those exogenous zeitgebers?

KEY STUDY 4.1

Night nurses are not all the same

- Hawkins and Armstrong-Esther studied 11 nurses during the first seven nights of a period of night duty.
- Performance was significantly impaired on the first night, but it improved progressively on successive nights. However, body temperature had not fully adjusted to night working even after seven nights.
- There were significant differences between individual nurses, with some appearing relatively undisturbed by working nights and others never really adjusting at all.

Source: Hawkins, L.H. and Armstrong-Esther, C.A., *Nursing Times*, 4 May, 49–52, 1978.

Coffey et al. (1988) examined the influence of day, afternoon, night and rotating shifts on the job performance and job-related stress of 463 female nurses at five U.S. hospitals.

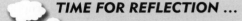

TIME FOR REFLECTION …

- Which shifts do you think produced (1) the highest job performance and (2) the most job-related stress?
- Give your reasons.

Using a structured questionnaire, Coffey et al. found that job performance was highest for nurses on the day shift, followed by the night, afternoon and rotating shifts. Rotating shift nurses reported the highest job-related stress, followed by afternoon, day and night shift nurses (Figure 4.1). These results contrast with those of mainly male factory workers, where individuals are doing essentially the same type of work regardless of the shift. But the type of work carried out by nurses differs considerably depending on their particular shift. So, performance by shift may be affected by the social organisation of hospital work, as well as circadian rhythm synchronisation.

Rotating shift nurses may suffer the most stress and have the least successful job performance due to both the disturbance of circadian rhythms and the fact that they often work with different colleagues and patients on each shift. This may make it more difficult to establish working relationships. Although day shift nurses suffer the least from circadian rhythm disruption, they are responsible for the instrumental activities of supervising patient preparation for diagnostic testing, treatment and therapy. The pace is rapid and the nurse

Figure 4.1 Night shift involves an enforced adjustment of sleep-wake cycles.

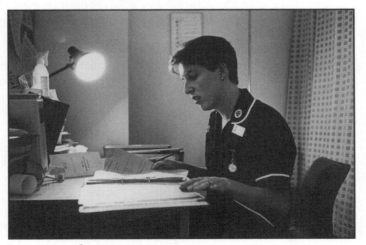

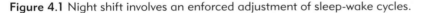

is interacting with the maximum number of colleagues, both nursing and non-nursing. This can all be very stressful.

Conversely, on the night shift the pace is slower and interaction with others considerably reduced, helping to reduce stress levels. Concentration is on the expressive activities of making patients comfortable and ensuring their rest and sleep. So, what about the afternoon shift? Circadian rhythm disruption is moderate, but nurses face the stress of both instrumental and expressive functions. They are responsible for continuing and monitoring the medical treatment initiated during the day shift, while dealing with the social and psychological aftermath of the medical regimen. This may account for their high stress levels (Coffey et al., 1988).

According to Singer (in Brown [1988]), who compared rota systems in different countries, there is a very high error and accident rate among people working an early morning shift that follows a late afternoon/evening shift. This combination should be avoided at all costs. Yet a late shift followed by an early shift is the staple diet of the internal rotation duty pattern in the United Kingdom (Brown, 1988).

Working with different staff, a new routine, and unnatural working hours were all sources of stress for me. And from 11 pm to 4 am the pace was the same as on day duty!

Life changes: The Social Readjustment Rating Scale

Holmes and Rahe (1967) examined 5000 patient records and made a list of 43 life events, of varying seriousness, which seemed to cluster in the months preceding the onset of their illness. Out of this grew the *Social Readjustment Rating Scale* (SRRS). Several studies have shown that people who experience many significant life changes (a score of 300 life change units [LCUs] or over) are more susceptible to physical and mental illness than those with lower scores. The range of health problems includes sudden cardiac death, heart attacks (non-fatal), tuberculosis, diabetes, leukaemia, accidents and even athletics injuries.

The amount of stress a person has experienced in a given period of time, say, 1 year, is measured by the total number of LCUs. These units result from the addition of the values (shown in the 'mean value' column of Table 4.1) associated with events the person has experienced during the target time period.

According to Holmes and Rahe (1967) the death of a close family member is high (5th) on the stress rating scale. It was Pauline, not Tom, who I confided that his parents had died recently within a few weeks of each other. Whether that triggered his ill-health we don't know, but encouraging Tom to talk about his feelings and offering bereavement counselling might help reduce future vulnerability.

Table 4.1 Selected items from the SRRS

Rank	Life event	Mean value
1	Death of spouse	100
2	Divorce	73
3	Marital separation	65
4	Jail term	63
5	Death of close family member	63
6	Personal injury or illness	53
7	Marriage	50
8	Fired at work	47
9	Marital reconciliation	45
10	Retirement	45
11	Change in health of family member	44
12	Pregnancy	40
13	Sex difficulties	39
16	Change in financial state	38
17	Death of close friend	37
18	Change to different line of work	36
22	Change in responsibilities at work	29
23	Son or daughter leaving home	29
28	Change in living conditions	25
30	Trouble with boss	23
31	Change in work hours or conditions	20
32	Change in residence	20
38	Change in sleeping habits	16
41	Vacation	13
42	Christmas	12
43	Minor violations of the law	11

Evaluation of the Social Readjustment Rating Scale

The SRRS assumes that *any* change is stressful by definition. But the *undesirable* aspects of events are at least as important as the fact that they change people's lives (Davison and Neale, 1994). A quick glance at Table 4.1 suggests that life changes have a largely negative feel about them (especially those in the top 10, which receive the highest LCU scores). So, the scale may be confusing 'change' and 'negativity'.

Similarly, life changes may be stressful only if they are unexpected and, in this sense, *uncontrollable*. In other words, it may not be change as such that is stressful but change we cannot prevent or reverse. Studies have shown that when people are asked to classify the undesirable life events on the SRRS as either 'controllable' or 'uncontrollable', only the latter are significantly correlated with subsequent onset of illness (Brown, 1986).

? RESEARCH QUESTION ...

- Why is it a mistake to infer that life events cause illness?
- Is it possible that (some) life events are caused by illness?
- What kinds of data are produced by studies that investigate the link between life events and illness?

Need for control

According to Parkes (1993), the *psychosocial transitions* that are the most dangerous to health are those that are sudden and allow little time for preparation. The sudden death of a relative from a heart attack, in an accident or as a result of crime is an example of the most stressful kinds of life changes (see Chapter 13).

Using Rotter's (1966) *Locus of Control Scale*, and devising a new scale (the *Life Events Scale*), Johnson and Sarason (1978) found that life events stress was more closely related to psychiatric symptoms (in particular, depression and anxiety) among people rated as high on *external* locus of control than among those rated as high on *internal* locus of control. In other words, people who believe that they do not have control over what happens to them are more vulnerable to the harmful effects of change than those who believe they do. This is related to Seligman's (1975) concept of *learned helplessness* (see Gross [2010]).

 Might being ill and helpless be more stressful for someone with an internal locus of control? Perhaps control is a significant factor for nurses too? Although night duty disturbs circadian rhythm most, Coffey et al. (1988) found job performance relatively high and Adam said he likes night duty as he feels more in charge of what he does.

Occupation-linked stressors

Along with social work, teaching and the police force, nursing is identified as a high-stress occupation. A study by Borrill et al. (1996) of 11,000 National Health Service (NHS) staff found nurses had the second-highest stress score among seven staff groups. The inherently stressful nature of shift work is common to all those working in the emergency services (police, fire, ambulance, emergency medical teams and mountain rescue) (Figure 4.2). They also share routine encounters with death, tragedy and horror deal with people in pain and distress and may face personal danger and injury.

Figure 4.2 High stress level, an occupational hazard for those workng in the emergency services.

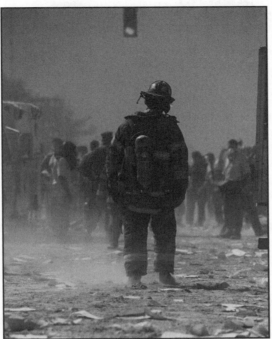

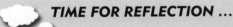

TIME FOR REFLECTION ...

- Thinking about areas of nursing that you have actually experienced as well as those you have not, which do you consider to be the most stressful?
- Are these sources of stress an inherent part of nursing or shared with other health professions? Try to think about both specific and more general aspects of the job.
- What specific sources of stress do student nurses experience? (Critical Discussion 4.1).

Apart from classes, I don't often meet with my student cohort as we're usually in different placements. However, some of us keep in touch by e-mail and texting, which does help.

Emotional labour of nursing

Intrinsic sources of stress (such as constantly having to deal with patients' pain, anxiety and death, as well as giving emotional support to patients' families) are made worse by the inadequate training received for handling such demands

CRITICAL DISCUSSION 4.1

It is tough at the bottom: Student nurse stress

- The fallout from the 'revolution' in nursing is starting to take its toll – the hours are longer and the emotional demands greater than for most other students. While they used to be part of a close-knit community living in heavily subsidised nurses' accommodation, today's students face rocketing rents and increasing isolation; they often have to travel long distances to split-site colleges or community placements.
- Although Project 2000 students were meant to be supernumerary, in practice this often did not happen. Traditionally trained staff may expect more from a student than he or she can deliver. These job demands, together with the academic ones, plus the financial hardships (which might mean students having to work night shifts before going to college) all add up to very high stress levels.
- Rocketing stress levels mean students are more prone to problems with drugs and alcohol (see Chapter 12).

Source: Snell, J., *Nursing Times*, 91(43), 55–58, 1995.

(Gaze, 1988). According to Mazhindu (1998), there has also been little research into the effects that *emotional labour* in nursing has on the quality of nursing practice and on nurses' personal lives.

The term emotional labour was first used by Hochschild (1983) in her study of flight attendants, who are able to maintain a cool, calm, caring and comforting exterior despite working in often quite deplorable and emotionally draining conditions. Being friendly, kind, courteous and smiling are all part of the job (and have financial value for the airline); hence, it is labour (rather than care). Hochschild (1983) defined emotional labour as 'the induction or suppression of feeling in order to sustain an outward appearance that produces in others a sense of being cared for in a convivial safe place'.

I hope I didn't reveal my feelings to Pauline; I tried hard not to. Adam **appeared** very controlled while dealing with Tom's sudden bleed; now I wonder if he really was feeling as calm and confident as he looked. If not, Hochschild (1983) argues, it would cost him, emotionally.

TIME FOR REFLECTION ...

- How much emotional labour do you consider you perform in your nursing role?
- Do you regard it as an inherent part of the job or is it something you do 'beyond the call of duty'?
- How does it affect you, compared with physical and technical work?
- How do you manage these effects?

Smith (1992) drew on Hochschild's work in her own study of student nurses' experiences of being socialised into nursing. She carried out her research on elderly care wards, an environment in which high-tech nursing tasks are few, but opportunities to listen to reminiscences (see Chapter 19), provide companionship and clip toenails are many. In such wards, 'the functioning hearing aid was just as much a lifeline to survival as the intravenous infusion to the post-operative patient in the acute surgical ward' (Smith, 1992). However, while the demands of emotional work can be as tiring and hard as physical and technical labour, they are not so readily recognised and valued – it may not be perceived as constituting 'real' work.

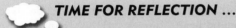 *Emotional care isn't a separate thing, is it? Adam's ability to combine them must have been demanding; he attended to Tom's physical needs, to Pauline's emotional needs and his professional duty to me. I think his actions were a good example of Schon's 'thinking in action' which Bulman quotes in Bulman and Schutz, 2008, page 3: 'Where we may reflect in the midst of action without interrupting it. Our thinking serves to reshape what we are doing while we are doing it.' Schon contrasts this to thinking (reflecting) on action as: 'Thinking back on what we have done in order to discover how our knowing in action may have contributed to an unexpected outcome.' (Schon, 1987, page 26)*

TIME FOR REFLECTION ...

- Are certain types of nursing inherently more stressful than others (such as coronary care units [CCUs], cancer wards/units, intensive care units [ICUs] and accident and emergency [A&E] departments)?
- To what extent is it the characteristics of the different patient groups that accounts for the difference (see Chapter 3)?

Stress related to different types of nursing work

Nurses in ICUs have to maintain high levels of concentration for long periods; they are often emotionally drained by continuous close contact with a distressed and frightened family, and the process of dying may not follow a natural course: technology (such as ventilators) and drugs may prolong it (Fromant, 1988). Staff working in A&E departments are in the front line at times of major disasters, such as the 1989 Hillsborough disaster and the July 2005 London bombings (Figure 4.3). However well prepared they may be practically, nothing can prepare them for the emotional demands (Owen, 1990).

This is recognised; victims of disasters have counsellors and students have mentors. I wonder if the needs of stressed nurses are also recognised?

Figure 4.3 Major disaster, major stress.

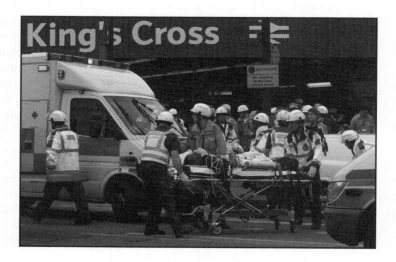

Mental health nurses

O'Donnell (1996) reported the findings of a survey in which nurses were asked about 16 different stressors. Overall, most of these stressors were perceived as being more extensive among mental health nurses (MHNs) than in nursing as a whole. 'Violence' was found to be substantially more extensive than average, as were 'job insecurity', 'not involved in decision-making' and 'career uncertainty'.

According to Sullivan (1993), all those professionals working in mental health may be at greater risk of stress than their colleagues working in physical health care. For example, psychiatrists have the highest suicide rate among doctors. MH nursing is often carried out against a background of risk-taking and uncertainty because of the volatile and potentially aggressive nature of some psychiatric patients (Cahill et al., 1991).

According to Burnard et al. (2000), psychological distress, emotional exhaustion and increased alcohol consumption are just some of the consequences of increased workplace stressors among community MHNs (CMHNs). They see themselves as overworked, struggling with too much paperwork and administration, having too many clients and having serious concerns about their client groups. As many as 20% feel they have no job security. These are among the key findings of a survey into stress among CMHNs in Wales, the largest of its kind in the United Kingdom. It included nurses working in a wide range of both urban and rural settings. What the findings describe is 'burnout' (Critical Discussion 4.2).

So, things like the high patient turnover, the current NHS changes and economic cuts all contributing to rising stress levels?

CRITICAL DISCUSSION 4.2

Burnout and HIV

- Maslach and Jackson (1981) define burnout as a combination of emotional exhaustion, depersonalisation (the usually brief experience in which everything that's normally familiar strikes us as strange and unreal) and a reduced sense of personal accomplishment. It is an 'occupational hazard' for a variety of health care professionals, especially those caring for the terminally ill (Hedge, 1995).
- For example, those working with HIV patients have to deal with profound physical and mental deterioration, which induces in staff a sense of helplessness, frustration and inadequacy at being unable to cure. They also experience anxiety, depression, feeling overworked, fatigued, stressed out, a fear of death and a decreased interest in sex (Hortsman and McKusick, 1986).

According to Hedge, many of the factors associated with burnout are experienced by workers in other fields (such as oncology and cystic fibrosis). But Bennett et al. (1991) found that the increased nurse–patient contact and emotional intensity of the work in HIV units increase stress levels. Nurses who identify closely with their patients will experience a grief reaction (see Chapter 13), but older, more experienced nurses are less likely to suffer from burnout. Perhaps they are better able to maintain professional boundaries to reduce emotional stress while expressing warmth and empathy.

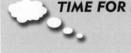 Adam agreed with Bennett et al. (1991) about this. His term for professional detachment – which he emphasised **didn't** mean not caring – was 'arm's length nursing'; he pointed out that total emotional involvement might adversely affect competence and efficiency.

TIME FOR REFLECTION ...

- How might the care patients receive be affected by nurse burnout?
- Try to identify some of the stressors experienced by patients coming into hospital and how these might be influenced by nurse stress.

Stress related to hospitalisation and different medical procedures

For many people, patients and relatives alike, hospitals and other health care settings can be unpleasant, frightening and even bewildering places. The environments within a hospital that are designed to help those with the most life-threatening conditions are also likely to evoke the most extreme negative reactions in both patients and staff. These extreme environments include CCUs, oncology (cancer) wards/units, ICUs and A&E departments.

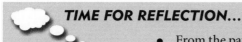

TIME FOR REFLECTION...

- From the patient's perspective, what do you consider are the most stressful aspects of being in a hospital?

Hospitalisation

Although hospitalisation in itself can greatly disrupt patients' lives, there has been little research into its impact from the adult patient's perspective (as opposed to the effects of painful medical procedures and critical illness). In contrast, in paediatric care there has been more interest in the experience of being in hospital as a stressful event in its own right (Smolderen and Vingerhoets, 2010).

Hospital admission is a stressor that produces severe anxiety in some form or another in 10%–80% of patients (Toogood, 1999). Smolderen and Vingerhoets (2010) cite frequently reported hospital stressors, across patient populations, including the following:

1. Aspects of the physical hospital environment (e.g., having to sleep in a strange bed, having machinery around)
2. Being separated from one's familiar environment or worries about one's family
3. Lack of control and loss of autonomy
4. Communication difficulties in staff–patient interaction
5. A lack of clear, understandable information about procedures, diagnosis and prognosis, leaving patients with many uncertainties about their stay, the treatments they have to undergo and the implications for their future

Although there is some overlap between hospital-related stressors for adult and child patients, research with children has identified some additional features that require special attention. Hospitalisation of children increases both their and their caregivers' levels of anxiety and this may, in different ways, extend well into post-discharge period (Leidy et al., 2005) (see the discussion on chronic childhood illness, pages 98, 99).

Repeated and lengthy hospitalisations, especially in the case of serious illness, may be a traumatic experience and can considerably interfere with normal cognitive and socio-emotional development. Making health care providers more aware of the possible harmful effects of hospitalisation and chronic illness on the child's development is a first and necessary step in this process (Smolderen and Vingerhoets, 2010). Adequate attention should be given to palliative care in children (see Chapter 13), as well as separation anxiety and homesickness (see Chapter 14), which are significant sources of distress for both the hospitalised child and his or her caregivers (Thurber and Walton, 2007).

According to Moos and Schaefer's (1984) *crisis theory*, illness, injury, hospitalisation or an unpleasant medical procedure throw up challenges that may represent a turning point in an individual's life; this may be associated with changes in identity, environment, role and social support and in prospects for the future. The crisis nature of illness may be exacerbated by factors such as inadequate information regarding the precise nature of the illness and uncertainty about its course. Patients will need to manage various disease-specific tasks, such as the following:

1. Dealing with pain, incapacity and other symptoms (see Chapter 3)
2. Dealing with the hospital environment and special treatment procedures
3. Developing and maintaining adequate relationships with health care staff

Alongside these, patients will face general tasks, such as (1) preserving a satisfactory self-image, (2) maintaining a sense of self-efficacy (see Chapter 3) and (3) sustaining relationships with family and friends and preparing for an uncertain future.

Pre-operative anxiety

In both children and adults, pre-surgical anxiety has an impact on post-operative anxiety. For example, pre-operative anxiety in particular can act as a possible barrier to post-operative recovery in children (McCann and Kain, 2001).

Although medication is often used to manage pre-operative anxiety (e.g., Carroll et al. [2012]), many nurses believe that reassurance and listening to patients' concerns are more beneficial. However, research suggests that nurses generally play a minor part in patients' psychological care, and the nurse–patient relationship on most surgical wards is task-related, short and to the point, with therapeutic discussion almost non-existent (Toogood, 1999).

Severe anxiety can affect a patient's ability to assimilate and retain information, while moderate anxiety can produce increased adrenaline and cortisol levels, inhibiting wound healing (Kiecolt-Glaser et al., 1998; Pediani, 1992; Toogood, 1999). It can also cause electrolyte imbalance and harm the body's immune response, leading to increased risk of wound infections (see Chapter 5).

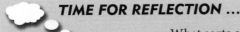 So there's good evidence to justify a nurse's role as patients' advocate in information giving; pre-operative assessment shouldn't be just about the physical aspects of surgery (and risks, which could be frightening for some patients) but also about many of the issues relating to hospital admission.

TIME FOR REFLECTION …

- What sorts of factors are likely to affect a pre-operative patient's anxiety level?

Personality (see Chapter 5), health status, age (see Chapters 15 and 19), cultural background and family role may all affect anxiety. Also, surgery that produces a change in body image (such as mastectomy, hysterectomy or amputation) may have a greater psychological impact (see Chapter 16).

Information giving

It is widely acknowledged that understanding helps reduce anxiety. If a situation cannot be interpreted, it cannot be dealt with and the individual experiences helplessness and anxiety (Lazarus and Averill, 1978). However, just giving information, though beneficial, is not enough. Even assuming the patient is able to understand the information sent before admission, it can actually *increase* stress (Salmon, 1993). What is needed is a careful assessment of a patient's needs and appropriate care. Nurses must bear in mind that patients' levels of intelligence and understanding vary and that one answer may not suit the needs of any two patients (Toogood, 1999).

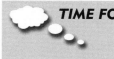

TIME FOR REFLECTION ...

● What non-medical methods could be used to reduce patients' pre-operative anxiety?

Boore (1978) compared a group of 'informed' patients with an 'uninformed' group, both groups receiving the same amount of 'nurse time' prior to surgery. The former had lower levels of steroids in their urine, suggesting that information allows patients to interpret and understand their surroundings and helps them to anticipate the events usually occurring in the post-operative period; this minimises feelings of helplessness and so lowers anxiety. Other studies have found that good psychological preparation can lead to earlier discharge from hospital, less need for analgesia, lower incidence of urinary retention and lower pulse rate and blood pressure (Pediani, 1992).

What these studies suggest is that good wound care is not just a matter of physical administration of dressings; it involves the need to prepare the patient psychologically (Pediani, 1992). Panda et al. (1996) suggest that patients value information from doctors most. But, in reality, nurses offer an emotional support service and are often required to fill in the gaps left by doctors, interpreting medical information that patients do not understand, so providing them with clear, detailed and logical explanations.

Although Clare (see case study 9, page 367) was given detailed medical information about her planned ileostomy operation, she asked the nurses several times to confirm what the doctors said and it was the nurses who supplied the much needed, continual emotional support.

Coronary care units

Admission to a CCU is a stressful experience for both patients and relatives. Vetter et al. (1977) found that patients with myocardial infarction (heart attack) who expressed extreme emotional upset often suffered complications related to poor prognosis. Consistent with this finding, arrhythmias and further ischaemia are related to catecholamine production and the increased coagulability of the blood (Taggart et al., 1972). This demonstrates the importance of alleviating anxiety – not to do so may prove fatal.

In some cardiac surgery units, patients may be invited to meet others who have recently undergone coronary bypass surgery and who are now recovering (North, 1988). This policy is supported by an American study by Kulik and Mahler (1989), who found that patients waiting for this surgery preferred to share a room with someone who had already had it rather than another patient waiting for the same operation. The preference seemed to be motivated by the need for information about the stress-inducing situation (see earlier).

The sudden onset of a life-threatening illness or high-risk surgery is obviously fear, and stress, inducing, so informed re-assurance would be more effective.

Cancer wards/units

Chemotherapy, an intense and cyclical treatment with many side-effects (such as hair loss, nausea, vomiting, diarrhoea and neuropathies [nerve-related pain; see Chapter 3]) is one of the most stressful treatments for cancer. The long periods of treatment, repeated hospitalisations and serious side-effects may cause a great deal of distress.

Approximately 25% of patients receiving anti-cancer chemotherapy experience anticipatory nausea and vomiting (ANV or *psychogenic emesis* [nausea and vomiting caused by psychological factors]). ANV is a conditioned response, acquired when anything that becomes associated with chemotherapy-induced emesis becomes capable of triggering it on its own (see Figure 4.4). This may include the mere sight of the hospital, the sign for the cancer ward/unit, an alcohol swab, a white coat or even a nurse! (Pandey et al., 2006). The process involved is classical conditioning and involves three steps or stages (see Box 2.2, page 23).

Figure 4.4 Classical conditioning of emesis.

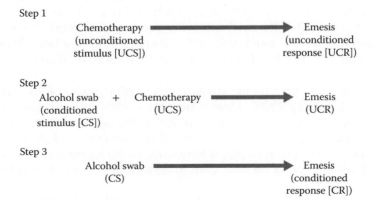

Step 1

Chemotherapy (unconditioned stimulus [UCS]) ⟶ Emesis (unconditioned response [UCR])

Step 2

Alcohol swab (conditioned stimulus [CS]) + Chemotherapy (UCS) ⟶ Emesis (UCR)

Step 3

Alcohol swab (CS) ⟶ Emesis (conditioned response [CR])

This explanation is supported by the finding that patients do not develop ANV unless they have first experienced post-treatment emesis (Weddington et al., 1984).

Many non-pharmacological approaches have been used to try to control the emesis associated with chemotherapy, with varying degrees of success. One of the most effective behavioural techniques is *systematic desensitisation*. The patient is first taught progressive relaxation techniques and is then asked to list those stimuli that trigger emesis, from the least to the most likely. Beginning with the least likely, and while in a relaxed state, the patient is asked to concentrate on each stimulus in the list for 20 seconds, then to imagine the stimulus fading away and dissolving. The aim is for the patient to be able to confront the actual stimulus without experiencing ANV. This method has been particularly effective when used with children and adolescents receiving chemotherapy (Zeltzer et al., 1984).

McIlfatrick et al. (2007) found that patients undergoing chemotherapy in a day hospital felt they were better able to maintain a sense of normality and resist the sick role; but on the negative side, they perceived themselves as being dehumanised by a factory-like system (see Box 4.1).

Sarah, a patient I knew in the community, told me she faints at the mere sight of a syringe. A painful steroid injection was the unconditioned stimulus (UCS); fainting was the unconditioned response (UCR). The next time she had her flu jab, the conditioned stimulus (CS) the syringe + injection (UCS) led to her fainting (UCR). Now when a syringe (CS) is produced she faints (CR). She now lies down prior to all injections!

Box 4.1 Impact on parents of PICU

- In contrast to their child's memory, parents' memory for events on PICU is often extraordinarily detailed; it is now well documented that a minority suffer clinically significant levels of distress in relation to these memories (Colville, 2012).
- While early studies tended to focus on how parents felt while their child was still on PICU, recent longitudinal studies indicate increased anxiety and PTSD for many months after discharge (Ballufi et al., 2004; Bronner et al., 2010) as well as a tendency to be rather overprotective, even where the child has made a good recovery (Colville et al., 2008). Parents' subjective sense of the degree to which their child's life was in danger is a much stronger determinant of their later distress than objective measures of severity of illness (such as time spent on a ventilator) (Ballufi et al., 2004).
- Parents often feel particularly vulnerable just after their child is transferred out of PICU (Colville et al., 2009). Having become reliant on the monitors and high staff ratios on PICU, they now become unnerved by the de-escalation of medical intervention; the need to get used to a new ward environment and staff group is stressful. Parents are also required to play a larger role in caring for a child who is much more aware of what is going on and, consequently, often more demanding as he or she recovers.

Another therapeutic treatment that is often offered to both adult and young oncology patients is bone marrow transplantation (BMT); this is used to treat several life-threatening conditions, including leukaemia, aplastic anaemia, lymphomas, multiple myeloma, immune deficiency disorders and some cases of solid tumours. Most studies have focused on long-term adjustment after BMT; however, it's the stressors related to hospitalisation – especially the initial hospitalisation (such as intensive therapy, isolation, inactivity, lack of information provided by medical staff, uncertainty regarding the future, family-related stress and side-effects) – that patients consider the most serious even several years post-treatment (Fife et al., 2000; Heinonen et al., 2005).

Intensive care units

Referral to an ICU generally implies critical or life-threatening conditions and, as such, the mere admission to an ICU can be considered a stressful life event (van de Leur et al., 2004). Apart from the condition itself, patients' unpleasant recollections are all related to feelings of discomfort: anxiety, pain (including painful medical interventions), thirst, sleeplessness, disorientation, shortness of breath, inability to move and the presence of an endotracheal tube (Granja et al., 2005; van de Leur et al., 2004). Patients who are amnesic for the early period of their critical illness may particularly be at risk of developing symptoms of post-traumatic stress disorder (PTSD) post-ICU admission (Granja et al., 2008). Patients diagnosed before admission to ICU with some form of mental disorder, and those who were given higher doses of benzodiazepines, are most likely to develop PTSD, as are females and younger patients (Smolderen and Vingerhoets, 2010).

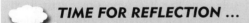

TIME FOR REFLECTION ...

- What do you understand by the term 'dehumanisation'?
- What is it about ICUs that might make patients feel dehumanised?

According to Calne (1994), some adult patients in ICU undergo a process of *dehumanisation*. The term is sometimes used to refer to situations where an individual loses his or her human identity and becomes (or is perceived as) machine- or animal-like. It can include the restriction or denial of attributes that contribute to an individual's self-identity and personality, leading to a loss of 'humanness'.

Typically, dehumanised patients have developed multiple organ failure and have been in ICU for a long time. They are always intubated and unable to communicate verbally, are mostly unresponsive and require complex technical monitoring. According to Calne (1994), the key factors that affect critically ill patients' freedom of self-expression are as follows:

- Reduced ability to communicate
- The distracting nature of the technical equipment
- Altered physical appearance
- Lack of personal belongings

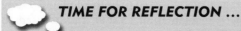

TIME FOR REFLECTION ...

- Take each of Calne's four factors in turn and consider (1) how they might affect the patient's self-identity and (2) how they are perceived by both nurses and relatives.

This doesn't just happen in ICU, does it? It's 'the objectification of self' I read about in Chapter 16 pages 368 and 379) in relation to Clare's surgery. Another instance was Sarah (in tears) telling me that when she had her immune-suppressing IV drug she was 'stuck on the end of a row of oncology outpatients having theirs, feeling like I was on a conveyor belt'.

Patients are dependent on the nurse's ability to interpret the fragmentary clues (such as change in the sound of the ventilator or in displayed patterns on their chart) that reveal their real fears and desires (Ashworth, 1990). Similarly, a sudden rise in heart rate, or a previously settled patient becoming agitated, would lead most nurses to infer that the patient is in pain, uncomfortable or frightened. At the same time, technical equipment can be a source of distraction, diverting attention away from the patient (Ashworth, 1980).

Changes in a critically ill patient's physical appearance can occur as a result of drug therapies, surgical interventions and altered physiology. These changes may include surgical wounds, extensive oedema, jaundice, anaemia, exaggerated skin loss, bruising from clotting disorders and loss of body mass. Their physical appearance may be so radically altered that even relatives do not immediately recognise the patient.

Calne (1994) cites several studies showing that ICU nurses may actually distance themselves, both psychologically and physically, from critically ill patients. They may protect themselves from emotional involvement with patients who are 'unlikely to survive'. Patients' physical appearance can be a source of stress for ICU staff, and non-task-related/non-invasive interaction is often limited.

Yet this is where the patient would depend heavily on the nurse to be an advocate. It's also a time of difficult emotional labour for health professionals who must suppress negative feelings while empathising with patients and relatives.

Clare (a young ileostomy patient) gripping my hand during her first dressing showed me how necessary physical touch can be. I've noticed the first thing many visitors do is hold the patient's hand.

Paediatric intensive care units

Over 18,000 children (most of them under 3 years old) are admitted to a paediatric intensive care unit (PICU) in the United Kingdom each year (PICANET, 2010). Also, until relatively recently, it was assumed that provided they were appropriately sedated, children in this situation were unaware of what was happening to them. However, new evidence is emerging that children can be

Sensory overload and sensory deprivation

According to Glide (1994), patients in ICUs experience both *sensory overload* and *sensory deprivation*. Noise levels are excessive, and long-term exposure to high noise levels can lead to increased tension and anxiety.

The most significant form of sensory deprivation patients experience appears to be the lack of human touch. Although ICU patients are often exposed to physical touch, this is mostly associated with technical intervention (task-related/invasive interaction) rather than personal, comforting physical contact. Clearly relatives can help to provide touch, but nurses can also help to reduce the sensory deprivation by allowing patients to wear glasses, hearing aids or dentures if at all possible. These also sustain the patient's dignity and ability to communicate.

troubled by disturbing memories of their treatment, of the circumstances that brought them into the unit, and of hallucinations they may have experienced during admission. These memories can, in turn, affect their longer term psychological recovery (Colville, 2012).

Children are admitted to PICU for a wide variety of emergency medical and surgical conditions, including end-stage cancer, meningitis, burns, fractures and respiratory problems, often relating to prematurity. Others are admitted electively for post-operative monitoring. Approximately 5% of children die during admission, and for the rest there continues to be an increased risk of death in the following year (PICANET, 2010). Although most survivors make a good physical recovery, some children are left with serious disfigurement, neurological difficulties or behaviour problems that may result from traumatic brain injury; others will have ongoing disabilities relating to congenital problems or prematurity (Colville, 2012).

Children's memories of their stay on the PICU are usually either patchy or non-existent: they commonly spend long periods unconscious or heavily sedated (e.g., Playfor et al., 2000). However, Colville et al. (2008) found that a third of their sample of 102 children reported bizarre nightmares and strange perceptual experiences early on in their recovery; these hallucinations were similar in content to those reported by adult ICU patients.

Consistent with the evidence for adult patients, there is growing evidence for longer term psychological symptomatology of children treated in PICUs: a significant minority reports high levels of PTSD symptoms for several months. These symptoms are not simply a function of the severity of their illness or injury (Colville, 2008; Davydow et al., 2010); they may also be distressed by witnessing the resuscitation or death of another patient. Also, children sedated for longer periods are more likely to report delusional experiences and suffer higher rates of PTSD symptoms (Colville et al., 2008).

Brown and Kulik (1982) (Gross, 2010, page 265) suggest emotion plays a significant role in triggering 'flashbulb memories' which would explain a parent's vivid recall of these times. The frightening nature of children's memories makes it even more important for parents (and nurses) to be a reassuring presence.

Accident and emergency

According to Hole (1998), advances in technology and treatment have increased the chances of surviving once-fatal injuries. However, the full impact of the trauma and surgery comes after the physiological effects have passed. While surgery may produce a marked cosmetic benefit to the injury, the medical staff may focus more on the cosmetic, functional progress than the patient's emotional state.

Since the severely injured patient loses much more than their health, a psychological approach is vital for preventing 'detrimental attitude formation, extreme psychopathology and various other treatment-related problems' (Badenhorst, 1990). Hole identifies three traumatic events experienced by the injured person:

1. The injury itself
2. The medical intervention to limit or rectify the anatomical and physiological effects
3. The road back to normality

The relatives of the severely injured person need to be included in their care and treatment. They too are victims of the traumatic event (Brown, 1991). Family members are crucial in the patient's reintegration into society, and they also need help to reintegrate.

However, it is not just relatives who need support. Nursing trauma patients can be harrowing. They are often young people with devastating and sometimes disfiguring injuries, whose lives have suddenly been thrown off course and who no longer have any idea what their future holds. Faced with trauma patients and their traumatised relatives,

> 'nurses have the normal human reactions of shock, horror, pity, sometimes even revulsion. But they have to overcome these feelings if they are to nurse the patient effectively'
>
> (Fursland, 1998).

Nurses might also feel guilty about being healthy and able-bodied in the face of the appalling injuries of their patients (a form of survivor guilt?). The grief reactions of seriously injured patients will include anger, which may be directed/displaced at nurses (see Chapter 13). They may be left feeling rejected and be unsure how to respond.

I have yet to face many of these situations; there is so much to learn before I can cope properly with them. However, from my experience with Gail, a young cancer patient in the community (case study 3, page 298), I understand the anger of grief and learned from my mentor's calm acceptance of it.

Psychosocial aspects of chronic illness

Rather than being seen as a passive response to biomedical factors, chronic illnesses (such as HIV/AIDS, cancer, coronary heart disease [CHD] and obesity) are better understood in terms of a complex interaction between physiological and psychological processes (Ogden, 2004). Health psychology has studied HIV, for example, in terms of attitudes towards HIV, changing these attitudes and examining predictors of behaviour (see Chapter 6). Similarly, children and young people with chronic conditions (such as widespread idiopathic chronic pain syndrome) are more likely to successfully manage the challenges presented by their medical condition if their health care addresses both their physical and psychological well-being.

HIV/AIDS

According to Hedge (1995),

> ... the uncertainty attached to the course of disease [HIV] and its poor prognosis frequently cause intense emotional reactions, even in those who are clinically well and asymptomatic. Good care addresses an individual's quality of life as well as its length: it aims to help people live with HIV infection rather than simply wait to die from it ...

Although people with HIV infection and AIDS develop mental health problems common to other life-threatening illnesses, they may experience psychological disorders that are specifically related to the following:

- Uncertainty surrounding disease progression and outcomes, the distressing nature of the symptoms themselves, and the knowledge that HIV is potentially fatal; related disorders include acute stress reactions (see Chapter 5), adjustment disorders, and functional psychoses (such as depression, schizophreniform disorders and suicidal ideas and attempts).
- The direct effects of the virus (Firn and Norman, 1995); these include a dementia-type illness characterised by progressive cognitive and/or motor impairment, which may be accompanied by behavioural disturbances (see Chapter 11).

Some of these reactions are related to the stigma associated with the disease, and anti-gay (and anti–drug user) prejudice and discrimination (see Chapter 7). This means that many people following a positive test result have to deal not only with the medical implications of the diagnosis but also with the potentially negative reactions of partners, friends, family and other social contacts. This is likely to exacerbate any existing mental health problems. Also, the continued spread of HIV and the improved treatment prophylaxis, which ensures that people with HIV live longer, mean that the incidence of HIV-related mental health problems is likely to increase (Firn and Norman, 1995).

TIME FOR REFLECTION ...

- In what ways do you think AIDS is potentially stigmatising?

People with it are often perceived as having engaged in activities that may be proscribed by society and, by implication, as belonging to a stigmatised group (such as gay men and drug users). These beliefs are often expressed in the language of blame, and even nurses who have chosen to work in specialist wards caring for AIDS patients can have difficulties in viewing them completely non-judgementally (see Chapter 7).

Prejudice and stigma are psychosocial dimensions that add even more stress for these patients; it reinforces the need for a biopsychosocial approach to caring for them.

Children and young people with chronic conditions

Almost 3 in 10 families will have a child diagnosed with a chronic illness (defined as a condition lasting longer than 3 months by the U.S. National Centre for Health Statistics) (Christie and Khatun, 2012). One in 10 children will have a chronic illness severe enough to substantially restrict his or her daily life and demand extended care and supervision (Yeo and Sawyer, 2005).

> Grasping the immediate and long-term implications of diagnosis is a complex process for the child or young person, parents and the wider family. Taking in the immediate demands of treatment can be confusing and frustrating. The realisation of the potential long-term impact of the illness on a young person's hopes, dreams and ambitions can be devastating.
> (Christie and Khatun, 2012).

Chronic illness has a substantial impact on emotional life, lifestyle, education, self-esteem and social relationships (such as isolation from peer groups and increased dependence on parents), as well as physical well-being (Yeo and Sawyer, 2005). For adolescents, chronic illness can both prevent the development of independence and impact what has already been achieved (Christie and Viner, 2009). Both parents and the young person may initially be angry with each other for causing the illness by passing on 'bad genes' or not having gone to the doctor early enough.

Janet, who already had two children, decided not to risk having a Down's syndrome baby (case study 10, page 128). I wonder if the possible impact on them contributed to her decision?

Grieving for how life used to be, and the future that cannot now happen, is also a common response to the diagnosis. One study found that parents of children with diabetes failed to fully 'accept' the diagnosis: although they adjusted to the management of the disease, they still described episodes of grief 7 years post-diagnosis (Lowes et al., 2005) (see Chapter 13).

According to the *risk-resistance adaptation model* (RRAM) (Wallander et al., 1989), when *risk factors* (disease/disability, functional independence, and psychosocial stressors) are excessive and *resistance factors* (intrapersonal and socio-ecological stress processing/coping strategies) are low, there are difficulties in emotional, physical and psychosocial function and adaptation.

How parents perceive the impact of the illness has been shown to influence adjustment. Mothers who became extremely overprotective of their diabetic children reported poor adjustment (Swift et al., 1967), and parents of children with asthma reported a greater impact on family life compared with those of diabetic children (Rydstrom et al., 2004). Mothers of diabetic children need to be always available for the sick child, making them (seem) less available for 'forsaken' partners and siblings. Siblings may experience guilt about remaining healthy, and they also often feel excluded and describe missing out on parental attention (Yeo and Sawyer, 2005).

According to Christie and Khatun (2012),

> ...all health care professionals have the opportunity to help families identify strengths, abilities and resources in order to contribute to positive adjustment and healthy outcomes. Health care professionals can also make a significant contribution to positive adjustment by ensuring they offer timely, thoughtful, effective and accurate information communicated at the time of diagnosis but also reviewed and repeated at different developmental stages. Ensuring successful adjustment is the responsibility of everyone in the young person's support network.

This analysis of stress has made me more aware of how widespread and variable the sources of stress are and that some of it is inevitable. Understanding its role in illness does highlight the need to reduce it where we can; Moos and Schaffer (1984) analyse the 'crisis' nature of ill health and hospitalisation and also suggest ways to reduce stress. Awareness of the need for emotional care by nurses is increasing, as shown by the recent input of Government funds into the NHS for that purpose; being identified as responsible for providing it is a bit daunting. However, reflecting on Adam's caring skills (thinking on action) I can see his knowledge and experience did allow him to manage his own 'emotional labour' and reduce everyone else's stress; after 12 years of experience he is what Schon calls a 'professional expert' who can 'think in action'. His confidence and skill I can only respect and aspire to!

CHAPTER SUMMARY

- *Stress* has been defined as a *stimulus* (corresponding to the *engineering model*), a *response* (corresponding to the *physiological model*) and as an *interaction* between an organism and its environment (corresponding to the *transactional model*).
- The physiological model is based on Selye's General Adaptation Syndrome (GAS).
- Potential causes of stress (*stressors*) include disruption of circadian rhythms (as in shift work), life changes (as measured by the Social Readjustment Rating Scale [SRRS]) and occupation-linked stressors.
- Nursing is a high-stress occupation, sharing many stressors with those working in the emergency services. Routinely dealing with death and people's pain and distress demands *emotional labour*, which may not be acknowledged or valued as readily as the more physical aspects of nursing.
- *Burnout* is an occupational hazard for a variety of health care professionals, especially those who work with terminally ill patients, such as in HIV units.
- Those hospital environments designed to help those with the most life-threatening conditions are also likely to evoke the most negative reactions, in both patients and staff. These extreme environments include CCUs, oncology (cancer) wards/units, ICUs (including PICUs), and A&E departments.
- Although hospitalisation in itself can seriously disrupt patients' lives (as reflected in Moos and Schaefer's *crisis theory*), there has been little research into its impact from their perspective; notable exceptions include the effects of painful medical procedures and critical illness, and paediatric care.
- Some adult patients in ICUs undergo a process of *dehumanisation*. Most experience both *sensory overload* and *sensory deprivation*.
- A significant minority of both adult and child patients treated in ICU/PICU report high levels of PTSD symptoms for several months.
- In both children and adults, pre-surgical anxiety influences post-operative anxiety. It can act as a possible barrier to post-operative recovery in children. Severe anxiety can affect a patient's ability to assimilate and retain information. In turn, understanding helps reduce anxiety.
- Rather than being seen as a passive response to biomedical factors, chronic illnesses (such as HIV/AIDS, cancer, CHD and obesity) are better understood as a complex interaction between physiological and psychological processes.
- For example, HIV/AIDS patients may develop psychological disorders that are specifically related to the stigma associated with the disease, as well as anti-gay (and anti–drug user) prejudice and discrimination.
- In relation to chronic conditions, the *risk-resistance adaptation model* (RRAM) predicts that when risk factors are excessive and resistance factors are low, there will be difficulties in emotional, physical and psychosocial function and adaptation.

5 Stress: Effects and methods of coping

Introduction and overview

As noted in Chapter 4, the *physiological model* of stress is primarily concerned with the *effects of stress*. As also noted in Chapter 4, Selye's General Adaptation Syndrome (GAS) provides an influential account of how stress affects us bodily. This, in turn, reflects the biomedical model (see Chapter 3). However, the GAS fails to take into account how the (autonomic) nervous and endocrine (hormonal) systems interact with the *immune system*, that is, it fails to recognise the *immunosuppressive effects* of stress, which are the focus of *psychoneuroimmunology* (PNI) (see Chapter 3).

According to the *transactional model*, it also fails to take the individual into account: we can only understand the effects of stress if we consider the individual *as a whole*. For example, personality, cultural background, gender and self-esteem represent *moderators/mediators* of stress, which may amplify or reduce the impact of a stressor. These same factors can help explain what constitutes a stressor in the first place: we cannot define stressors *separately* from the individual. Clearly, the transactional model is consistent with the biopsychosocial (BPS) model (again, see Chapter 3)

Similarly, the transactional model maintains that the question 'How do we cope with stress?' can only be satisfactorily answered in terms of an *interaction* between the individual and his/her environment. There are several different types of coping, associated with different short- and long-term benefits and consequences; many of these can be described, collectively, as ways in which we 'manage our stress'.

More formally, *stress management* refers to a range of psychological techniques used by professionals to help people reduce their stress. While these techniques have not been developed specifically to help reduce stress in hospitalised patients, they are used with good effect with this population. The chapter also discusses methods that have been designed or adapted for use with different groups of patients; these include *modelling*, *pre-exposure*, *distraction*, patient-controlled analgesia (PCA), *therapeutic touch* (TT) and *humour*. At the end of the chapter, we discuss how patients cope with being diagnosed with a chronic illness and the illness itself.

Effects of stress: How does stress make us ill?

 From my diary (16): Year 3/Elderly Care Ward

An upsetting day at work. I had worked a long day and was almost ready to go off duty when Charlie, a frail, 91-yr-old patient and a favourite of mine asked me for the commode. The night HCA helped me get him on to it and I gave him his bell, made sure the curtain was closed and went outside. A short time later I came back to check and Charlie was lying on the floor. I thought he'd fallen but then saw his face was bluish and his eyes open and staring and realised, with a huge sense of shock, he'd had a cardiac arrest. I rang the emergency bell, then felt for a carotid pulse and there was none. I was pulling the commode out of the way when two staff nurses arrived; one said, 'Go and dial 2222 – don't forget to say the ward,' and as they began cardiac resuscitation the other said, 'Get the crash trolley!' I thought, 'phone first', flew up the ward and met the HCA, who must have heard, bringing the crash trolley. When I got back the HCA and I moved the bed and commode out of the way so they had space to work and pulled the curtains round the other beds. By this time the F1 and F2 had arrived, followed a few seconds later by the site co-ordinator and the medical registrar (Helen), all out of breath.

I hadn't seen a cardiac arrest before and at first it seemed chaotic – they all seemed to be frantically doing their own thing, intubating him, putting up an IV, drawing up solutions and talking, but very quickly Helen took charge and was directing the action which calmed everything down. And then I thought about the other patients and went to speak to them, but the HCA was there so I went back to Charlie.

General Adaptation Syndrome

According to Selye (1956), GAS represents the body's defence against stress. The body responds in the same way to any stressor, whether it is environmental or arises from within the body itself. GAS comprises three stages: the *alarm reaction*, *resistance* and *exhaustion*.

Alarm reaction

When a stimulus is perceived as a stressor, there is a brief, initial *shock phase*. Resistance to the stressor is lowered. But this is quickly followed by the *countershock* phase. The sympathetic branch of the autonomic nervous system (ANS) is activated, which, in turn, stimulates the *adrenal medulla* to secrete increased levels of adrenaline and noradrenaline (*catecholamines*).

The catecholamines are associated with sympathetic changes, collectively referred to as the *fight-or-flight syndrome* (or response [FOFR]): the individual's instinctive, biological preparation for confronting danger or escaping it. The catecholamines mimic sympathetic arousal (*sympathomi-metics*), and noradrenaline is the transmitter at the synapses of the sympathetic branch of the ANS. Consequently, noradrenaline from the adrenals prolongs the action of noradrenaline released at synapses in the ANS. This prolongs sympathetic arousal after the stressor's removal. This is referred to as the *ANS-adrenal-medulla system* (or *sympatho-adrenomedullary* [SAM] *axis*).

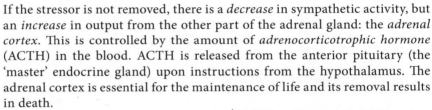 Selye's physiological model explains my own 'alarm' response to Charlie's cardiac arrest. My own heart seemed to stop and then start again, thumping so hard it almost hurt and, I experienced a surge of panic. I wasn't thinking clearly at all.

Resistance

If the stressor is not removed, there is a *decrease* in sympathetic activity, but an *increase* in output from the other part of the adrenal gland: the *adrenal cortex*. This is controlled by the amount of *adrenocorticotrophic hormone* (ACTH) in the blood. ACTH is released from the anterior pituitary (the 'master' endocrine gland) upon instructions from the hypothalamus. The adrenal cortex is essential for the maintenance of life and its removal results in death.

The effect of ACTH is to stimulate the adrenal cortex to release *corticosteroids* (or *adrenocorticoid hormones*), one group of which are the *glucocorticoid hormones* (chiefly, corticosterone, cortisol and hydrocortisone). These control and conserve the amount of glucose in the blood (*glucogenesis*), which helps to resist stress of all kinds. The glucocorticoids convert protein into glucose, make fats available for energy, increase blood flow and generally stimulate behavioural responsiveness. In this way, the *anterior pituitary-adrenal cortex system* (or *hypothalamic-pituitary-adrenal* [HPA] *axis*) contributes to the FOFR.

Exhaustion

Once ACTH and corticosteroids are circulating in the bloodstream, they tend to inhibit the further release of ACTH from the pituitary. If the stressor is removed during the resistance stage, blood sugar levels will gradually return to normal. But when the stress situation continues, the pituitary-adrenal excitation will continue. The body's resources are now becoming depleted, the adrenals can no longer function properly, blood glucose levels drop and, in extreme cases, hypoglycaemia could result in death.

It is at this stage that *psychophysiological disorders* develop, including high blood pressure (hypertension), heart disease (coronary artery disease), coronary heart disease (CHD), asthma and peptic (stomach) ulcers. Selye called these the *diseases of adaptation* (see Figure 5.1).

Figure 5.1 Summary diagram of the three stages of the General Adaptation Syndrome and their relationship to the physiological changes associated with (i) the ANS – adrenal medulla and (ii) anterior pituitary – adrenal cortex systems.

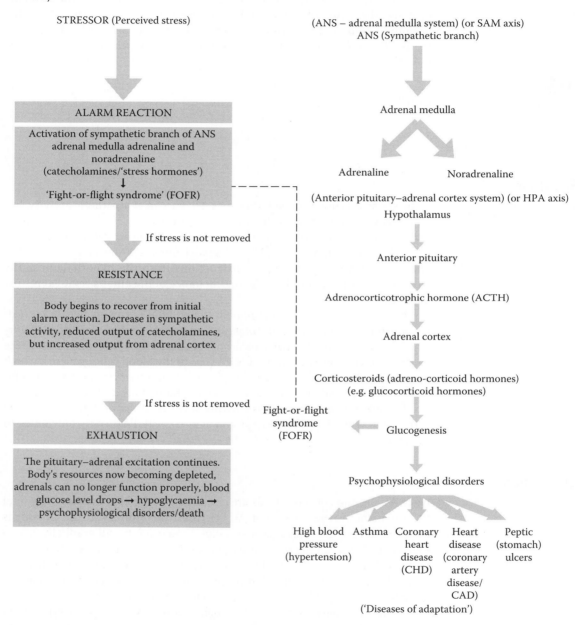

The crash team all ran to the ward and I ran to the phone so this was literally a 'flight' reaction. After I got back and used some more physical energy, I felt a bit less shaky; this may have been due to 'using up' blood glucose.

Evaluation of GAS

- Lazarus (1999) cites a study of patients dying from injury or disease. Post-mortem examination showed that those who remained unconscious had normal levels of corticosteroids, while the opposite was true for those who were conscious (presumably aware they were dying). Lazarus infers from this that 'some psychological awareness – akin to a conscious perception appraisal – of the psychological significance of what is happening may be necessary to produce the adrenal cortical changes of the GAS'.
- Selye helped us understand how stressors affect the body. But to understand what makes a psychological event stressful, we must put the person into the equation. In effect, says Lazarus, 'it takes both the stressful stimulus conditions and a *vulnerable person* to generate a stress reaction'. In other words, stressors do not exist objectively but reflect the transactional model's view of stress.

This is a good example of why we need to put the O (organism/person) between the S (stimulus) and R (response) (see Chapter 2). Probably the crash team, the ward nurses and certainly I, perceived the situation differently according to our roles and varying degrees of ability to carry them out.

- Research conducted since Selye's pioneering work has supported the role of the (autonomic) nervous and endocrine systems in how the body responds to stress. However, the GAS fails to take into account the interaction between these two systems and the immune system (see pages 107, 108). While Selye's GAS reflects the biomedical model of health and illness, research into the interaction between the ANS and the immune system is better accommodated by the BPS model of health and illness (see Chapter 3).
- While the three stages of the GAS implies that stressors can last shorter or longer periods of time, it fails to make explicit a crucial distinction between *acute* (immediate, short-term) and *chronic* (persistent, long-term) stress. This distinction can help us understand the conditions under which stress makes us ill, by:
  - Distinguishing, in turn, between evolutionarily basic stressors (those that threaten our very physical survival) and modern stressors (that are psychosocial in nature rather than physical or biological)
  - Explicitly identifying the role of the central (as opposed to the autonomic) nervous system (in particular, the brain) in determining what will be perceived as stressful in the first place

Both the preceding points are better accommodated by the BPS model than the biomedical model.

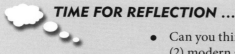

TIME FOR REFLECTION …

- Can you think of some examples of (1) evolutionarily basic stressors and (2) modern stressors?
- How does the distinction between these two types of stressor relate to the distinction between acute and chronic stress? (see Box 5.1).

Box 5.1 Evolutionarily basic and modern stressors, acute and chronic stress and the pre-frontal cortex

- The sympathetic branch of the ANS responds as a unit, producing a state of generalised, undifferentiated arousal. This was probably of crucial importance in our evolutionary past, when our ancestors were frequently confronted by life-threatening dangers (very acute stress!). This is precisely what the FOFR is for.
- While an increase in heart rate may be necessary for supplying more blood to the muscles when facing a hungry-looking sabre-toothed tiger, it may be quite irrelevant to most of the stressors we face in modern life.
- Modern stressors involve a far higher psychosocial element and *do not* pose any physical threat. But our nervous and endocrine systems have evolved in such a way that we typically react to stressors *as if* they did. Most everyday stressors are either common daily hassles (such as traffic jams and bad weather) or long-term chronic stressors.
- A special feature of the human brain is that it can look back and learn from the past *and* look ahead, planning for the future. Unfortunately, this often leads to ruminating about the past and worrying about the future – especially in the case of the more important stressors, such as problems in relationships, income and health. Humans, therefore, are able to think about stressors in their absence (in space or time); this is sufficient to produce the same potentially harmful physiological effects as our ancestors experienced in life-threatening situations. Chronic stress responses are probably a rather recent – and unique – human 'invention' (Thayer and Brosschot, 2010).
- This cognitive representation of stressors, before or after their occurrence, is called *perseverative cognition* (PC) (Brosschot et al., 2006; Watkins, 2008). A key area of the brain involved in PC is the pre-frontal cortex (PFC), the area immediately behind the forehead that serves as the control centre that mediates our highest cognitive abilities (including concentration, planning, decision-making, insight, judgement and the ability to retrieve memories). The PFC is the part of the brain that evolved most recently (see Chapter 2) and it can be extremely sensitive to even temporary everyday anxieties and worries (Arnsten et al., 2012).
- Recent research demonstrates that acute, uncontrollable stress triggers a series of chemical events that weaken the influence of the PFC while strengthening the dominance of the brain's older parts, in particular the amygdala; this is involved in the control of emotional behaviour (see Chapter 2).

… As the older parts take over, we may find ourselves either consumed by paralysing anxiety or else subject to impulses that we usually manage to keep in check: indulgence in excesses of food, drink, drugs … Quite simply, we lose it. (Arnsten et al., 2012)

When I first realised Charlie had arrested I did freeze momentarily before acting. The crash team were all in a state of arousal and there was a sense of panic – or perhaps it was urgency – initially; the registrar was most in control of herself, and the situation. I became increasingly emotional and distressed, so when Helen eventually said 'Stop', I was glad it was all over for Charlie. I cried all the way home; I suppose that was the effect of a weakened PFC?

Stress and the immune system

The immune system is a collection of billions of cells, which travel through the bloodstream and move in and out of tissues and organs, defending the body against invasion by foreign agents (such as bacteria, viruses and cancerous cells). These cells are produced mainly in the spleen, lymph nodes, thymus and bone marrow. The study of the effect of psychological factors on the immune system is called *psychoneuroimmunology* (PNI) (see Chapter 3 and Figure 5.2).

People often catch a cold soon after a period of stress (such as final exams) because stress seems to reduce the immune system's ability to fight off cold viruses (we are 'run down'). Goetsch and Fuller (1995) refer to studies that show decreases in the activity of *lymphocytes* among medical students during their final exams (e.g. Kiecolt-Glaser et al., 1984). Lymphocytes ('natural killer cells') are a particular type of white blood cells, which normally fight off viruses and cancer cells. Levels of immunoglobulin A increase immediately after an oral exam (if it appeared to go well), but *not* after written exams (suggesting that the stress is not relieved until much later – when the results come out!) (Petit-Zeman, 2000).

Of course, none of these findings means that stress actually *causes* infections. Stress makes us more susceptible to infectious agents by temporarily suppressing immune function (the *immunosuppressive effects* of stress). Stressors that seem to have this effect include exams and the death of a spouse (see Chapter 13). For example, Schliefer et al. (1983) found that the immune systems of men whose wives had died from breast cancer functioned less well than before their wife's death.

Soon after tissue damage has occurred, *interleukin-b* is produced, helping to remodel connective tissue in wounds and to form collagen (scar tissue). Kiecolt-Glaser et al. (1995) compared the rate of wound healing in two groups: (1) a group of 13 'high-stress' women, caring for relatives with Alzheimer's disease and (2) a 'stress-free' matched control group. All the women underwent a 3.5-mm full thickness punch biopsy on their non-dominant forearm. Healing took significantly longer in the caregivers than in the controls (48.7 vs. 39.3 days) (see Key Study 5.1 and Critical Discussion 5.1).

KEY STUDY 5.1

Using psychological techniques to boost the immune system

Norton (2000) reports on a study in which women with breast cancer were encouraged to visualise their white blood cells waging war against the cancer cells. This was intended to boost their immune system in a way that could help them fight the disease.

This *guided imagery* was combined with progressive muscle relaxation as well as standard surgery, chemotherapy and radiotherapy.

Compared with women in a control group (given only the medical treatment), those who used the psychological techniques had higher numbers of mature T-cells, activated T-cells and cells carrying T-cell receptors (see Figure 5.2). These are important for attacking malignant cells.

At the end of the 9-month study, these women also had higher levels of lymphokines (activated killer cells), which help prevent the disease from spreading. The women reported a better quality of life and fewer side-effects from medical treatments.

Source: Norton, C., *Independent on Sunday*, 16 April, 12, 2000.

I wish we could have used this with Pat, a 68-year-old woman who seemed to have a lifetime of stress. I met her on my community placement when she had a mastectomy for breast cancer followed by radiotherapy. A wound abscess was excised and the wound left open to heal by 'secondary intention'. As she needed daily dressings I got to know Pat well.

This is a 'double whammy' situation – the prolonged GAS response makes us ill in specific ways, like heart attacks and strokes (see Chapter 5), while the suppression of the immune system makes us prey to any illness that comes along. Like Pat's cancer.

Moderators and mediators of stress

Moderator variables are antecedent conditions (such as personality, ethnic background and gender) that interact with exposure to stress to affect health outcome. *Mediator variables* intervene in the link between stress exposure and health outcome – for example, appraisal (Folkman and Lazarus, 1988). If they *reduce* the impact of a stressful event, they are called 'protective' or 'buffering' variables – they soften or cushion the impact (Bartlett, 1998).

Personality

What is now referred to as the *Type A behaviour pattern* (TABP) was originally called 'Type A personality' – a stable personality trait (Friedman and

Figure 5.2 Immune system. (Adapted from Hayward, S., Stress, health and psychoneuroimmunology, *Psychology Review*, 5(1), 16–19, 1998.)

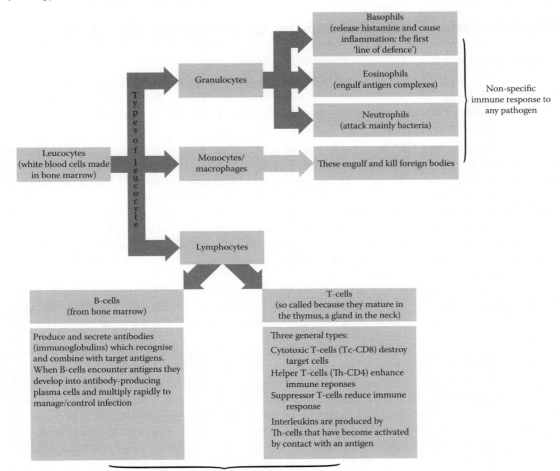

Specific immune response to individual antigens

Rosenman, 1974). TABP is now conceptualised as a stereotypical set of behavioural responses, including the following:

- Competitiveness and achievement orientation
- Aggressiveness and hostility
- Sense of time urgency

Many early studies showed that people who display TABP were at much greater risk of high BP and CHD, compared with 'Type Bs' (the opposite of Type As). However, these risks are only *relative*: the vast majority of 'Type As' *do not* develop CHD and many Type Bs *do* (Davison and Neale,

CRITICAL DISCUSSION 5.1

Allostatic load: When the immune system fails to protect us

While the immune system is so vital, Sternberg and Gold (1997) warn that

> its responses are so powerful that they require constant regulation to ensure that they are neither excessive nor indiscriminate and yet remain effective. When the immune system escapes regulation, autoimmune and inflammatory diseases or immune deficiency syndromes result.

As we have seen, the GAS involves the release of cortisol (one of the major glucocorticoids) into the bloodstream. But the immune system, too, is capable of triggering this stream of biological events: it has a direct line to the hypothalamus. When the immune system is activated to fight an infection, it sends a signal to the hypothalamus to produce its stress hormones (including cortisol). The flow of hormones, in turn, *shuts off* the immune response. This ingenious *negative feedback loop* allows a short burst of immune activity, but prevents the immune system from getting carried away. In this way, a little stress is 'good for you'. But *chronic* stress produces such a constant flow of cortisol that the immune system is dampened down too much; this helps explain how stress makes us ill (Sternberg, 2000).

This account of how the immune system can be shut down in the face of chronic stress is consistent with the concept of *allostatic load*. The *allostatic load model* (Sterling and Eyer, 1998) aims to explain why biological changes designed to *protect* the organism can also be *harmful*.

Allostasis is contrasted with *homeostasis* (derived from the Greek *homos* – meaning 'same' and *stasis* – meaning 'stoppage'); the term was coined by Cannon (1929) to refer to the process by which an organism maintains a fairly constant internal (bodily) environment, that is, how body temperature, blood sugar level, salt concentration in the blood and so on are kept in a state of relative balance or equilibrium. In the cases of allostasis, physiological parameters must be maintained outside the normal range to match chronic demands (either physical or psychological), essentially altering the normal homeostatic 'set point' for all physiological systems (Sterling and Eyer, 1998). While homeostatic changes (such as ANS response to acute threat) may be adaptive, maintaining an allostatic state in the long term causes physiological wear and tear, leading to pathology (LeMoal, 2007).

For example, while the increased heart rate and blood pressure associated with the FOFR are essential for ensuring sufficient oxygen and energy supply to the muscle and brain, repeated or prolonged episodes of these changes can cause damage to the heart and blood vessels. Restricted blood flow contributes to the risk of stroke and heart attack, as well as contributing to insulin resistance, abdominal obesity and development of type 2 diabetes (Clow, 2001; McEwan and Seeman, 1999).

McEwan and Seeman (1999) also explain how the impact of stress mediators can also be both protective (allostatic) and harmful (allostatic load). Adrenal steroids promote allostasis together with other catecholamines by helping to move immune cells ('trafficking') to organs and tissues where they are needed to fight infection. But chronic overactivity of these same mediators produces immunosuppressive effects.

1994). Also, most studies have found that TABP assessed immediately following a heart attack *does not* predict future attacks. This suggests that TABP *is not* a distinct risk for CHD in those already at risk of the disorder (Penny, 1996).

However, there seem to be clear physiological differences between Type As and Bs in response to stress – even when the person is not conscious (Fletcher, 1995). Krantz et al. (1982) found that, compared with Type Bs, Type A patients undergoing coronary bypass surgery showed greater BP changes while anaesthetised (by as much as 30 mmHG) and were much more likely to have complications during surgery that could be attributed to enhanced sympathetic nervous system activity.

According to Temoshok (1987), *Type C personalities* are cancer-prone. The Type C personality has difficulty expressing emotion and tends to suppress or inhibit emotions, particularly negative ones such as anger. While there is no clear-cut evidence that these personality characteristics can actually cause cancer, it does seem likely that they influence the progression of cancer and, hence, the survival time of cancer patients (Weinman, 1995).

Greer and Morris (1975) found that women diagnosed with breast cancer showed significantly more emotional suppression than those with benign breast disease (especially among those under 50). This had been a characteristic for most of their lives (see Key Study 5.2). Cooper and Faragher (1993) reported that experiencing a major stressful event is a significant predictor of breast cancer in women who did not express anger but used denial as a form of coping.

KEY STUDY 5.2

Beating breast cancer

- Greer et al. studied women who had a mastectomy after being diagnosed with breast cancer.
- Those who reacted either by *denying* what had happened ('I'm being treated for a lump, but it's not serious') or by showing *fighting spirit* ('This is not going to get me') were significantly more likely to be free of cancer 5 years later than women who stoically accepted it ('I feel an illness is God's will …') or were described as 'giving up' ('Well, there's no hope with cancer, is there?').
- A follow-up at 15 years (Greer, 1991; Greer et al., 1990) found that survival was almost three times lower in the stoical or 'giving up' women. This difference was obtained independently of factors such as age, menopausal status, clinical stage, type of surgery, tumour size and post-operative radiotherapy.

Source: Greer, S., *Psychological Medicine*, 21, 43–49, 1991; Greer, S. et al., *The Lancet*, 13, 785–787, 1979.

? RESEARCH QUESTION …
- Why was it important to control for these factors?
- What crucial independent variable were the researchers investigating?

Pat was a 'Type C' personality. She had a tragic history, starting at eight years old when her mother died. Her second baby was badly deformed (Pat had taken thalidomide) and died soon after birth. The drug damaged Pat's liver – she was hospitalised and separated from her other child for six months; he became a heroin addict. When she was 40 her husband died suddenly of a heart attack. However, a few years ago she met her present partner; they are happy together but aren't married. A year ago she discovered a lump in her breast which she ignored for too long; she told Sally (the Community nurse) she'd never discussed her problems with anyone except her 'as what was the point'?

According to Hegarty (2000), 'Such research … appears to give scientific support to the advice … "to think positive" in the face of a diagnosis of cancer. It suggests the value of having psychological resources which will allow individuals to adapt to, rather than succumb to, a severe threat to their well-being. It might even be possible to teach such strategies to people who neither have nor use them.'

Pat's feelings about her illness were all negative; she told Sally she felt sexually unattractive, hated the messiness of the wound and worried the malignancy would progress. Her attitude was 'stoical' – resigned to her illness as the last in a long line of misfortunes. According to Greer et al.'s (1990) study, this could affect her prognosis.

Another protective personality variable is *hardiness* (Kobasa, 1979; Kobasa et al., 1982). Hardiness comprises the three Cs:

- *Commitment*: A tendency to involve oneself in whatever one is doing and to approach life with a sense of curiosity and meaningfulness.
- *Control*: This is related to Rotter's (1966) *locus of control* (LOC), that is, individual differences in people's beliefs regarding what controls events in their everyday lives. Hardy individuals have a *high internal* LOC; they believe that they are in control, rather than being at the mercy of environmental events (including other people). Those who hold this latter view have a *high external* LOC.
- *Challenge*: A tendency to believe that change, as opposed to stability, is normal in life, and to anticipate change as an incentive to personal growth and development rather than a threat to security.

According to Funk (1992), hardiness seems to moderate the stress–illness relationship by reducing cognitive appraisals of threat and reducing the use of regressive coping (see pages 114 through 117).

Gender and personality

Interestingly, a Danish study has claimed that high levels of daily stress *reduce* the chances of women developing breast cancer in the first place by 40%. The study involved 6500 women followed over an 18-year period. It seems that sustained high stress levels (as in career women) may reduce levels of oestrogen (the female hormone), which is known to affect the development of breast cancer (Laurance, 2005).

In men, the combined tendency to internalise or deny their emotions and putting work/career before their marriage and family (often to the detriment of the latter) are associated with an *increased* risk of developing prostate cancer (Hill, 2007).

These two examples seem contradictory at first; all the successful career women I know could also be described as having 'hardiness' which would perhaps effectively mediate their stress. Interesting it affects the sexes differently – women physiologically and men psychologically.

Self-esteem

The study of community mental health nurses (CMHNs) in Wales described in Chapter 4 found that those with high self-esteem/self-worth used a wide range of coping skills to deal with work stress. However, 40% of respondents reported low self-esteem and felt others had little respect for them. Low self-esteem scores were associated with higher levels of psychological distress, greater emotional exhaustion, lower use of coping skills and increased alcohol consumption.

Research has shown a significant *inverse* relationship between self-esteem and symptoms of depression (the lower the former, the greater the latter) (Pearlin and Lieberman, 1979). Carson et al. (1997) believe it is reasonable to predict that nurses with high self-esteem will have lower levels of stress and burnout and better coping skills than those with low self-esteem.

The Claybury community psychiatric nurse study (Carson et al., 1997) was a survey of stress, coping and burnout in 245 mental health nurses (MHNs) and 323 ward-based nurses in five large mental hospitals and two district hospital psychiatric units. A range of standardised measures was used, including the modified Rosenberg Self-Esteem Scale (see Chapter 16), the General

TIME FOR REFLECTION ...

- Can you think of ways in which sexism might adversely affect women's health?
- Do women have access to protective factors that men do not?

Health Questionnaire (a well-validated measure of psychological distress) and the Maslach Burnout Scale (Maslach and Jackson, 1986). Overall, the results confirmed the prediction that levels of stress, burnout and use of coping skills are related to levels of self-esteem in MHNs.

Isn't it important to know *why* they had low self-esteem? Pat's seems to stem partly from feeling sexually unattractive, while not knowing what to do in new situations (like Charlie's cardiac arrest) immediately lowers my self-esteem.

Coping with stress

What do we mean by coping?

Lazarus and Folkman (1984) define coping as 'constantly changing cognitive and behavioural efforts to manage external and/or internal demands that are appraised as taxing or exceeding the resources of the person'. (This mirrors the definition of stress as the individual's belief that his/her available biological, psychological and social resources are not sufficient to meet the demands of the situation.)

This definition clearly reflects the transactional model (see Chapter 4), which explicitly acknowledges the ongoing interactions between a person and his/her environment. In other words,

> … stressful experiences are construed as person-environment transactions created initially by an individual's appraisal of the stressor and subsequently influenced by ongoing appraisals of available coping resources, effectiveness of coping behaviours and so forth …. (Smyth and Filipkowski, 2010)

When faced with an environmental event or situation, we evaluate its potential threat; this *primary appraisal* represents our judgement about whether the event/situation is (potentially) threatening (i.e. it is a stressor) or not (it is benign or irrelevant). If we judge that it is a stressor, we then assess our coping resources (a *secondary appraisal*) (Lazarus and Folkman, 1984) (see Figure 5.3).

Actual *coping efforts* will follow these appraisal processes and, in turn, shape the outcome of the coping process. According to Smyth and Filipkowski (2010),

> … In a broad sense, any behavior could be considered coping – the key is that an individual engages in that behavior in some attempt to manage stress and its consequences … coping is a dynamic process in which the demands of the environment, available resources

Figure 5.3 Primary and secondary appraisal. (From Smyth, J.M. and Filipkowski, K.B., *Individual Differences and Personality*, London, Longman, 2010.)

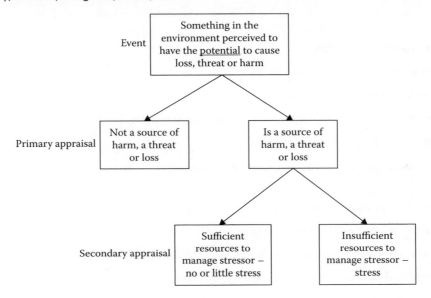

and characteristics of the event/stressor are constantly evolving and influencing each other. Thus, coping is not a one-time response to dealing with a stressor, but a balance of situational and personal factors that unfold over time.

Which is why Helen coped best with the cardiac arrest, what to her, is a familiar situation. She was also the most knowledgeable one.

Different kinds of coping

According to Roger and Nash (1995), the term 'coping' conjures up ideas about being able to handle any situation that comes our way. But in relation to stress, they distinguish between *maladaptive* and *adaptive* coping styles, as follows:

- *Maladaptive* styles involve failing to adjust appropriately to our environment and experiencing misery and unhappiness as a result. They can take the form of *emotional* and *avoidance* coping styles.
- *Adaptive* styles involve an appropriate adjustment to the environment and gaining from the experience. These can be either *detached* or *rational*.

In fact, the term 'maladaptive coping' is a contradiction in terms (see Table 5.1). Cohen and Lazarus (1979) have classified all the coping strategies that a person might use into five general categories.

Table 5.1 Maladaptive and adaptive coping and their short- and long-term consequences

Maladaptive coping
Emotional
Feeling overpowered and helpless
Becoming miserable, depressed and angry
Taking frustrations out on other people
Preparing for the worst possible outcome and seeking sympathy from others
Short-term benefits: Expression of emotion
Long-term consequences: Increasingly overwhelmed by problem
Avoidance
Sitting tight and hoping it all goes away
Pretending there is nothing the matter if people ask
Thinking about something else and talking about it as little as possible
Trusting in fate and believing things will sort themselves out
Short-term benefits: Temporary relief as problem blocked out
Long-term consequences: Blocking out cannot be sustained
Adaptive coping
Detached
Not seeing the problem or situation as a threat
Keeping a sense of humour
Taking nothing personally and seeing the problem as separate from yourself
Resolving the issue by getting things into proportion
Short-term benefits: Able to stand back and take stock of problem
Long-term consequences: Prevents overidentification with problem
Rational
Using past experience for working out how to deal with the situation
Taking action to change things
Taking one step at a time and approaching the problem with logic
Giving the situation full attention and treating it as a challenge to be met
Short-term benefits: Logic determines resolution of problem
Long-term consequences: Problems put into perspective
Source: Adapted from Roger, D, Nash, P. *Nurs. Times*, 91, 42–43, 1995.

1. *Direct action response*: The individual tries to directly change or manipulate his/her relationship to the stressful situation, such as escaping from/removing it.
2. *Information-seeking*: The individual tries to understand the situation better and to predict future events that are related to the stressor.
3. *Inhibition of action*: Doing nothing. This may be the best course of action if the situation is seen as short term.
4. *Intrapsychic or palliative coping*: The individual reappraises the situation (e.g. through the use of psychological defence mechanisms – see Chapter 2) or changes the 'internal environment' (through drugs, alcohol, relaxation or meditation).
5. *Turning to others* for help and emotional support.

 Pat apparently 'coped' with several crises in her life by suppressing her emotions and 'soldiering on'. Whether or not this contributed to her cancer can't be known, but avoidance coping might adversely affect her recovery.

TIME FOR REFLECTION ...

- Which of these coping responses best describes your typical response to stressful situations?
- How about your best friend or partner?
- Does the way you cope depend on the nature of the stressor?

These five categories of coping overlap with the distinction between *problem-focused* and *emotion-focused* coping (Lazarus and Folkman, 1984).

Pat used avoidance and emotional coping at first; she wouldn't look at her scar, discuss her cancer or go out in case her wound leaked through the dressing. She'd told Sally she felt 'helpless and hopeless'. Sally used the 'rational' approach to manage Pat's problems, concentrating first on the wound. She used effective padding and measured the wound healing weekly to promote optimism. It was a good induction for me into adaptive coping.

Which I forgot when Charlie collapsed; my emotional response was maladaptive. The crash team, the staff nurses and the HCA used rational (and some also detached) coping skills and worked together efficiently. I wish now I'd been more rational and detached when observing them and learned more.

Stress management

Much of what we have said about coping with stress refers to what people do in a largely *spontaneous* way. In this informal sense, we all 'manage our stress' more or less effectively. But, more formally, *stress management* refers to a range of psychological techniques used in a quite deliberate way, in a professional setting, to help people reduce their stress. These techniques may be used singly or in combination.

- In the case of *biofeedback* (discussed in Chapter 3 in relation to pain control), the focus is on treating the symptoms of stress rather than the stressor itself.
- The same is true of a number of procedures used to bring about a state of relaxation, in particular *progressive muscle relaxation* – such as the Alexander technique (see Maitland and Goodliffe, 1989) – meditation and hypnosis.
- *Cognitive restructuring* refers to a number of specific methods aimed at trying to change the way individuals think about their life situation and self, to change their emotional responses and behaviour. This approach is based largely on the work of Beck (*the treatment of automatic thoughts*) and Ellis (*rational emotive therapy*), two major forms of *cognitive behaviour therapy* (CBT) (see Chapter 3 and Gross, 2010). This approach provides information to reduce uncertainty and to enhance people's sense of control.

Reducing stress in hospitalised patients

A wide variety of psychological interventions (including those described in the section on 'Stress management' and in Chapter 3 in relation to pain management) are available to help patients cope with stressful medical procedures. Several have been shown to be effective across a range of health outcomes, ranging from patient satisfaction and levels of anxiety and distress to pain reduction, decreased use of medication and reduced hospital stay (Smolderen and Vingerhoets, 2010). Unfortunately, the relative effectiveness of individual interventions is difficult to determine, because they are very often combined in treatment 'packages'.

Smolderen and Vingerhoets (2010) identify three broad types of coping:

- *Appraisal-focused coping* refers to attempts to understand the illness and searching for meaning (such as logical analysis and mental preparation).
- *Problem-focused coping* involves dealing with the problem and redefining or reconstructing it as manageable (such as learning specific procedures and behaviours during a diagnostic procedure).
- *Emotion-focused coping* involves managing emotions and maintaining emotional equilibrium (such as maintaining hope when dealing with a stressor [affective coping], venting feelings [emotional discharge] and coming to terms with inevitable outcomes of an illness (resigned acceptance) (see Chapter 13 and Table 5.1).

Sally's problem-focused coping helped Pat to cope emotionally in spite of avoiding (as far as we could tell) any kind of appraisal-focused coping.

Information, social support and skills training

According to Smolderen and Vingerhoets (2010), providing information, social support and skills training (including relaxation techniques) are the most frequently applied and best-evaluated techniques.

Preparatory information and patient education have the capacity to decrease anxiety levels in adult patients undergoing surgery (McDonald et al., 2004) or diagnostic procedures (Galaal et al., 2007). (Information-giving in relation to pre-surgical anxiety is discussed in Chapter 4).

Evidence also exists showing that increasing patient comfort can be beneficial over and above the benefits provided by specific techniques. For example, Lang et al. (2000) conducted a randomised trial comparing the benefits of (i) standard care with those of (ii) structured attention and self-hypnotic relaxation in a sample of patients undergoing percutaneous vascular and renal procedures. The latter produced both greater anxiety reduction and lower use of medication and significantly shorter procedure times.

RESEARCH QUESTION
- What do you understand by a 'randomised trial'?

In another randomised trial, one group of coronary bypass patients provided with a combination of an educational and supportive intervention pre-surgery benefited in terms of both quality of life and post-operative length of stay compared with a group receiving just standard care (Arthur et al., 2000).

Children represent a special vulnerable group within the hospital setting: they may lack the ability to understand the necessity and objectives of hospitalisation and medical procedures. Since pain and anxiety are often inter-related (see Chapter 3), interventions specially designed for children address both aspects (Smolderen and Vingerhoets, 2010).

As with adult care, the provision of information about procedures to children can be offered as a tailor-made intervention; this can alleviate distress in unfamiliar situations because it increases predictability and feelings of control. With children, it is also important to distinguish between *procedural information* (focusing on the details of the procedures) and *sensory information* (addressing the experiences associated with the procedures). The latter is primarily intended to reassure the child that particular (painful) sensations are normal and do not mean that there is something wrong. Also helpful are suggestions about how to deal best with such negative experiences and discomfort: information about swallowing techniques, which position to take or how to breathe are examples of coping instructions that may be given in the context of unpleasant medical procedures (Smolderen and Vingerhoets, 2010).

In the context of the paediatric intensive care unit (PICU), individualised story books – illustrated books written in developmentally appropriate language by the psychologist about the patient's condition and treatment – may help children make sense of their experience once they begin to recover. Such books may also facilitate a more open discussion about what has happened with other family members (Colville, 2012). However, PICU staff may also benefit from psychoeducation and support, particularly given the high levels of burnout in this staff group (Embriaco et al., 2007) (see Chapter 4).

Modelling can be considered a way of providing information and educating children about hospitalisation and painful medical procedures. This may take the form of a video, in which a child actor (the model) undergoes the same procedure as the patient and displays a non-fearful response to it. This may be especially beneficial for patients undergoing invasive procedures that require them to stay awake and focused (O'Halloran and Altmaier, 1995). Being of the same/similar age and gender helps the patient to identify with the model. Alternatively, children may benefit from observing a fellow patient (live model) undergoing the same procedure (Smolderen and Vingerhoets, 2010). Modelling is related to *social learning theory* (e.g. Bandura, 1971) or *social cognitive theory* (e.g. Bandura, 1989) (see Gross, 2010).

Behavioural strategies and regulation of emotions

As we saw in Chapter 4 when discussing cancer wards/units, anticipatory nausea and vomiting (or *psychogenic emesis*) can be explained in terms of classical conditioning. The acquisition of these kinds of conditioned responses can be prevented by *pre-exposure*, based on the principle of *latent inhibition*. So, for example, a child is exposed to the treatment room and the medical staff under neutral conditions. For those children who become very distressed by a wide variety of stimuli following a painful procedure, this pre-exposure may take the form of a positive emotional exposure (such as a play situation in which the child plays the role of the doctor, examining and treating a doll or pet: Van Broeck, 1993). The interventions and medical procedures applied to their 'patients' are those the child is familiar with and, if possible, real medical equipment/materials are used (such as thermometers, empty medicine bottles, syringes [without needle] and bandages). Especially in 4–9-year-olds, this kind of play contributes to a kind of 'natural' desensitisation. When systematic desensitisation (SD) is used as a form of behaviour therapy (see Chapter 2), the child or adult is exposed in a safe, gradual and controlled way to the feared object or situation; this is usually carried out first in the imagination and then with actual objects or situations.

Play therapy can also be helpful in coming to terms with children's painful experiences; it may enable them to express emotions, both positive and negative (including aggression and revenge, sadness, powerlessness, frustration, pity and tenderness), which might have otherwise been inhibited. Therapeutic play can be used in conjunction with modelling interventions. While play therapy is widely used in hospitals, there is hardly any systematic research into its effects (Smolderen and Vingerhoets, 2010).

In a small way, I used procedural information and play therapy (above) with Lucy when we pretended to bandage our ears to familiarise her with post-op procedures (see Chapter 15) However, for some things, I can see the use of books and videos could be more time efficient and expert sources of information.

Based on research with adults, *hypnosis* has also been reported as a successful technique for reducing children's distress during painful or frightening medical procedures (e.g. Butler et al., 2005).

Favourable effects of hypnosis have been supported by a systematic review of psychological interventions for needle-related procedural pain with children and adolescents. Hypnosis was one of the most effective single strategies for reducing pain and distress (Uman et al., 2006).

Recent reviews further demonstrate that *distraction* is one of the most promising techniques for reducing pain and distress. This may vary from simple counting aloud, blowing a party blower, playing with toys to using multimedia including virtual reality (VR); VR is very promising even in the case of very painful wound-care procedures in burn patients (Blount et al., 2006; Uman et al., 2006).

Hypnosis would need the services of a psychologist or psychiatrist, whereas learning to use distraction techniques is easily included in nurse training and may be enough for most patients.

Patient control and optimising comfort

Providing patients undergoing medical procedures with more control may have a positive effect on their well-being and distress. *Patient-controlled analgesia* (PCA) is a relatively new technique currently used routinely as an analgesic post-operative strategy. Patients can administer opioids intravenously through a specially designed programmable pump. Patients receiving PCA tend to use somewhat higher doses of medication, but this procedure generally provides better pain control and increased patient satisfaction compared with conventional methods (Hudcova et al., 2006) (see Chapter 3).

While PCA may not be appropriate for children, those of 8 years and over with chronic conditions may be offered the opportunity to start and stop an often repeated medical procedure and to allow pauses (Van Broeck, 1993).

According to Lorentz (2006), therapeutic touch (*TT*) and *humour* are two examples of mind–body interventions that nurses can use in conjunction with conventional daily nursing practice to help reduce patients' stress (see Box 5.2).

Charlie used to joke a lot – I suspect to cover up his fear of going into a nursing home; and I've noticed how often patients' families use 'therapeutic touch'; it seems almost instinctive.

TIME FOR REFLECTION …

- How do you think the use of humour might benefit the nurse and other health professionals – both with patients and between themselves?
- What sort of factors should nurses and other health professionals consider when using humour with their patients?

Box 5.2 Therapeutic touch and humour

- TT is a process of energy modulation in which nurses use their hands with the intention of helping or healing their patients (Krieger, 2002). The most important factor in TT is intention: this refers to the nurse being compassionate and focusing attention on the patient exclusively.
- TT also denotes healing and not curing. While curing involves removing all signs and symptoms of a disease, TT aims at facilitating a relationship or a connection between the patient's mind, body and spirit to promote a state of harmony or peace.
- *Humour* is regarded by nurses as an interaction or communication that leads to laughing, smiling or a feeling of amusement (Smith, 2002). It can be used effectively in highly stressful situations to help patients overcome their anxieties as well as provide a safe atmosphere that enables patients to express their thoughts, feelings and emotions.
- Humour can also be thought of as a defence mechanism for dealing with stress (see Chapter 2). It has been shown to be very effective for helping patients deal with fear and anxiety as well as increasing their pain threshold (Smith, 2002). Most importantly, humour may bring hope and joy to the situation, which helps relieve stress and speed recovery (Smith, 2002).

Source: Based on Lorentz, M.M., *Altern. J. Nurs.*, 11, 1–11, 2006.

Patient diaries and follow-up clinics

Two forms of intervention currently being trialled in adult ICUs are patient diaries and follow-up clinics. A patient diary in this context refers to a daily record of the patient's ICU stay, written in everyday language, usually by nursing staff at the bedside but with contributions from other health professionals and visiting relatives. Content would usually include the reason for admission and details of significant events during the stay on and off the ward, for example, extubation, the first time the patient managed to sit up, or an important family event (such as a birthday) (Colville, 2012).

The use of diaries has been well received anecdotally: they help to fill in the 'memory gap' that many adult patients find disturbing (Griffiths and Jones, 2001). Two recent randomised control trials have provided evidence that the use of diaries is associated with lower depression, anxiety and post-traumatic stress disorder in adult ICU patients at follow-up (Jones et al., 2010; Knowles and Tarrier, 2009). Dedicated follow-up clinics, at which issues specific to recovery after critical illness can be addressed, are growing in popularity (Colville, 2012); to date, these have been described largely in adult settings. The NICE (2009a) guidelines on rehabilitation after intensive care have recommended that formal follow-up is offered more routinely, in order that the patient's physical and psychological recovery can be more closely monitored. However, the only large-scale randomised control trial evaluating the impact of a nurse-led follow-up clinic (focusing primarily on physical rehabilitation) found no evidence of psychological or physical benefit to patients at 1 year (Cuthbertson et al., 2009).

It seems the fact physical rehabilitation isn't enough is being recognised. In a recent article by James Gallagher on post-ICU psychological disorders Dr David Howell, the clinical director of critical care, said: 'It is fair to say there hasn't been enough focus on the psychological aspects of recovery in intensive care and afterwards.' Doctors now want to trial reducing stress and altering drugs in intensive care (BBC News 14.10.12).

Coping with illness

According to Leventhal et al.'s (1997) *self-regulatory model of illness cognitions*, people go through the following three stages of 'problem solving' when faced with their own illness:

1. *Interpretation* involves making sense of the illness, giving meaning to symptoms or a doctor's diagnosis by accessing their illness cognitions. This is likely to be accompanied by changes in emotional state (such as anxiety), and any coping strategies have to relate to both illness cognitions and the emotional state.
2. *Coping* involves dealing with the illness to regain a state of equilibrium. This can take the form of either (a) approach coping (such as taking pills, going to the doctor, resting and talking to friends about the anxiety) or (b) avoidance coping (such as denial or wishful thinking).
3. *Appraisal* involves evaluating the effectiveness of the coping strategies and deciding whether to continue with this strategy or opt for an alternative.

This process must take time. However it appeared, Pat's perception of her illness must have changed dramatically when her 'lump' was diagnosed as malignant. And as I saw, her ability to cope was very much influenced by Sally's attitude and care.

Coping with a diagnosis

According to Shontz (1975), based on observations of hospital patients, people go through a series of stages following diagnosis of a chronic illness (see Box 5.3).

Box 5.3 Stages of coping with a diagnosis

- *Shock*: Stunned, bewildered, behaving in an automatic way, with feelings of detachment
- *Encounter reaction*: Disorganised thinking and feelings of loss, grief, helplessness and despair
- *Retreat*: Denial of the problem and its implications, retreat into the self. This is only a temporary stage, as denial cannot last forever. It represents a launch pad for a gradual reorientation towards reality.

Source: Shontz, F.C., *The Psychological Aspects of Physical Illness and Disability*, Macmillan Co, New York, 1975.

Shontz's model focuses on the *immediate* changes following a diagnosis, suggesting that the desired outcome of any coping process is to face up to reality and that reality orientation is an adaptive coping mechanism (Ogden, 2004). At the same time, we should not underestimate the impact that diagnosis can have, in both the short-term and long-term – especially when a life-threatening disease is involved. Indeed, according to Moos and Schaefer's (1984) *crisis theory*, physical illness can be considered a crisis, a turning point in the individual's life, which produces certain inevitable changes.

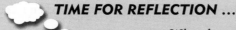

TIME FOR REFLECTION …

- What do you think some of these changes might be?

- Change in identity: for example, 'breadwinner' to 'person with illness'/'patient'
- Change in location: for example, becoming bedridden or hospitalised
- Change in role: for example, from independent adult to passive dependant
- Change in social support: for example, isolation from friends and family
- Changes to 'the future': for example, a future involving children, career or travel can become uncertain

Crisis theory is meant to account for the impact of *any* form of disruption to an individual's established personal and social identity. A good example of such disruption is bereavement, and the changes described in the preceding list are consistent with the concept of the *assumptive world*: 'everything that we assume to be true on the basis of our previous experience … the internal model of the world that we are constantly matching against incoming sensory data in order to orient ourselves, recognise what is happening, and plan our behaviour accordingly' (Parkes, 1993).

Like the loss of a loved one through death (see Chapter 13), being diagnosed with a serious illness represents a *psychosocial transition* that threatens the patient's assumptive world. However, according to crisis theory, psychological systems are driven to the maintenance of homeostasis or equilibrium (in the same way as physical systems). Any crisis is self-limiting, as the individual will find a way of returning to a stable state: people are self-regulators.

Pat's mother, baby and husband dying and her son's addiction were all crises for Pat and being diagnosed with cancer is the latest psychosocial transition to threaten her health – and her happiness.

While this may be true in general terms, there are often factors specific to illness, such as unpredictability, lack of clear information/ambiguity (especially about cause, seriousness and prognosis), the need for quick decisions (e.g. regarding treatment options and what to tell people) and limited prior experience ('I've never had cancer before, what should I do next?') (Ogden, 2004).

📄 *Charlie's death was a traumatic incident for me. My first reactions were shock and panic; later, I was sad and upset. However, it was good that in spite of feeling scared, I used the experience I already had to help as much as I could and (eventually) thought about reassuring the other patients. I became upset but accept it was because I cared so much about Charlie; it was my most difficult 'emotional labour' so far.*

Objectively the experience has increased my confidence; having observed the cardiac arrest procedures for real will help reduce (although not prevent!) my stress in a similar situation. I find the Roger and Nash (1995) theory of coping particularly helpful; I will certainly try to use 'information seeking' and 'rational' methods of coping in future. Exploring the theory of coping with illness and reflecting on Sally's care of Pat makes me more aware of the potential of nurses' mediating role in helping patients cope with the stress of illness.

CHAPTER SUMMARY

- Selye's General Adaptation Syndrome (GAS) comprises the *alarm reaction, resistance* and *exhaustion.*
- The alarm reaction involves changes in the sympathetic branch of the ANS, which are collectively called the *FOFR* (or *response*). This is associated with the *ANS-adrenal-medulla system* (or *SAM axis*).
- Resistance is associated with the *anterior pituitary-adrenal cortex system* (or *HPA axis*).
- Exhaustion is related to *psychophysiological disorders* ('diseases of adaptation').
- The GAS fails to distinguish between evolutionarily basic and modern stressors, which are related to acute and chronic stress respectively; chronic stress responses are probably a recent – and unique – human 'invention'. Even temporary everyday anxieties can weaken the influence of the *Pre-frontal cortex* (*PFC*), the most recently evolved brain region that mediates our highest cognitive abilities
- The GAS (which reflects the *biomedical model* of health and illness) also fails to recognise the interaction between (1) the ANS and endocrine systems and (2) the immune system (the *immunosuppressive* effects of stress). This interaction is the focus of *psychoneuroimmunology* (*PNI*) and reflects the *BPS model* of health and illness.
- The explanation of how the immune system can be shut down in the face of chronic stress is consistent with the concept of *allostatic load*. Sterling and Eyer's *allostatic load model* aims to explain how biological changes designed to *protect* the organism (*allostatic*) can also be *harmful* (*allostatic load*).
- *Personality* represents an important *moderator* of stress. Relevant examples include *Type A Behaviour Pattern* (*TABP*), *Type C personality* and *hardiness*. These have been studied in relation to CHD, cancer and the stress–illness relationship in general, respectively. While TABP and Type C represent *risk* factors, hardiness is *protective*.

- Positive and resilient *self-esteem* represents another protective factor.
- If we judge a situation/event to be a stressor (based on our *primary appraisal*), a *secondary appraisal* assesses our coping resources. This is followed by actual *coping efforts*.
- Cohen and Lazarus distinguish five categories of coping: *direct action response, information-seeking inhibition of action, intrapsychic/palliative coping* and *turning to others*. These overlap with the distinction between *problem-focused* and *emotion-focused* coping.
- Roger and Nash distinguish between *maladaptive* and *adaptive* coping styles, each having short-term benefits and long-term consequences.
- *Stress management* represents the *formal* provision of methods for dealing with stress provided by trained professionals. Methods include *biofeedback* and *cognitive restructuring* (based on Beck and Ellis's versions of CBT).
- Others include provision of information (including psychoeducation), social support, skills training, *systematic desensitisation* (SD), hypnosis, *patient-controlled analgesia* (PCA), *therapeutic touch* (TT), humour, patient diaries and follow-up clinics.
- While these methods can be used with all age groups, methods used mainly with children include *modelling, pre-exposure*, and *distraction*.
- These psychological interventions (and others used to treat pain) are used to help patients cope with stressful medical procedures. While several have been shown to be effective, they are often combined in treatment 'packages'; this makes it difficult to assess the relative effectiveness of individual methods.
- Moos and Schaefer's *crisis theory* has been used to explain how patients cope with a diagnosis of chronic illness.

6 Attitudes and attitude change

Introduction and overview

The study of attitudes has undergone many important changes since Gordon Allport (1935) claimed that 'The concept of attitudes is probably the most distinctive and indispensable concept in contemporary American social psychology'. According to Stainton Rogers et al. (1995), psychologists have tried to answer the following fundamental questions over the last 70 years:

1. Where do attitudes come from? How are they moulded and formed in the first place?
2. How can attitudes be measured?
3. How and why do attitudes change? What forces are involved and what intrapsychic mechanisms operate when people shift in their opinions about particular 'attitude objects'?
4. How do attitudes relate to behaviour? What is it that links the way people think and feel about an attitude object and what they do about it?

In this chapter, the emphasis is on some of the answers that have been offered to questions 3 and 4. This discussion is also relevant to prejudice, considered as an extreme attitude (see Chapter 7).

During the 1940s and 1950s, the focus of research was on attitude change, in particular *persuasive communication*. Much of the impetus for this came from the use of propaganda during the Second World War, as well as a more general concern over the growing influence of the mass media, especially in the United States. This period also saw the birth of a number of theories of attitude change, the most influential of these being Festinger's *cognitive dissonance theory* (CDT).

The 1960s and 1970s was a period of decline and pessimism in attitude research, at least partly due to the apparent failure to find any reliable relationship between measured attitudes and behaviour (Hogg and Vaughan, 1995).

However, the 1980s saw a revival of interest, stimulated largely by the cognitive approach, so attitudes represent another important aspect of *social cognition* (see Chapter 10).

 From my diary (10): Year 2/Surgical Ward

We had a termination of pregnancy today. Janet, 42, elected to have an abortion after an amniocentesis showed slightly raised alpha-protein levels indicating a small risk of a baby with Down's syndrome. She appeared very composed throughout but just before she went home I found her crying in the bathroom. I stayed with her and asked if she was sad at 'losing' her baby. She said yes, but mostly she felt guilty. I tried to reassure her that, too, was a natural part of the grief reaction (see Chapter 13), but she said no, that wasn't it. She then told me that she'd recently re-trained as a hairdresser, her children were 10 and 13, her marriage was 'rocky' and she just couldn't have another baby at her age. The Down's syndrome threat was 'a good excuse' but, although she didn't regret it, she felt she'd done wrong. I tried to comfort her and then reported it to Caroline (Ward Manager). She said she'd explain to Janet her follow-up appointment would include an opportunity for counselling.

What are attitudes?

Allport (1935) regarded the study of attitudes as the meeting ground for the study of social groups, culture and the individual. Festinger (1950) also emphasised the integral interdependence of individual and group. But, with a few notable exceptions, attitude research has focused on *internal* processes, ignoring the influence of groups on attitude formation and change (Cooper et al., 2004).

Warren and Jahoda's (1973) definition is probably the most 'social': '… attitudes have social reference in their origins and development and in their objects, while at the same time they have psychological reference in that they inhere in the individual and are intimately enmeshed in his behaviour and his psychological make-up.'

According to Rosenberg and Hovland (1960), attitudes are 'predispositions to respond to some class of stimuli with certain classes of response'. These classes of response are as follows:

- *Affective*: what a person feels about the attitude object; how favourably or unfavourably it is evaluated.
- *Cognitive*: what a person believes the attitude object is like, objectively.
- *Behavioural* (sometimes called the '*conative*'): how a person actually responds, or intends to respond, to the attitude object.

This *three-component model*, which is much more a model of attitude *structure* than a simple definition (Stahlberg and Frey, 1988), is shown in Figure 6.1. It sees an attitude as an intervening/mediating variable between observable stimuli and responses, illustrating the influence that behaviourism was still having, even in social psychology, at the start of the 1960s (see Chapter 2). A major problem with this multi-component model is the assumption that the three components are highly correlated (see pages 131 through 133).

Figure 6.1 Three-component view of attitudes. (From Rosenberg, M.J. and Hovland, C.I., Cognitive, affective and behavioural components of attitude. In M.J. Rosenberg, C.I. Hovland, W.J. McGuire, R.P. Abelson and J.W. Brehm (eds.), *Attitude Organisation and Change: An Analysis of Consistency Among Attitude Components*, New Haven, CT, Yale University Press., 1960; Stahlberg, D. and Frey, D., Attitudes 1: Structure, measurement and functions. In M. Hewstone et al. (eds.), *Introduction to Social Psychology*, Oxford, Blackwell, 1988.)

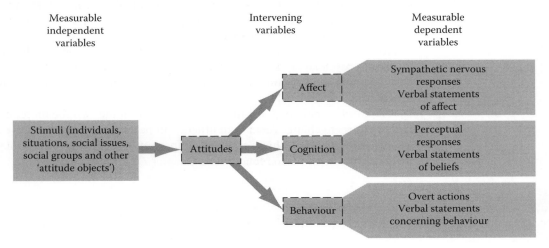

Attitudes, beliefs and values

An attitude can be thought of as a blend or integration of beliefs and values. Beliefs represent the knowledge or information we have about the world (although these may be inaccurate or incomplete) and, in themselves, are *non-evaluative*. To convert a belief into an attitude, a 'value' ingredient is needed. Values refer to an individual's sense of what is desirable, good, valuable, worthwhile, and so on. While most adults will have many thousands of beliefs, they have only hundreds of attitudes and a few dozen values.

> ### TIME FOR REFLECTION …
>
> - Try to identify some of your most cherished values (there should be a relatively small number of these).
> - Then try to identify some related attitudes, which are less abstract than values.

Using Rosenberg and Hovland's (1960) classification, my attitude to abortion is – I **feel** uncomfortable at the idea of it but within the circumstances outlined in the Abortion Act 1967 (and 1990 amendments), I **believe** it is sometimes justified. Behaviourally, **I would have a 'justified' abortion**. But at handover this morning, Bridie (another student) made her disapproval clear and, as a practising Catholic, refused to be involved.

What are attitudes for?

According to Hogg and Vaughan (1995), attitudes provide us with ready-made reactions to, and interpretations of, events, just as other aspects of our cognitive 'equipment' do, such as stereotypes (see Chapter 7). Attitudes save us energy, since we do not have to work out how we feel about objects or events each time we come into contact with them.

However, not all attitudes serve the same function. Katz (1960), influenced by Freud's psychoanalytic theory (see Chapter 2), believes that attitudes serve both conscious and unconscious motives. He identified four major functions of attitudes (see Table 6.1).

Katz's functional approach implies that some attitudes will be more resistant to efforts to change them than others – in particular, those that serve an *ego-defensive function*. This is especially important when trying to account for prejudice and attempts to reduce it (see Chapter 7).

Knowing her reasons I saw nothing ethically wrong with Janet's decision so didn't question it. I'm wondering now if that is serving an adjustive (wanting approval) function. It must have taken courage (a value-expressive function) for Bridie to speak out in front of the staff.

Table 6.1 Four major functions of attitudes.

Knowledge function	We seek a degree of predictability, consistency and stability in our perception of the world. Attitudes give meaning and direction to experience, providing frames of reference for judging events, objects and people.
Adjustive (instrumental or utilitarian) function	We obtain favourable responses from others by displaying socially acceptable attitudes, so they become associated with important rewards (such as others' acceptance and approval). These attitudes may be publicly expressed, but not necessarily believed, as in *compliance* (see Chapter 8).
Value-expressive function	We achieve self-expression through cherished values. The reward may not be gaining social approval, but confirmation of the more positive aspects of our self-concept, especially our sense of personal integrity.
Ego-defensive function	Attitudes help protect us from admitting personal deficiencies. For example, *prejudice* helps us to sustain our self-concept by maintaining a sense of superiority over others. Ego defence often means avoiding and denying self-knowledge.

Source: Katz, D., *Public Opinion Quarterly*, 24, 163–204, 1960.

The measurement of attitudes

- An attitude cannot be measured directly, because it is a *hypothetical construct*. Consequently, it is necessary to find adequate attitude indicators, and most methods of attitude measurement are based on the assumption that they can be measured by people's beliefs or opinions about the attitude object (Stahlberg and Frey, 1988). Most attitude scales rely on verbal reports and usually take the form of standardised statements that clearly refer to the attitude being measured. Such scales make two further assumptions:

  1. The same statement has the *same meaning* for all respondents, and more fundamentally
  2. Subjective attitudes, when expressed verbally, can be *quantified* (represented by a numerical score)

  One of the most widely used scales is the Likert scale (1932), which if applied to abortion would require the participant to indicate how much she/he agrees or disagrees with the following statement:

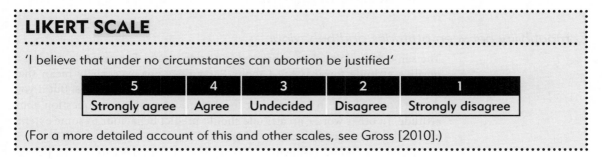

LIKERT SCALE

'I believe that under no circumstances can abortion be justified'

5	4	3	2	1
Strongly agree	Agree	Undecided	Disagree	Strongly disagree

(For a more detailed account of this and other scales, see Gross [2010].)

 On this scale I would have ticked 1 (perhaps 2); Bridie, I'm sure, would have ticked 5!

The relationship between attitudes and behaviour

- Once we've established people's attitudes, can we then accurately predict how they'll behave? Rosenberg and Hovland's (1960) three-component model (see pages 128 and 129) implies that the behavioural component will be highly correlated with the cognitive and affective components.

TIME FOR REFLECTION ...

- Do people's expressed attitudes (cognitive and affective components) necessarily coincide with their overt actions (behavioural component)?
- Do we always act in accordance with our attitudes?

Influences on behaviour

- It is generally agreed that attitudes form only one determinant of behaviour. They represent *predispositions* to behave in particular ways, but how we actually act in a particular situation will depend on the immediate consequences of our behaviour, how we think others will evaluate our actions, and habitual ways of behaving in those kinds of situations. In addition, there may be specific *situational factors* influencing behaviour. Sometimes, we experience a conflict between our attitudes, and behaviour may represent a compromise between them.

Janet feels her situation justifies her action but her feeling of guilt suggests she fears disapproval from some source – perhaps her family or friends? Would I have an abortion if it meant being socially ostracised?

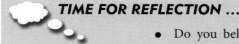

TIME FOR REFLECTION ...

- Do you believe it is right for nurses and other health professionals to take industrial action, even if this is aimed at improving patient care?

Compatibility between attitudes and behaviour

The same attitude may be expressed in various ways. For example, having a positive attitude towards the Labour Party does not necessarily mean that you actually become a member or that you attend public meetings. But if you do not vote Labour in a general or local election, people may question your attitude. In other words, an attitude should predict behaviour to some extent, even if this is extremely limited and specific.

Indeed, Ajzen and Fishbein (1977) argue that attitudes can predict behaviour, provided that both are assessed at the same level of generality: there needs to be a high degree of *compatibility* (or *correspondence*) between them. They argue that much of the earlier research suffered from either trying to predict specific behaviours from general attitudes, or vice versa, and this accounts for the generally low correlations. A study by Davidson and Jaccard (1979) tried to overcome this limitation (see Key Study 6.1).

Ajzen and Fishbein (1977) are saying (and I've indicated) that, in spite of my expressed attitude, predicting whether I'd have an abortion without knowing the specific circumstances would be difficult.

According to Ajzen and Fishbein (1977), every single instance of behaviour involves four specific elements:

1. A specific action
2. Performed with respect to a given target
3. In a given context
4. At a given point in time.

KEY STUDY 6.1

Attitudes can predict behaviour if you ask the right questions

- Davidson and Jaccard analysed correlations between married women's attitudes towards birth control and their actual use of oral contraceptives during the 2 years following the study.
- When 'attitude towards birth control' was used as the attitude measure, the correlation was 0.08 (very low correspondence).
- But when 'attitudes towards oral contraceptives' were measured, the correlation rose to 0.32, and when 'attitudes towards using oral contraceptives' were measured, the correlation rose still further, to 0.53.
- Finally, when 'attitudes towards using oral contraceptives during the next two years' was used, it rose still further, to 0.57. Clearly, in the last three cases, *correspondence* was much higher.

Source: Davidson, A.R. and Jaccard, J., *Journal of Personality & Social Psychology*, 37, 1364–1376, 1979.

According to the *principle of compatibility*, measures of attitude and behaviour are compatible to the extent that the target, action, context and time element are assessed at identical levels of generality or specificity (Ajzen, 1988). For example, a person's attitude towards a 'healthy lifestyle' specifies only the target, leaving the other three unspecified. A behavioural measure that would be compatible with this global attitude would have to aggregate a wide range of health behaviours across different contexts and times (Stroebe, 2000).

Janet seemed to be anti-abortion, but (reflecting Ajzen and Fishbein's four elements above), she had an abortion because 1) she had a new career, 2) she had two children already, 3) she felt too old to have another baby and 4) her marriage was 'rocky'. If she wasn't working, or if she had been happier in her marriage or younger she may have decided differently.

The reliability and consistency of behaviour

Many of the classic studies that failed to find an attitude–behaviour relationship assessed just single instances of behaviour (Stroebe, 2000). But because behaviour depends on many factors in addition to the attitude, a single instance of behaviour is an unreliable indicator of an attitude (Jonas et al., 1995). Only sampling many instances of the behaviour will by the influence of specific factors 'cancel out'. This *aggregation principle* (Fishbein and Ajzen, 1974) has been demonstrated in a number of studies (see Figure 6.2).

According to Hogg and Vaughan (1995), what emerged in the 1980s and 1990s is a view that attitudes and overt behaviour are not related in a simple

Figure 6.2 A demonstration of attitude–behaviour consistency that amazed the world; a pro-democracy Chinese student stands up for his convictions and defies tanks sent in against fellow rebels in Tiananmen Square, Beijing, China. Some 2000 demonstrators died in the subsequent massacre and the student was tried and shot a few days later.

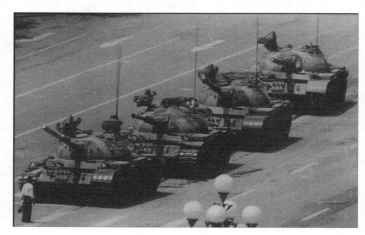

one-to-one fashion. In order to predict someone's behaviour, it must be possible to account for the interaction between attitudes, beliefs and behavioural intentions, as well as how all these connect with the later action. One attempt to formalise these links is the *theory of reasoned action* (TRA) (Ajzen and Fishbein, 1970; Fishbein and Ajzen, 1975; see Chapter 10).

Eight years ago Janet might not have terminated another pregnancy as her circumstances appear to have been very different then.

The strength of attitudes

Most modern theories agree that attitudes are represented in memory and that an attitude's *accessibility* can exert a strong influence on behaviour (Fazio, 1986). By definition, strong attitudes exert more influence over behaviour, because they can be *automatically activated*. According to the MODE model – 'motivation and opportunity as determinants' (Fazio, 1986, 1990) – spontaneous/automatic attitude–behaviour links occur when people hold highly accessible attitudes towards certain targets; such attitudes spontaneously guide behaviour, partly because they influence people's selective attention and perceptions of a particular target or situation.

So are they a shortcut to decision-making – like stereotypes? The TRA emphasises the importance of subjective norms derived from our social context (see Chapter 10). Bridie was brought up in a rural, Catholic community; presumably her religious convictions would 'automatically activate' her decision-making.

One factor that seems to be important is *direct experience*. For example, Fazio and Zanna (1978) found that measures of students' attitudes towards psychology experiments were better predictors of their future participation if they had already taken part in several experiments than if they had only read about them.

MODE acknowledges that, in some situations, people engage in *deliberate, effortful* thinking about their attitudes when deciding how to act (forming behavioural intentions). For example, a student deciding which university to go to will probably scrutinise his/her attitudes before making a choice. But research conducted under MODE focuses on automatic processing (Cooper et al., 2004). The *theory of planned behaviour* (TPB) (Ajzen, 1991), which built on the TRA, was designed to explain the relationship between attitudes and behaviour when deliberate, effortful processing is required. According to TPB, it is behavioural *intentions*, rather than attitudes, that directly influence behaviour (see Chapter 10).

The TPB sees intentions as strategies to achieve particular goals (see figure 10.3, page 233); one of Janet's is more financial security for her children and herself.

Social influence and behaviour change

Persuasive communication

According to Laswell (1948), in order to understand and predict the effectiveness of one person's attempt to change the attitude of another, we need to know 'who says what in which channel to whom and with what effect'. Figure 6.3 Similarly, Hovland and Janis (1959) say that we need to study:

- *The source* of the persuasive communication – that is, the communicator (Laswell's 'who')
- *The message* itself (Laswell's 'what')
- *The recipient* of the message or the audience (Laswell's 'whom')
- *The situation* or *context* (see Figure 6.4)

The basic paradigm in laboratory attitude-change research involves the following three steps or stages:

1. Measure people's attitude towards the attitude object (*pre-test*)
2. Expose them to a *persuasive communication* (manipulate a source, message or situational variable, or isolate a recipient variable as the independent variable)
3. Measure their attitudes again (*post-test*)

If there's a difference between pre- and post-test measures, then the persuasive communication is judged to have 'worked'.

Figure 6.3 Different kinds of attempts to change people's attitudes and behaviour. These range from professional help for emotional and behavioural problems, through inevitable features of social interaction/social influence, to deliberate attempts to manipulate and control others for the benefit of the manipulator.

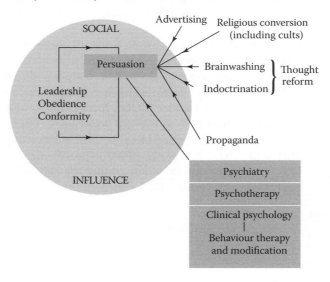

Figure 6.4 The four major factors involved in persuasive communication (arrows between boxes indicate examples of interaction between variables).

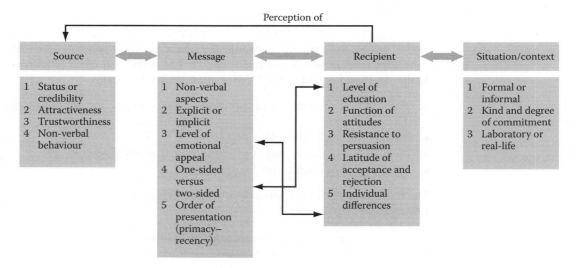

It's likely the attitude of most of the nursing staff wouldn't be changed by Bridie's 'message': she was of low authority professionally, the message was religiously motivated (one-sided) and most nurses would be professionally resistant to such persuasion.

Fear and persuasion

A famous early attempt to induce attitude change through the manipulation of fear was made by Janis and Feshbach (1953) (see Key Study 6.2).

Similar results were reported by Janis and Terwillinger (1962), who presented a mild and strong fear message concerning the relationship between smoking and cancer.

These studies suggest that, in McGuire's (1969) terms, you can frighten people into attending to a message, comprehending it, yielding to it and retaining it, but not necessarily into acting upon it. Indeed, fear may be so great that action is *inhibited* rather than facilitated. However, if the audience is told how to avoid undesirable consequences and believes that the preventative action is realistic and will be effective, then even high levels of fear in the message can produce changes in behaviour. The more specific and precise the instructions, the greater the behaviour change (the *high availability factor*).

KEY STUDY 6.2

Fear of the dentist as a means to healthier teeth

- Janis and Feshbach randomly assigned American high-school students to one of four groups (one control and three experimental).
- The message was concerned with dental hygiene, and degree of fear arousal was manipulated by the number and nature of consequences of improper care of teeth (which were also shown in colour slides). Each message also contained factual information about the causes of tooth decay, and some advice about caring for teeth.
- The *high fear condition* involved 71 references to unpleasant effects (including toothache, painful treatment and possible secondary diseases, such as blindness and cancer). The *moderate fear condition* involved 49 references, and the *low fear condition* involved just 18. The control group heard a talk about the eye.
- Before the experiment, participants' attitudes to dental health, and their dental habits, were assessed as part of a general health survey. The same questionnaire was given again immediately following the fear-inducing message, and 1 week later.
- The results show that the stronger the appeal to fear, the greater their anxiety (an index of attitude change). But as far as actual changes in dental *behaviour* were concerned, the high fear condition proved to be the *least* effective. Eight per cent of the high-fear group had adopted the recommendations (changes in tooth brushing and visiting the dentist in the weeks immediately following the experiment), compared with 22 per cent and 37 per cent in the moderate- and low-fear conditions, respectively.

Source: Janis, I. and Feshbach, S., *Journal of Abnormal & Social Psychology*, 48, 78–92, 1953.

'One certain reason for the increase in abortion is that women use less hormonal contraception than they used to … Media myths about contraceptives can frighten people and they lose confidence in their use' (Tschudin, 2003: 125). For some women then, the fear of the effects of hormonal contraception is greater than the fear of getting pregnant. However, if abortion were still illegal, would more women risk hormonal contraception?

TIME FOR REFLECTION …

- Can you relate the high availability factor to one of the principles we identified when discussing the measurement of attitude–behaviour correlations?

According to Stroebe (2000), mass-media campaigns designed to change some specific health behaviour should use arguments aimed mainly at changing beliefs relating to that *specific* behaviour – rather than focusing on more general health concerns. This is another example of the compatibility principle. For example, to persuade people to lower their dietary cholesterol, it would not be very effective merely to point out that coronary heart disease (CHD) is the major killer and/or that high levels of saturated fat are bad for one's heart. To influence diet, it would have to be argued that very specific dietary changes, such as eating less animal fat and red meat, would have a positive impact on blood cholesterol levels, which, in turn, should reduce the risk of developing CHD.

To persuade Janet to use more reliable contraception it wouldn't be any good pointing out that unprotected sex can lead to pregnancy! It would be more effective to discuss (at the follow-up appointment) specific contraceptive methods suitable for her and specify where they can be obtained and when she would start using them.

In situations of minimal or extreme fear, the message may fail to produce any attitude change, let alone any change in behaviour. According to McGuire (1968), there is an inverted U-shaped curve in the relationship between fear and attitude change (as shown in Figure 6.5).

In segment 1 of the curve, the participant is not particularly interested in (aroused by) the message: it is hardly attended to and may not even register. In segment 2, attention and arousal increase as fear increases, but the fear remains within manageable proportions. In segment 3, attention will decrease again, but this time because defences are being used to deal with extreme fear: the message may be denied ('it couldn't happen to me' – see Chapter 10) or repressed (see Chapter 2). Despite evidence of defensive processing, Stroebe (2000) maintains that

> …the overwhelming majority of studies on fear appeals has found that higher levels of threat resulted in greater persuasion than did lower levels. However, the effectiveness of high-fear messages appeared to be somewhat reduced for respondents who feel highly vulnerable to the threat.

Figure 6.5 Inverted U curve showing relationship between attitude change and fear arousal. (Based on McGuire, W.J., *Handbook of Personality: Theory and Research*, Chicago, IL, Rand-McNally, 1968.)

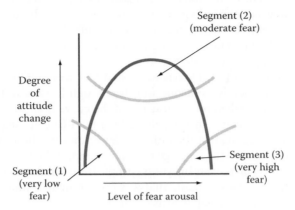

Figure 6.6 Part of an anti-smoking commercial based on the appeal to fear.

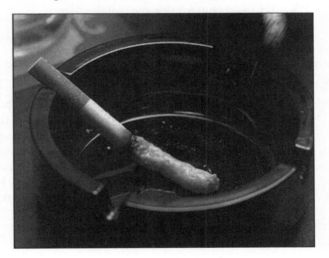

Despite the millions of pounds spent by the U.K. government in 2005 on hard-hitting campaigns (see Figure 6.6) aimed at reducing smoking rates to under 21 per cent by 2010, the proportion of adults who smoke fell just 3 per cent (to 25 per cent) between 1998 and 2004. And rates among younger age groups, considered as more susceptible to such advertising campaigns, have *risen* (Frith, 2006). At the Royal College of Nursing's 2006 annual conference, a resolution was debated suggesting that funds would be better spent on treating patients and targeting the most at-risk groups.

...such as providing contraceptive information and free condoms for teenagers as they did at Josh's school (see case study 8, page 400) which was one way to target that particular 'at-risk' group.

The importance of feeling vulnerable

In order to arouse fear, it is not enough that a health risk has serious consequences: the individual must also feel personally at risk (i.e., vulnerable). There is some evidence that unless individuals feel vulnerable to a threat, they're unlikely to form the intention to act on the recommendations in the message (Kuppens et al., 1996).

Feeling vulnerable relates to what McGuire (1968) calls the *initial level of concern*. Clearly, someone who has a high level of initial concern will be more easily pushed into segment 3 of the curve than someone with a low level. The former may be overwhelmed by a high-fear message (in which case defences are used against it), while the latter may not become interested and aroused enough for the message to have an impact. While the government is focusing efforts on preventing young people from starting to smoke, anecdotal evidence from nurses suggests that it is predominantly middle-aged smokers who are now seeking help (Carlisle, 2012).

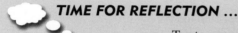

TIME FOR REFLECTION …

- Try to account for this anecdotal evidence.

Janet, having experienced a traumatic pregnancy, will certainly have a higher initial level of concern.

Fear appeals are also most likely to be effective for individuals who are unfamiliar with a given health risk. For example, when the dangers involved in unprotected anal intercourse among homosexuals became known in the early 1980s, the information appeared to produce an enormous reduction in such practices. But there was a hard core of men who were unaffected by the information, illustrating that simply repeating the dangers of HIV infection does not achieve risk reduction with such individuals (Stroebe, 2000; see also Chapter 10).

These men are either using defences, such as denial, against a high fear level – or might they be unconcerned about the consequences?

Theories of attitude change

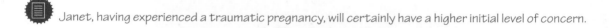

The most influential theories of attitude change have concentrated on the principle of *cognitive consistency*. Human beings are seen as internally active information processors, who sort through and modify a large number of cognitive elements in order to achieve some kind of cognitive coherence. This need for cognitive consistency means that theories such as Festinger's *CDT* (1957) are not just theories of attitude change, but are also accounts of human motivation.

Cognitive dissonance theory

According to CDT, whenever we simultaneously hold two cognitions that are psychologically inconsistent, we experience *dissonance*. This is a negative drive state, a state of 'psychological discomfort or tension', which motivates us to reduce it by achieving consonance. Attitude change is a major way of reducing dissonance. Cognitions are 'the things a person knows about himself, about his behaviour and about his surroundings' (Festinger, 1957), and any two cognitions can be consonant (A implies B), dissonant (A implies not-B) or irrelevant to each other.

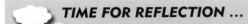 Janet was in a state of cognitive dissonance; her true attitude to abortion was that it was wrong; she had done something she didn't approve of.

TIME FOR REFLECTION ...

- How might someone who smokes try to reduce dissonance?

The cognition 'I smoke' is psychologically inconsistent with the cognition 'smoking causes cancer' (assuming that we don't wish to get cancer). Perhaps, the most efficient (and certainly the healthiest!) way to reduce dissonance is to stop smoking, but many people will work on the other cognition. For example, they might

- Belittle the evidence about smoking and cancer (e.g., 'The human data are only correlational')
- Associate with other smokers (e.g., 'If so-and-so smokes, then it can't be very dangerous')
- Smoke low-tar cigarettes
- Convince themselves that smoking is an important and highly pleasurable activity

These examples illustrate how CDT regards human beings as *rationalising* (not rational) creatures: attempting to *appear* rational, both to others and to oneself.

Just as Diana (case study 2, pages 216 and 226) used the 'stress reducing' excuse to continue smoking, Janet used the risk of a baby with Down's syndrome to rationalise, or justify, her decision to herself.

Research into CDT has focused on three major areas: (1) dissonance following a decision; (2) dissonance resulting from effort (both discussed by Gross [2010]); and (3) engaging in counter-attitudinal behaviour.

Engaging in counter-attitudinal behaviour

This aspect of CDT is of most relevance to our earlier discussion of the relationship between attitudes and behaviour (see Key Study 6.3).

TIME FOR REFLECTION …

- How would CDT explain these findings? (You first need to ask yourself who experienced the greater dissonance.)

The large, 20-dollar incentive gave those participants ample justification for their counter-attitudinal behaviour, and so they experienced very *little* dissonance. But the 1-dollar group experienced considerable dissonance: they could hardly justify their counter-attitudinal behaviour in terms of the negligible reward (hence, the change of attitude to reduce the dissonance).

So if Janet had been told her baby **would** have Down's syndrome, or a known defect, she would suffer less cognitive dissonance – and less guilt?

An evaluation of CDT

- Festinger and Carlsmith's findings have been replicated by several studies in which children are given either a mild or severe threat not to play with an attractive toy (Aronson and Carlsmith, 1963; Freedman, 1965). If children

KEY STUDY 6.3

The '1 dollar/20 dollar' experiment

- College students were brought, one at a time, into a small room to work for 30 minutes on two extremely dull and repetitive tasks (stacking spools and turning pegs).
- Later, they were offered either 1 dollar or 20 dollars to try to convince the next 'participant' (in fact, a female stooge) that the tasks were interesting and enjoyable.
- Common sense would predict that the 20-dollar students would be more likely to change their attitudes in favour of the tasks (they had more reason to do so), and this is also what *reinforcement/incentive theory* (Janis et al., 1965) would predict (the greater the reward/incentive, the greater the attitude change).
- However, as predicted by CDT, it was in fact the 1-dollar group that showed the greater attitude change (the *less-leads-to-more effect*).

Source: Festinger, L. and Carlsmith, J.M., *Journal of Abnormal & Social Psychology*, 58, 203–210, 1959.

obey a *mild* threat, they will experience *greater* dissonance, because it is more difficult for them to justify their behaviour than for children given a severe threat. So, the mild threat condition produces greater reduction in liking of the toy.

- However, dissonance occurs only when the behaviour is *volitional* (voluntary): if we believe we had no choice, there's no dissonance, and hence no attitude change. A study by Freedman (1963) shows that dissonance and reinforcement theory are not mutually exclusive; instead, they seem to apply to voluntary and involuntary behaviour, respectively.

- According to Bem's *self-perception theory* (SPT) (1965, 1967), the concept of dissonance is both unnecessary and unhelpful. Any self-report of an attitude is an *inference* from observation of one's own behaviour and the situation in which it occurs. This is because we do not have 'privileged access' to our own thoughts and feelings, but find out them in the same way as we learn about other people (for a detailed discussion of SPT, see Gross, 2010).

- According to some *impression management theorists* (e.g., Schlenker, 1982; Tedeschi and Rosenfield, 1981), many dissonance experiments might not reflect genuine cases of 'private' attitude change (a drive to be consistent). Rather, they reflect the need to *appear* consistent, and hence to avoid social anxiety and embarrassment, or to protect positive views of one's own identity. So, the 1-dollar group's attitude change is genuine, but is motivated by *social* (rather than *cognitive*) factors.

- Despite challenges and reconceptualisations, Hogg and Vaughan (1995) maintain that

> … cognitive dissonance theory remains one of the most widely accepted explanations of attitude change and many other social behaviours. It has generated over one thousand research studies and will probably continue to be an integral part of social psychological theory for many years.

Experiencing Janet's cognitive dissonance made me re-think my own attitude to abortion. Rosenberg and Hovland's (1960) 'classes of response' model of attitude helped me analyse it rather than accept it on the basis of its legality. Perhaps the underlying value of the sanctity of human life is at odds with my expressed attitude and my need for 'very good reasons' for abortion an attempt to justify it. Again by obtaining empirical knowledge (theory) and aesthetic knowledge (experimental), I'm now considering it as more than one individual's decision; the social, ethical and emotive debate surrounding abortion broadens it further.

Ajzen and Fishbein's (1977) view on predicting behaviour helps me understand that Janet's decision to have this termination didn't necessarily reflect her true attitude; consistent behaviour is a more convincing indication. Reflecting on this incident, I may have modified my attitude slightly, or perhaps my perception of it is clearer? In any case, it's not sufficient to change my behaviour at work.

CHAPTER SUMMARY

- The *three-component model* of attitude structure sees attitudes as comprising *affective*, *cognitive* and *behavioural* components. Attitudes have much in common with beliefs and values, but they need to be distinguished.
- Katz identifies the *knowledge, adjustive, value-expressive* and *ego-defensive functions* of attitudes.
- Early research into the *relationship between attitudes and behaviour* showed that attitudes are very poor predictors of behaviour. But attitudes represent only one of several determinants of behaviour, including situational factors.
- Attitudes can predict behaviour, provided there's a close correspondence between the way the two variables are defined and measured (the *principle of compatibility*). Also, measures of a representative sample of behaviours relevant to the attitude must be made (the *aggregation principle*).
- *Persuasive communication* has traditionally been studied in terms of the influence of four interacting factors: the *source* of the persuasive message, the *message* itself, the *recipient* of the message and the *situation/context*.
- *Theories of systematic processing* see the impact of persuasive messages as dependent on a sequence of processes, including *attending* to the message, *comprehending* it, *accepting* its conclusions, *retaining* it and *acting* as a result.
- People can be frightened into attending to, comprehending, accepting and retaining a message, but the *high availability factor* is necessary for any behaviour change to take place.
- People also need to feel personally *vulnerable* if fear appeals are to have any impact. There appears to be an inverted U-shaped curve in the relationship between fear and attitude change.
- The major theories of attitude change share the basic principle of *cognitive consistency*. The most influential of these is Festinger's *CDT*.
- *Dissonance* is most likely to occur after making a very *difficult choice/decision*, when putting ourselves through *hardship* or making a *sacrifice* only to find it was for nothing, or when engaging *voluntarily* in *counter-attitudinal behaviour*.
- Bem's *SPT* claims that we infer our attitudes from observing our own behaviour, just as we do other people's attitudes.
- *Impression management theory* stresses the *social* rather than the *cognitive* motivation underlying attitude change.

7 Prejudice and discrimination

Introduction and overview

While genocide – the systematic destruction of an entire cultural, ethnic or racial group – is the most extreme form of discrimination, the prejudice that underlies it is essentially the same as that which underlies less extreme behaviours. Prejudice is an *attitude* that can be expressed in many ways or that may not be overtly or openly expressed at all. Like other attitudes, prejudice can be regarded as a *disposition* to behave in a prejudiced way (to practise *discrimination*). So, the relationship between prejudice and discrimination is an example of the wider debate concerning the attitude–behaviour relationship (see Chapter 6).

Theories of prejudice and discrimination try to explain their origins: how do people come to be prejudiced and to act in discriminatory ways? Answers to these questions potentially answer the further question: how can they be reduced or even prevented altogether? This, of course, has much greater practical significance for people's lives.

Perhaps for nurses and other health professionals, the key issues are

- Being aware of their own (often unconscious) prejudices
- Recognising how this may affect their professional practice (again, something that often goes unnoticed by the professionals themselves)

Patients may be from a different ethnic/cultural background to the nurse, they may be gay or lesbian, they may have HIV/AIDS (see George, 1995; McHaffie, 1994), they may be transsexual (see Rees, 1993; Thomas, 1993) or obese (see Whyte, 1998), or even the victim of rape (see Donnelly, 1991). In all these cases, they may become the victims of the nurse's prejudice and discrimination.

From my diary (14): Year 2/Elderly Care Ward

A patient made me angry today. Mrs Maitland (she declined to be called by her first name) – an overweight, 68-year-old woman with poorly controlled diabetes and atherosclerotic peripheral arterial disease – had been admitted with a tiny ulcer on her toe. When Rasheed (the Asian F1) examined her she looked disgruntled and answered in monosyllables. Afterwards I asked her if she was happy with everything he'd told her; she replied in a very disparaging way that she didn't know what she'd been told, she couldn't understand a word he said. I protested that Rasheed spoke excellent English and she said, 'That's as may be, but he's got that funny, foreign accent. Why can't that nice young doctor see to me?' (He was white and from another ward.) Trying to be patient, I started to explain what Rasheed said, but she interrupted me with, 'Never mind – I'll wait till I can see a proper nurse.' I bit my tongue and walked away, thinking I wouldn't bother any more with her and as I went heard her whisper to her neighbour, 'They're everywhere, aren't they?' Minutes later I felt even angrier as I saw her smiling and talking to Rachel, a (white) HCA. I wondered what she'd think if she knew Rachel was gay!

Prejudice as an attitude

As an *extreme* attitude, prejudice comprises the three components common to all attitudes:

1. The cognitive component is the *stereotype*.
2. The affective component is a strong feeling of hostility.
3. The behavioural component can take different forms.

Allport (1954) proposed five stages of this component:

1. *Antilocution* – hostile talk, verbal denigration and insult, and racial jokes
2. *Avoidance* – keeping a distance but without actively inflicting harm
3. *Discrimination* – exclusion from housing, civil rights and employment
4. *Physical attack* – violence against the person and property
5. *Extermination* – indiscriminate violence against an entire group (including genocide)

'Discrimination' is often used to denote the behavioural component, while 'prejudice' denotes the cognitive and affective components. But just as the cognitive and affective components may not necessarily be manifested behaviourally, so discrimination does not necessarily imply the presence of cognitive and affective components. People may discriminate if the prevailing social norms dictate that they do so and if their wish to become or remain a member of the discriminating group is stronger than their wish to be fair and egalitarian. According to Fiske (2004), the affective component is crucial. This is illustrated by the findings that individual differences in emotional prejudice correlate with discrimination better than stereotypes do (Dovidio et al., 1996), and affective reactions to gay men predict discrimination far better than stereotypes do (Talaska et al., 2003).

Although the relationship between prejudice and discrimination is moderate, it is comparable to the general attitude–behaviour relationship (Fiske, 2004; see also Chapter 6).

Mrs M's disparaging remarks border on antilocution, and her not wanting to talk to me a kind of avoidance; I perceived both as revealing an underlying prejudice.

Stereotypes and stereotyping

Stereotypes can be thought of as a special kind of *implicit personality theory*, that is, ready-made beliefs about how individuals' characteristics 'belong together'; what makes them special is that they relate to an entire social group. The term 'stereotype' was introduced into social science by Lippmann (1922), who defined stereotypes as 'pictures in our heads'. Other definitions include the following:

> ... the process of ascribing characteristics to people on the basis of their group memberships .... (Oakes et al., 1994)

> ... widely shared assumptions about the personalities, attitudes and behaviour of people based on group membership, for example ethnicity, nationality, sex, race and class .... (Hogg and Vaughan, 1995)

Nurses constitute another 'group membership'.

Traditional view of stereotypes: Are they inherently bad?

For most of the time that psychologists have been studying stereotypes and stereotyping, they have condemned them for being both false and illogical, and dangerous, and people who use them have been seen as prejudiced and even pathological.

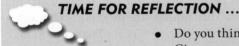

TIME FOR REFLECTION ...

- Do you think that stereotypes/stereotyping are inherently bad/wrong?
- Give reasons for your answer.

One of the earliest studies of ethnic/racial stereotyping was Katz and Braly's (1933) study of undergraduates at Princeton University in the United States. It was intended to trace the link between stereotypes and prejudice: stereotypes are public fictions arising from prejudicial influences 'with scarcely any factual basis'. So, should they be dismissed as completely unacceptable?

According to Allport (1954), most stereotypes do contain a 'kernel of truth'. This can be understood in terms of McCauley and Stitt's (1978) claim that what 'typical' seems to mean is *characteristic* – that is, true of a higher percentage of the group in question than of people in general. Stereotypes, then, seem to be *schemas* about what particular groups are like relative to 'people in general'. They *are not* exceptionless generalisations.

Sherif (1966) also argued that stereotypes are not in themselves deficient, but serve to reflect the reality of intergroup relations. Instead of asking if they are objectively true or accurate, stereotypes need to be understood in this *intergroup* context. To this extent, they are highly flexible, since changes in the relationship with other groups will result in changes to the stereotyped images of those groups. However, according to Operario and Fiske (2004), it is precisely this broader context of stereotypes, reflected in social hierarchy and history, that defines their truly insidious nature.

So it is the image of the stereotype that alters, reflecting social changes, rather than the cognitive process of stereotyping. After more than fifty years in a multiracial society, we might expect acceptance of the idea of multiracial medical and nursing staff.

Stereotyping as a normal cognitive process

If stereotypes are 'categories about people' (Allport, 1954; Brislin, 1981), and categories in general – and stereotypes in particular – are shortcuts to thinking, then from a purely cognitive point of view, there is nothing unique about stereotypes. According to Brislin (1993), stereotypes 'reflect people's need to organise, remember, and retrieve information that might be useful to them as they attempt to achieve their goals and to meet life's demands …'.

Lippmann (1922) also argued that stereotypes serve a crucial *practical* function:

> … the real environment is altogether too big, too complex, and too fleeting for direct acquaintance. We are not equipped to deal with so much subtlety, so much variety, so many permutations and combinations. And although we have to act in that environment, we have to reconstruct it on a simpler model before we can manage it.

According to the *cognitive miser* perspective (Fiske and Taylor, 1991), stereotypes are resource-saving devices. They simplify the processing of information about other people. As Fiske (2004) says, '… under the busy conditions of ordinary interaction, people can save cognitive resources by using stereotype-consistent information …'.

'Big, complex and fleeting' describes many caring situations, so it's tempting to justify stereotyping as a time-saving cognitive process. However, as health professionals, we are committed to treating people **not** as stereotypes, but individuals.

Stereotypes, expectations and behaviour

Our expectations of people's personalities or capabilities may influence the way we actually treat them, which in turn may influence their behaviour in such a way that confirms our expectation (the *self-fulfilling prophecy*). This illustrates how stereotypes can (unwittingly) influence our behaviour towards others, and not just our perception and memory of them.

📃 I don't know how Rasheed felt about Mrs Maitland's behaviour but my initial reaction was not to care about her – or for her.

Stereotypes and nurses' behaviour

In a small, ethnographic study of midwives' stereotypes of Asian women, Bowler (1993) suggested that these relate to four main themes: communication problems, failure to comply with care, making a fuss about nothing and a lack of normal (Western) maternal instinct. Bowler points to several instances where care was less than optimal, because the midwives relied on their stereotypes. After observing the deliveries of six Asian women, she noted that only one was offered pain relief. The midwives may have found it too difficult to explain pain relief options to women who spoke little English, or perhaps they thought that the women did not need (or deserve) pain control because of their known 'low pain thresholds' (Bowler 1993; see also Chapter 3 and Key Study 7.1).

So, it would seem that it is not stereotypes themselves that are dangerous or objectionable, but how they affect behaviour. According to Operario and Fiske (2004), '… stereotypes are both (a) basic human tendencies inherent within our mental architecture; and (b) potentially damaging belief systems, depending on the power of the situation …'.

📃 This is disturbing, but I'm learning how such things happen and communication problems are again a factor. Apart from showing how dangerous stereotypical assumptions are, it shows how accurate assessment of patients' needs must take account of culture.

KEY STUDY 7.1

Gender and ethnic stereotyping and analgesic administration

- An American study by McDonald aimed to discover whether nurses provide greater amounts of narcotic analgesics (1) to men than to women and (2) to white patients than to those from minority ethnic communities.
- The sample consisted of 180 patients (79 women, 101 men), aged 18–64, all with non-perforated appendicitis with subsequent uncomplicated appendectomy. None had a criminal or drug addiction history.
- The ethnic composition was 2% Asian, 12% African American, 8% Hispanic, and 78% white.
- Males received significantly more analgesics than females for the initial post-operative dose. This suggests that, if stereotyping occurs, it may not be extensive or prolonged.
- However, members of ethnic majorities received significantly more than members of minority groups for the total post-operative dose. McDonald finds this latter finding more difficult to explain.
- In addition to nurses' stereotypes, minority patients may have been less likely to express their pain, more reluctant to receive analgesics, or their complaints may have been given less credibility.

Source: McDonald, D.D., *Research in Nursing and Health, 17*(1), 45–49, 1994.

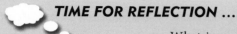

TIME FOR REFLECTION ...

- What images of 'the nurse' do you think are held by members of the general public (as portrayed in the media, for example)?
- What effect are these stereotypes likely to have on patients' impressions of nurses?
- How might they be challenged/overcome?

For most, nurses are female (see Critical Discussion 7.1), self-sacrificing angels, handmaidens ('the good woman serving the doctor'), battleaxes or sex kittens (O'Dowd, 1998).

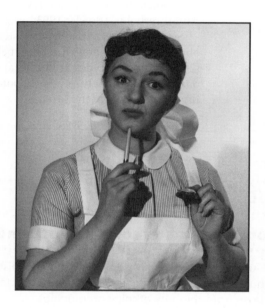

Two elderly women, waiting for angiograms, have said to me that they don't want the male Staff Nurse ('that man') looking after them. Yet they're quite happy for male doctors to examine them! And most male patients seem quite happy to be cared for by female nurses.

TIME FOR REFLECTION ...

- How do you feel about men becoming midwives?
- Is this an 'inappropriate' area of nursing for men?
- Are there any other 'inappropriate' areas?
- Should patients have the right to choose the gender of the nurses who care for them?

CRITICAL DISCUSSION 7.1

Nursing: a suitable profession for a man?

- A typical candidate is in his early 20s and no one in his immediate family has a medical background. He would not have thought about becoming a nurse in school and will probably have been in a totally unrelated job since 16 or 18. He will have stumbled on nursing after a couple of unfulfilling years career-wise. Despite the misgivings of friends and family, he then decides it is the career for him (Mason, 1991).
- While wanting to care for people is the prime reason given by men for entering nursing (as it is for females), in psychiatric nursing, the need for physical strength to restrain patients has led to male/female ratios closer to 50:50 (Mason, 1991).
- The perceived link between male nursing and homosexuality rests on the belief that gay men are more caring than straight men. But this assumption commands little support, even among gays. And although most acknowledge that a male nurse has to be able to work well with women, there is no evidence that gay men are any better in this respect than other men (Mason, 1991).
- The subject of young female mental health patients falling in love with male nurses has always been a sensitive, but often unacknowledged, issue (Holyoake, 1998). While cases of male psychiatric nurses abusing female patients are dealt with stringently by the UKCC (1992), there are also cases of women patients making overt moves towards male nurses, who may feel embarrassed or compromised (Stanley, 1998).

Definitions of prejudice

Most definitions of prejudice stress the hostile, negative kind of prejudice (it can also be positive), as does the research that tries to identify how prejudice arises and how it might be reduced.

The definitions in Table 7.1 locate prejudice squarely *within the individual* – it is an attitude that represents one aspect of social cognition. However, Vivian and Brown (1995) prefer to see prejudice as a special case of *intergroup conflict*, which occurs when 'people think or behave antagonistically towards another group or its members in terms of their group membership and seem motivated by concerns relating to those groups'.

Mrs M's wanting others to care for her showed positive prejudice towards white staff. It was also a form of avoidance of Rasheed and me – and discriminatory.

Defining prejudice in terms of intergroup conflict 'lifts' it to the social plane. Consistent with this is Fernando's (1991) distinction between 'racial prejudice' and 'racism': the former denotes an attitude possessed by an individual, while

Table 7.1 Some definitions of prejudice and discrimination

'… an antipathy based on faulty and inflexible generalisation directed towards a group as a whole or towards an individual because he is a member of that group. It may be felt or expressed' (Allport, 1954)

'Prejudice is an attitude (usually negative) toward the members of some group, based solely on their membership in that group …' (Baron and Byrne, 1991)

'Prejudice is a learned attitude towards a target object that typically involves negative affect, dislike or fear, a set of negative beliefs that support the attitude and a behavioural intention to avoid, or to control or dominate, those in the target group … Stereotypes are prejudiced beliefs … when prejudice is acted out, when it becomes overt in various forms of behaviour, then discrimination is in practice …' (Zimbardo and Leippe, 1991)

the latter refers to a political and economic ideology, which is a characteristic of society. Strictly, then, it is societies (or institutions, such as the police or the armed forces) that are racist and individuals who are racially prejudiced.

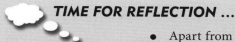 Mrs M's attitude suggested she was racially prejudiced towards Rasheed and me. When I discussed it with Maggie, my mentor, she said we can't control patients' attitudes, but the NHS couldn't allow discrimination; if it did, it would be a racist institution. She asked me if I wanted to report it and I said no. After all, it wasn't unusual, I couldn't prove it and I didn't want to make a fuss.

TIME FOR REFLECTION …

- Apart from racism, what other 'isms' are there that meet these criteria for being social, rather than individual, phenomena?

Until quite recently, most of the theory and research into prejudice and discrimination was concerned with racism, 'the quite specific belief that cultural differences between ethnic groups are of biological origin and that groups should be ranked in worth' (Littlewood and Lipsedge, 1989). However, gender (as in *sexism* – see Gross, 2010), sexual orientation or preference (as in *heterosexism* – see discussion on pages 155 and 156 and Figure 7.1) and age (as in *ageism* – see Chapter 19) can all be targets for hostility and discrimination. Other examples include *sizeism* (hostility and discrimination against people who are obese – and '*HIV/AIDS-ism*' (independently of the perceived link with homosexuality).

My first reaction to Mrs M was hostility. I must confess that as I walked away I thought 'if you weren't so careless at controlling your diet and so overweight, you probably wouldn't be here!' When I'd calmed down I was ashamed I'd allowed her to trigger an aggressive attitude in me; I do know better. What's more – it revealed my 'sizeist' prejudice, didn't it?

Figure 7.1 Sexual orientation is a target for hostility and discrimination in a heterosexist society.

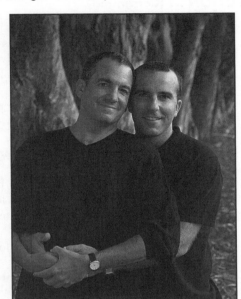

TIME FOR REFLECTION ...

- Are you a racist?
- While most people would automatically say 'no', the question is not as simple as it seems. Racism can stem from ignorance, both of what it is and what can be done to combat it.
- A questionnaire (Nursing Times, 1990) aimed to help nurses explore how much they really know about racial discrimination in the workplace.
- The Race Relations Act 1976 outlawed discrimination in the workplace against anyone on racial grounds. But what do you understand by the term 'racial grounds'? Does it refer to (1) colour, (2) nationality, (3) ethnic or national origin and (4) race?
- Direct discrimination in the workplace occurs when a person treats another person less favourably on racial grounds. Which of the following scenarios do you think are examples of direct discrimination?
  - a. Hospital management decides not to promote a nurse because 'the consultant won't work with an Asian ward sister'.
  - b. An inner-city mental health team advertises for an Afro-Caribbean Registered Mental Nurse (RMN) to work with the Afro-Caribbean clients.
  - c. A Turkish applicant for a staff nurse post is rejected because the previous year there was a Turkish nurse in the ward who was constantly taking time off work because of her children.
  - d. A Nigerian auxiliary (health care assistant [HCA]) is dismissed for theft of hospital property.

(Continued)

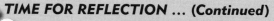

TIME FOR REFLECTION ... (Continued)

- Indirect discrimination is more insidious. It refers to the way in which health authority policies on such issues as recruitment and advertising for promotion discriminate, possibly inadvertently, against people from different racial groups. Which of the following might constitute examples of indirect discrimination?

    a. Refusing to employ a Pakistani nurse who, because of her Muslim beliefs, will not wear a nurse's uniform – although she offers to wear matching trousers and top.

    b. A job advertisement that requires that English must be the applicant's mother tongue.

    c. An applicant for an auxiliary (HCA) post is turned down on the grounds that she has been unemployed for over 2 years. The management argues that it would be difficult to obtain references in such a case.

    d. A young Kenyan girl is refused entry for Registered Nurse training because she does not have five GCSEs.

    - Racial grounds' includes all of these (Commission for Racial Equality [CRE], 1983).

    - Both (a) and (c) constitute direct discrimination (CRE, 1989).

    - Both (b) and (c) constitute indirect discrimination (CRE, 1985, 1989). Neither (a) nor (d) is clear-cut (see Nursing Times, 1990).

Prejudice and discrimination in health care

Institutionalised racism within the NHS

If this truly exists, then both nurses themselves and patients can become victims. According to Kroll (1990),

> ... The NHS was created with the philosophy of providing care for all, irrespective of race, colour or creed. It is assumed that NHS staff are free from prejudice and knowledgeable about the needs of a multiracial society. However, most experts believe that racism is embedded in the organisational culture of the NHS, which is run predominantly by white, middle-class professionals.

Black and minority ethnic nurses account for about 20% of the U.K. nursing profession, but new figures indicate that they experience disturbing levels of bullying and racism. A survey of 9000 Royal College of Nursing (RCN) members working in the NHS and the independent sector revealed that 45% of African-Caribbean nurses had been bullied or harassed in the previous year

(RCN, 2005). Of these, 61% said the bullying was racially motivated and 43% that it was linked to their nationality. This contrasted with just 21% of the white British and 24% of the Asian nurses who responded. Perhaps most disturbing of all is the finding that 30% of the bullying came from other nursing colleagues and 45% from supervisors or senior managers.

The CRE is keen to dispel the myth that racism is just about colour prejudice. Snell (1997) describes claims of discrimination against Irish nurses, who make up the largest group in Europe applying to go on the UKCC register.

This is acknowledged by The NHS Direct Dignity at Work Policy (Bullying and Harassment) 24 April 2012. It states that the Human Rights Act 1988 came into force in October 2000 and covers all infringements of human rights regardless of gender, disability, ethnic identity, sexuality or class. It includes – 'the right to freedom from unfair discrimination (including religious discrimination) in the enjoyment of these rights'. (www.nhsdirect.nhs.uk/.../OurPoliciesAndProcedures/.../...)

According to Kroll (1990), racism is endemic in midwifery. She identifies four major features of antenatal clinics that may make them seem alienating, racially prejudiced places to women from non-white ethnic groups:

- The language barrier.
- Lack of awareness by ethnic minorities of the availability of certain services (e.g. most African-Caribbean women still know very little about sickle cell anaemia).
- Midwives know very little about the spiritual beliefs and customs of the different cultural groups within their health authorities.
- Midwives rarely consult the groups and advisory centres that exist in the various ethnic communities.

For instance, on a post-natal ward, Asian Muslim women couldn't eat the food provided because of their strict dietary laws and their families weren't allowed to bring them in cooked food, while other women had take-away burgers and chips brought in for them. This discrimination wasn't noticed, or was perhaps overlooked, until a Muslim midwife pointed out the inconsistency (Schott and Henley, 1999).

Anti-gay and lesbian prejudice and discrimination

According to Rose and Platzer (1993), the attitudes of many nurses are grounded in their assumptions about people's heterosexual nature and their lack of knowledge about different lifestyles and how these affect people's health. Ignorance about how lesbians and gay men live can lead nurses to ask inappropriate questions during assessments, resulting in mistaken judgements.

For example, one lesbian patient who was receiving a cervical smear test was asked if she was sexually active. After saying she was, she was asked what contraceptive she used and replied 'none'. She was then asked if she was trying to become pregnant, which she was not. She had to disclose her lesbianism to ensure that health professionals did not make incorrect assumptions about her, which could have led to an incorrect diagnosis.

James et al. (1994) cite several studies showing that many nurses and doctors are homophobic. The research also indicates that lesbians and gay men fear homophobia from health care providers, are anxious about the consequences of revealing their sexual orientation and breaches of confidentiality and are concerned about facing hostility and even physical harm.

According to the UKCC Code of Professional Conduct (1992), nurses are required to respect patients or clients *unconditionally*. Homophobia is clearly a breach of this obligation. In describing the results of a survey of lesbian nurses, Rose (1993) states that nurses must also demonstrate this respect for each other. Nurses may believe that homosexuality is wrong, but when faced with working with openly gay colleagues, they may experience cognitive dissonance (see also Chapter 6).

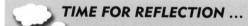 Admitting a patient, I asked a woman who her next of kin was; she said 'my partner' and gave another woman's name. I put it down but felt flustered as I was surprised, which probably showed. I didn't like to ask if she was married (a civil marriage would have made it legal) so I asked for another next of kin. Did this indicate cognitive dissonance – that I thought I accepted homosexuality but my behaviour indicated I wasn't comfortable with it?

TIME FOR REFLECTION ...

- How might a homophobic nurse deal with such cognitive dissonance?

Institutionalised prejudice and discrimination

The preceding discussion illustrates that a great deal of prejudice and discrimination is unconscious, reflected in basic, stereotyped assumptions that we make about others. These assumptions influence our behaviour towards them, which may not necessarily be overtly hostile or 'anti'. It is this pervasive form of prejudice and discrimination that is perhaps the most difficult to break down, because we are unaware of it and because it reflects institutionalised heterosexism, racism and so on.

Both Cochrane (1983) and Littlewood and Lipsedge (1989) show how ethnic minorities in England are more often hospitalised for mental illness than non-black English people. This is interpreted as reflecting an implicit, unwitting prejudice against minority groups that pervades the NHS as an institution. This definition of 'institutionalised racism' as 'unwitting' was included in the government report (1999) on the behaviour of the police in their investigation of the murder of the black London teenager, Stephen Lawrence (in Horton, 1999) (see Figure 7.2).

Underlying racism is the deep-seated and widely held belief that people resembling each other in obvious physical ways (such as skin colour and hair texture) belong to a 'race' that represents a genetically distinct human type. It is now widely accepted that 'race' has no scientific meaning. For example, Wetherell (1996) argues that 'race' is a *social* as opposed to a natural (biological) phenomenon.

Figure 7.2 Stephen Lawrence. (1974–1993)

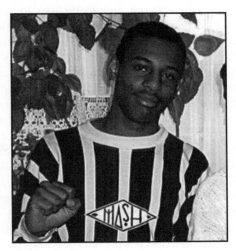

Doesn't reliance on classification, whether social or biological, threaten our perception of people as individuals? The first component of the Roper-Logan-Tierney model of nursing is 'activities of living'. Included in this is a socio-cultural factor, which influences the way individual patients perform those activities. So consideration of ethnic differences should be ensured in our nursing assessment (Roper et al., 1996, in Alexander et al., 2006).

Theories of prejudice and discrimination

Attempts to explain prejudice and discrimination fall into three broad categories:

1. Those that see prejudice as stemming from *personality variables* and other aspects of the psychological make-up of individuals
2. Those that emphasise the role of *environmental factors* (sometimes called the *conflict approach*)
3. Those that focus on the effects of the mere fact of *group membership*

Each approach may be important to a complete understanding of the causes of intergroup conflict and prejudice and to their reduction (Vivian and Brown, 1995).

Prejudice and personality

Authoritarian personality

Adorno et al. (1950) proposed the concept of the *authoritarian personality* (in a book of the same name), someone who is prejudiced by virtue of specific personality traits that predispose them to be hostile towards ethnic, racial and other minority or out-groups.

Adorno et al. began by studying anti-Semitism (AS) in Nazi Germany in the 1940s and drew on Freud's theories to help understand the relationship between 'collective ideologies' (such as fascism) and individual personality (Brown, 1985). After their emigration to the United States, studies began with college students and other native-born, white, non-Jewish, middle-class Americans (including school teachers, nurses, prison inmates and psychiatric patients). These involved interviews concerning their political views and childhood experiences and the use of *projective tests* designed to reveal unconscious attitudes towards minority groups. In the course of their research, Adorno et al. constructed a number of scales: *AS scale, (Ethnocentrism (E) scale* (which measures the belief in the superiority of one's own ethnic group); *Political and Economic Conservatism (PEC) scale*; and *Potentiality for Fascism (F) scale* (intended to measure *implicit* authoritarian and anti-democratic trends in personality, making someone with such a personality susceptible to explicit fascist propaganda).

Adorno et al. concluded from the correlations between scores on the different scales that people who are anti-Semitic are also likely to be hostile towards 'Negroes', 'Japs' and any other minority group or 'foreigner' (all *out-groups*): the authoritarian personality is prejudiced in a very *generalised* way.

Typically, authoritarians are hostile to people of inferior status, servile to those of higher status and contemptuous of weakness. They are also rigid and inflexible, intolerant of ambiguity and uncertainty, unwilling to introspect feelings and upholders of conventional values and ways of life (such as religion). This belief in convention and intolerance of ambiguity combine to make minorities 'them' and the authoritarian's membership group 'us'; 'they' are by definition 'bad' and 'we' are by definition 'good'.

Evaluation of the authoritarian personality theory

- While some evidence is broadly consistent with the theory, there are a number of serious methodological and other problems that make it untenable. For example, if prejudice is to be explained in terms of individual differences, how can it then be manifested in a whole population, or at least a vast majority of that population (Brown, 1988)? In pre-war Nazi Germany, for example (and in many other places since), consistent racist attitudes and behaviour were shown by hundreds of thousands of people, who must have differed on most other psychological characteristics.

- It is assumed that authoritarianism is a characteristic of the *political right*, implying that there is no equivalent authoritarianism on the left. According to Rokeach (1960), 'ideological dogmatism' refers to a relatively rigid outlook on life and intolerance of those with opposing beliefs. High scores on the *dogmatism scale* reveal (1) closedness of mind, (2) lack of flexibility and (3) authoritarianism, regardless of particular social and political ideology. Dogmatism is a way of *thinking*, rather than a set of beliefs (Brown, 1965).

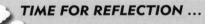 Mrs M is conventional, wanted to be addressed formally, seemed intolerant of both Rasheed and me and see us as 'them' (i.e. black). She wanted the white doctor – an assumption that black doctors aren't as able as white doctors? I don't know if she's authoritarian; her notes show that, until a year ago, she lived in a small Somerset village and so may be very uncertain and apprehensive in a multiracial city hospital. Her behaviour may be an instinctive, 'prejudged' response to seeing people who were 'different'.

Scapegoating: The frustration–aggression hypothesis

According to Dollard et al.'s (1939) *frustration–aggression hypothesis*, frustration always gives rise to aggression and aggression is always caused by frustration (see Gross, 2010). The source of frustration (whatever prevents us from achieving our goals) might often be seen as a fairly powerful threat (such as parents or employers) or may be difficult to identify. Drawing on Freudian theory, Dollard et al. claim that when we need to vent our frustration but are unable to do this directly, we do so *indirectly* by displacing it onto a substitute target (we find a *scapegoat*) (see Figure 7.3).

TIME FOR REFLECTION …

● Can you see any connections between the frustration–aggression hypothesis and certain parts of Adorno et al.'s theory?

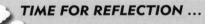 I recognise my aggressive feeling came from having my goal of wanting to care for Mrs M frustrated – by her! As yet I haven't been tempted to find a scapegoat, but I recognise scapegoating as one of Freud's defence mechanisms (see Chapter 2).

The choice of scapegoat is not usually random. In England during the 1930s and 1940s, it was predominantly the Jews, who were replaced by West Indians

Figure 7.3 According to the frustration–aggression hypothesis, discrimination against outsiders (in this case eastern European asylum seekers) is a form of displaced aggression.

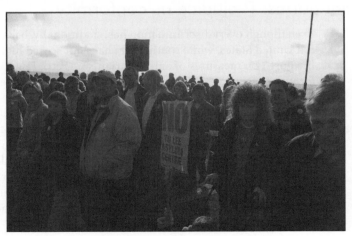

during the 1950s and 1960s and during the 1970s, 1980s and 1990s by Asians from Pakistan. In the southern United States, lynchings of blacks from 1880 to 1930 were related to the price of cotton: as the price dropped, so the number of lynchings increased (Hovland and Sears, 1940). While this is consistent with the concept of displaced aggression, the fact that whites chose blacks as scapegoats rather than some other minority group suggests that there are usually socially approved (legitimised) targets for frustration-induced aggression.

Limitations of the personality approach

- Several researchers (e.g. Billig, 1976; Brown, 1988; Hogg and Abrams, 1988) have argued that any account of prejudice and discrimination in terms of individuals (*intrapersonal behaviour*) is *reductionist*. In other words, the *social* nature of prejudice and discrimination requires a *social* explanation (in terms of *intergroup behaviour*).
- Adorno et al. (1950) imply that racism is the product of the abnormal personality of a small minority of human beings, rather than a social and political ideology. This distinction is of great practical as well as theoretical importance, because what is considered to be the cause of prejudice has very real implications for its reduction. Indeed, Adorno et al. (1950) recognised that *society* provides the content of attitudes and prejudice and defines the out-groups.
- According to Brown (1985), 'cultural or societal norms may be much more important than personality in accounting for ethnocentrism, out-group rejection, prejudice and discrimination'.

 This explains why getting rid of an authoritarian leader (as in Iraq) hasn't stopped intergroup conflict.

Role of environmental factors

Impact of social norms: Prejudice as conformity

Even though overt discrimination has, traditionally, been greater in the southern United States, white southerners have not scored higher than whites from the north on measures of authoritarianism (Pettigrew, 1959). So, clearly, *conformity to social norms* can prove more powerful as a determinant of behaviour than personality factors.

Pettigrew (1971) also found that Americans in the south are no more anti-Semitic or hostile towards other minority groups than those from the north (as the authoritarian personality explanation would require). In other words, prejudice *is not* the generalised attitude that Adorno et al. claimed. According to Reich and Adcock (1976), the need to conform and not be seen as different may cause milder prejudices. But active discrimination against, and ill-treatment of, minorities reflects a prejudice that already exists and that is maintained and legitimised by conformity.

So if the NHS is a racist institution, it reflects wider social norms that are accepted as legitimate, in which case it's a very good reason we are encouraged to challenge practice. This makes me feel guilty. Should I change my mind and challenge Mrs M's behaviour after all?

Realistic group conflict theory

According to Sherif's (1966) *realistic group conflict theory* (RGCT), intergroup conflict arises as a result of a conflict of interests. When two groups want to achieve the same goal but cannot both have it, hostility is produced between them. Indeed, Sherif claims that conflict of interest (or competition) is a *sufficient* condition for the occurrence of hostility or conflict. He bases this claim on the 'Robber's Cave' experiment, which Brown (1986) describes as the most successful field experiment ever conducted on intergroup conflict (see Gross, 2010).

This experiment was about the hostility that developed between two groups of boys at a summer camp, who were 'set up' by experimenters to compete for prizes (which supports the 'competing for scarce resources' concept). It helps explain remarks like 'they come over here and take our jobs' – the reason given for prejudice against 'foreign' workers in the NHS and elsewhere.

An evaluation of RGCT

- According to Fiske (2004), RGCT is the most obvious explanation for prejudice and discrimination, but it has received only limited and inconsistent support, and the *perceived, symbolic threat* posed by out-groups matters more than any real or tangible threat. For this reason, the 'realistic' may as well be dropped from its name and the theory renamed 'perceived group conflict theory'.
- Perceived conflict *does* predict negative attitudes towards out-groups (Brown et al., 2001; Hennessy and West, 1999), and conflict matters only when people identify with their in-groups. More importantly, in-group identification *by itself* can account for intergroup hostility, even in the absence of competition (Brewer and Brown, 1998). Intangible outcomes (such as group recognition, status and prestige) produce conflict far more often than do tangible resources. Even when the conflict appears to involve resources, often the real pay-off is pride in one's own identification with a group capable of winning them. This is related to *social identity theory* (SIT) (see discussion, pages 162 and 163).
- It seems, then, that 'competition' may not be a sufficient condition for intergroup conflict and hostility after all. If we accept this conclusion, the question arises, 'can hostility arise in the *absence* of conflicting interests?'

It doesn't explain prejudice against black people in general, or homosexuals, or religious groups. White racists believe they are superior to black people, in any circumstances. However, prejudice exists also between Asian and African-Caribbean people, and what about the professional rivalry between health professionals – traditionally doctors and nurses?

Influence of group membership

Minimal groups

According to Tajfel et al. (1971), the *mere perception* of another group's existence can produce discrimination. When people are arbitrarily and randomly divided into two groups, knowledge of the other group's existence is a sufficient condition for the development of pro-in-group and anti-out-group attitudes. These artificial groups are known as *minimal groups*.

Before any discrimination can occur, people must be categorised as members of an in-group or an out-group (making categorisation a *necessary* condition). More significantly, the very act of categorisation produces conflict and discrimination (making it also a *sufficient* condition).

An evaluation of minimal group experiments

- In more than two dozen independent studies in several countries, using a wide range of experimental participants of both genders (from young children to adults), essentially the same result has been found: the mere act of allocating people into arbitrary social categories is sufficient to elicit biased judgements and discriminatory behaviours (Brown, 1988).
- Wetherell (1982) maintains that intergroup conflict *is not* inevitable. She studied white and Polynesian children in New Zealand and found the latter to be much more generous towards the out-group, reflecting cultural norms that emphasised cooperation.
- The minimal group paradigm has been criticised on several methodological and theoretical grounds, especially its artificiality and *meaninglessness* (e.g. Schiffman and Wicklund, 1992). But Tajfel (1972) argues that it is precisely the need to find meaning in an 'otherwise empty situation' (especially for the *self*) that leads participants to act in terms of the minimal categories.

Social identity theory

Tajfel (1978) and Tajfel and Turner (1986) explain the minimal group effect in terms of *SIT*. According to SIT, an individual strives to achieve or maintain a positive self-image. This has two components: *personal identity* (the personal characteristics and attributes that make each person unique) and *social identity* (a sense of who we are, derived from the groups we belong to).

In fact, each of us has several social identities, corresponding to the different groups with which we identify. In each case, the more positive the image of the group, the more positive will be our own social identity, and hence our self-image. By emphasising the desirability of the in-group(s) and focusing on those distinctions that enable our own group to come out on top, we help to create for ourselves a satisfactory social identity. This can be seen as lying at the heart of prejudice.

Some individuals may be more prone to prejudice because they have an intense need for acceptance by others and feelings of personal inadequacy. Their personal and social identities may be much more interconnected than for those with a lesser need for social acceptance.

Does Tajfel's (1972) argument (above) help explain the rapid growth of gang culture: are the members looking for meaning, acceptance – and identity – in their 'empty lives'?

Evaluation of SIT

- While there is considerable empirical support for the theory, much of this comes from minimal group experiments. Not only have they been criticised, but SIT was originally proposed to explain the findings from those experiments. So, there is a *circularity* involved, making it necessary to test SIT's predictions in other ways.

- Stemming from Allport's (1954) claims that stereotypes are 'categories about people' and that 'the human mind must think with the aid of categories' (see discussion in pages 146 and 147), Tajfel (1969) (Tajfel et al., 1971) saw the process of *categorisation* as a basic characteristic of human thought. SIT implies that intergroup hostility is natural and built into our thought processes as a consequence of categorisation. Although there is abundant evidence of intergroup discrimination, this appears to stem from raising the evaluation of the in-group, rather than denigrating the out-group (Vivian and Brown, 1995). Indeed, SIT suggests that prejudice consists largely of liking 'us' more than disliking 'them': favouring the in-group is the core phenomenon, *not* out-group hostility (Brewer, 1999; Hewstone et al., 2002). However, one form that in-group favouritism can take is 'modern' or *symbolic* racism (see Box 7.1).

Using cognitive 'shortcuts' such as stereotyping doesn't justify denigrating other groups, does it? Taking pride in being a nurse doesn't mean devaluing other health professionals; we work as a team.

Box 7.1 Modern (or symbolic) racism and subtle prejudice

- According to Fiske (2004), most estimates put 70%–80% of whites as relatively high on *modern/subtle* forms of racism; these are 'cool' and indirect, automatic, unconscious, unintentional, ambiguous and ambivalent. This is in sharp contrast with the crude and blatant racist abuse associated with Allport's 'antilocution' (page 146).

- Subtle prejudice is not a uniquely American, white-on-black phenomenon (Pettigrew, 1998; Pettigrew and Meertens, 1995). In Europe, there are French/North Africans, British/South Asians and Germans/Turks.

- Symptomatic of this form of racism (or perhaps a variety of it) is the belief that 'one is not a racist' while simultaneously engaging in racist talk. A recent, much-publicised example (2011) is the case of the ex–England football captain, John Terry, and Anton Ferdinand. In another example, Pat Bottrill (MBE) resigned (in 2002) from her job as chair for the RCN's governing council after making a remark perceived as racist. She said,

   Although I did not intend any offence, I am stepping down as a sign of my own and the RCN's commitment to tackling any form of racism… the RCN has stated that it will not tolerate racism – even if it is unintentional.

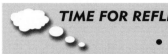 Mrs M would probably deny being racist too.

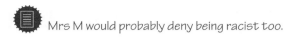

TIME FOR REFLECTION ...

- What do the major theories we have discussed imply about how prejudice and discrimination could be reduced – or prevented?

Reducing prejudice and discrimination

- The *authoritarian personality theory* implies that, by changing the personality structure of the prejudiced individual, the need for an ego-defensive 'prop' such as prejudice is removed. By its nature, this is practically very difficult to achieve, even if it is theoretically possible.
- According to the *frustration–aggression hypothesis*, preventing frustration or providing people with ways to vent their frustration in less antisocial ways than discrimination are possible solutions. However, this would involve putting the historical clock back or changing social conditions in quite fundamental ways.
- RGCT makes it very clear that removing competition and replacing it with superordinate goals and cooperation will remove or prevent hostility (this is discussed further in pages 166 and 167).
- SIT implies that if intergroup stereotypes can become less negative and automatic, and if boundaries between groups can be made more blurred or more flexible, then group memberships may become a less central part of the self-concept, making positive evaluation of the in-group less inevitable.

We're unlikely to change Mrs M's (authoritarian?) personality, but by coming into this hospital a degree of social change has been imposed on her, however briefly.

Contact hypothesis

Probably the first formal proposal of a set of social-psychological principles for reducing prejudice was Allport's (1954) *contact hypothesis* (CH) (as it has come to be called), according to which

> Prejudice (unless deeply rooted in the character structure of the individual) may be reduced by equal status contact between majority and minority groups in the pursuit of common goals. The effect is greatly enhanced if this contact is sanctioned by institutional supports (i.e. by law, custom or local atmosphere) and

provided it is of a sort that leads to the perception of common interests and common humanity between members of the two groups.

Most programmes aimed at promoting harmonious relations between groups that were previously in conflict have operated according to Allport's 'principles', in particular, *equal status contact* and the pursuit of *common (superordinate) goals*.

Boundaries are more blurred between doctors and nurses than in the past which encourages teamwork towards the superordinate goal of good health care, and the more equal status of nursing has been instrumental in achieving it.

Equal status contact

When people are segregated, they are likely to experience *autistic hostility* – that is, ignorance of others, which results in a failure to understand the reasons for their actions. Lack of contact means there is no 'reality testing' against which to check our own interpretations of others' behaviour, and this in turn is likely to reinforce negative stereotypes. By the same token, ignorance of what 'makes them tick' will probably make 'them' seem more dissimilar from ourselves than they really are. Bringing people into contact with each other should make them seem more familiar, and at least offers the possibility that this negative cycle can be interrupted, and even reversed.

Related to autistic hostility is the *mirror-image phenomenon* (Bronfenbrenner, 1960), whereby enemies come to see themselves as being in the right (with 'God on our side') and the other side as in the wrong. Both sides tend to attribute to each other the same negative characteristics (the 'assumed dissimilarity of beliefs'). Increased contact provides the opportunity to disconfirm our stereotypes. The out-group loses its strangeness, and group members are more likely to be seen as unique individuals, rather than an 'undifferentiated mass' (see Figure 7.2). This represents a reduction in the *illusion of out-group homogeneity* ('they all look the same').

Mrs M has had to face the reality of Rasheed as her doctor. If he (or I) can gain her confidence, it may begin to challenge her attitude to all black people.

How effective is equal status contact?

It is generally agreed that increased contact *alone* will not reduce prejudice. Despite evidence that we prefer people who are familiar, if this contact is between people who are consistently of *unequal status*, then 'familiarity may breed contempt'. Aronson (1980) points out that many whites (in the United States) have always had a great deal of contact with blacks – as dishwashers, toilet attendants, domestic servants and so on. Such contacts may simply reinforce the stereotypes held by whites of blacks as being inferior. Similarly, Amir

Figure 7.4 Summary of how the negative cycle of lack of contact/segregation between racial/ethnic groups and reinforcement of negative stereotypes can be broken by direct contact (as advocated by Allport's contact hypothesis).

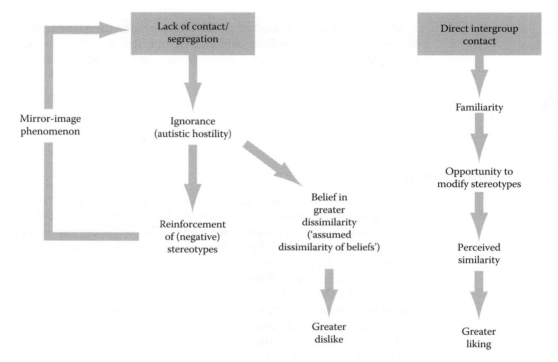

(1994) argues that we need to ask, 'Under what conditions does intergroup contact have an impact, for whom, and regarding what outcomes?'

A case in point are the findings of Stouffer et al. (1949) and Amir (1969) that interracial attitudes improved markedly when blacks and whites served together as soldiers in battle and on ships, but relationships were not so good at the base camp.

Mrs M will see many black people in lower-status jobs in the hospital which could confirm her opinions. However, she will also be cared for, inevitably, by many Asian and African-Caribbean trained nurses and doctors.

Pursuit of common (superordinate) goals

In a *cooperative* situation, the attainment of one person's goal enhances the chances of attainment of the goals of other group members; this is the reverse of a competitive situation (Brown, 1986).

One influential attempt to realise both mutual cooperation and equal status contact is Aronson et al.'s (1978) *jigsaw method*. This is a highly structured method of interdependent learning, in which children are assigned to six-person, interracial learning groups. According to Aronson (1992, 2000), the jigsaw method consistently enhances students' self-esteem, improves academic performance, increases liking for classmates and improves some interracial perceptions, compared with children in traditional classrooms.

However, although the children of different racial/ethnic groups who had actually worked together came to like each other better as individuals, their reduced prejudice did not *generalise* to those ethnic groups as a whole. This may be partly accounted for by the fact that most experiments of this type are small-scale and relatively short-term interventions. The jigsaw method also works best with young children, before prejudiced attitudes have an opportunity to become deeply ingrained (Aronson, 1992).

If it reduces some prejudice towards others it's a start, isn't it? Health care provides a natural programme to promote harmony; the whole health care team is interdependent. Mrs M can see many different (multiracial and professional) 'groups' working with equal status and collaborating to achieve a common goal: her successful recovery. Hopefully, it will change her attitude.

Do common goals always work?

The imposition of superordinate goals may sometimes even *increase* antagonism towards the out-group – if the cooperation fails to achieve its aims. Groups need distinctive and complementary roles to play, so that each group's contributions are clearly defined. When this does not happen, liking for the other group may actually *decrease*, perhaps because group members are concerned with the integrity of the in-group (Brown, 1988).

Maintaining group boundaries – *mutual differentiation* (Fiske, 2004) – is essential for promoting generalisation from the particular out-group members to the whole out-group (Hewstone, 2003). But is not there the danger that emphasising group/category boundaries during contact will *reinforce* perceptions of group differences and increase intergroup anxiety? It certainly should not be done in the initial stages of contact, especially when intergroup relationships are very negative. According to Hewstone (2003), the best approach is 'to promote contact that is simultaneously both "interpersonal" (e.g. involving personal exchange within a close relationship) and "intergroup" (i.e. both members are still aware that they belong to different groups) …'.

The definition of competency boundaries is necessary for accountability (see case study 6, page 72) However, if something went wrong with Mrs M's recovery, she might look for her scapegoat among the black staff, I suppose. Alternatively, if she sees me as an Asian nurse who cares well for her, she is more likely to have a favourable impression of all Asian nurses.

An evaluation of the contact hypothesis

- Contact can 'work' through more subtle processes than generalisation (Hewstone, 2003). For example, it can help reduce the 'almost automatic fear' caused by interacting with members of out-groups – 'intergroup awe' (Stephan and Stephan, 1985). Contact has been shown to play a crucial mediating role in reducing anxiety between Hindus and Muslims in

Bangladesh and between Catholics and Protestants in Northern Ireland (Hewstone, 2003). According to Pettigrew (1998), generating affective (emotional) ties (including anxiety reduction) is the key mechanism involved in contact. Forming close friendships with out-group members appears to be the most effective in reducing prejudice and is certainly more effective than the rather superficial contact that occurs in the neighbourhood or at work.

- In a meta-analysis ('study of studies') of over 500 studies, Pettigrew and Tropp (2006) found that the greater the contact between groups, the lower the prejudice expressed. Only about 6% showed the reverse effect. Pettigrew and Tropp concluded that Allport's original contact conditions are not necessary for positive contact effects to occur, but they are *facilitating* conditions likely to make contact more effective. They concluded, emphatically, that 'contact works'.

- Pettigrew and Tropp (2006) proposed a reformulation of the CH. Instead of conditions necessary for positive contact, they identified negative conditions that must be *avoided* to prevent positive contact effects being erased. Contact opportunities should:
  a. occur often enough
  b. not include threat or anxiety
  c. encourage the development of cross-group friendships
  This reformulation provides a much more optimistic view than the original CH: preconditions for positive effects can now be met more easily (Kessler and Mummendy, 2008).

- The CH does not apply only to relationships between members of different ethnic/racial groups. The positive effects of contact have also been shown with attitudes towards psychiatric patients, gay men and disabled children (Hewstone, 2003).

And presumably working closely together as a team is the best way to break down barriers between different health care groups, however categorised.

Conclusions: What to do with stereotypes?

According to Brislin (1993), 'In many cultures, stereotypes of certain groups are so negative, so pervasive, and have existed for so many generations that they can be considered part of the culture into which children are socialised …'.

As we have seen, stereotypes represent a way of simplifying the extraordinarily complex social world we inhabit by placing people into categories. This alone would explain why they are so resistant to change. But they also influence selective attention and selective remembering, processes that are to a large extent outside conscious control. However, these automatic stereotyped reactions (one of the authors of this book is still 'guilty' of inferring that 'doctor' denotes 'he') can be seen simply as habits that can be broken. Prejudice reduction is a *process*, which involves learning to inhibit these automatic reactions and deciding that prejudice is an inappropriate way of relating to others (Devine and Zuwerink, 1994). But trying to suppress your stereotypes may actually *strengthen* their automaticity. Hogg and Abrams (2000) argue that 'The knack would seem to be to get people to have insight into their stereotypes – to understand them and see through them rather than merely to suppress them'.

To reflect adequately on this piece I would have to use Gibbs' framework for its emphasis on feelings and Goodman's level three consideration of the social, political and ethical context of prejudice. My experience with Mrs M revealed some subtle aspects of prejudice; the theory in this chapter has revealed the complexity of the factors influencing it and it has given me insight into my own. It has also made me aware of the political aspects of the NHS. In the future, I'll be much more aware of the socio-cultural aspect of patient behaviour and respectful of other ethnic groups and not so quick to judge. I felt I wanted to challenge Mrs Maitland's behaviour in my own way. As I do believe that developing a warm, trusting relationship with others is a powerful way to reduce prejudice my goal is to achieve this with Mrs M. I'm supported in this by the ward manager who agrees that to uphold anti-discrimination principles I should have maximum opportunity to care for her. I hope it works!

CHAPTER SUMMARY

- As an extreme attitude, *prejudice* comprises *cognitive* (stereotype), *affective* (hostility) and *behavioural* components. *Discrimination* usually refers to any kind of prejudiced behaviour.
- Most definitions of prejudice identify it as the characteristic of an individual, but it is often associated with *intergroup conflict*. Racism, sexism, heterosexism, ageism, sizeism and 'HIV/AIDS-ism' can all be regarded as *ideologies*, which are characteristics of society, not individuals.
- The most influential 'individual' theory of prejudice is the *authoritarian personality*. Adorno et al. argued that the authoritarian personality is prejudiced in a generalised way.
- Rokeach's theory of *ideological dogmatism* identifies authoritarianism as an extreme way of thinking (the 'closed mind'), rather than a particular political persuasion.
- According to the *frustration–aggression hypothesis*, frustration-induced aggression is often displaced onto minority groups, which act as *scapegoats*.
- According to realistic group conflict theory (*RGCT*), competition between groups for scarce resources is a sufficient condition for intergroup hostility.
- *Minimal group experiments* demonstrate that intergroup conflict can occur without competition; the mere *categorisation* of oneself as belonging to one group rather than another is sufficient for intergroup discrimination.
- The *minimal group effect* is explained in terms of social identity theory (*SIT*), according to which we try to increase self-esteem by accentuating the desirability of our in-group(s). Prejudice can be seen as part of the attempt to boost self-image.

- An important framework for attempts to reduce prejudice is Allport's contact hypothesis (*CH*), which stresses the need for *equal status contact* and the pursuit of *common* (superordinate) *goals* between members of different ethnic groups.
- Group segregation can produce *autistic hostility* and the related *mirror-image phenomenon*, with the likely reinforcement of negative stereotypes. Unequal status contact can also reinforce stereotypes.
- In *equal status situations*, there needs to be a balance between mutual group differentiation (which maintains intergroup contact) and interpersonal contact.
- There is considerable support for the CH, including the *jigsaw method of learning*. The key mechanism involved seems to be creating affective ties, including the reduction of *intergroup awe*.
- *Stereotypes* are very resistant to change, because they often form part of the culture.
- They can be activated automatically/unconsciously, but may be broken if people are encouraged to focus on the unique characteristics of individuals.

8

Conformity and group influence

Introduction and overview

It is impossible to live among other people and not be influenced by them in some way. According to Allport (1968), social psychology as a discipline can be defined as 'an attempt to understand and explain how the thoughts, feelings and behaviours of individuals are influenced by the actual, imagined, or implied presence of others'.

Sometimes, other people's attempts to change our thoughts or behaviour are very obvious, as when, for example, a ward manager tells a student nurse to attend to a particular patient. If we do as we are told, we are demonstrating *obedience*, which implies that one person (in this example, the ward manager, an authority figure) has more social power than others (student nurses). Obedience is discussed in Chapter 9. In common with obedience, other forms of *active social influence* involve deliberate attempts by one person to change another's thoughts or behaviour.

However, on other occasions, social influence is less direct and deliberate and may not involve any explicit requests or demands at all. For example, sometimes the mere presence of other people can influence our behaviour, either inhibiting or enhancing it.

Another form of indirect or passive social influence occurs when, for instance, your taste in music is affected by what your friends listen to. This is *conformity*. Your peers (equals) exert pressure on you to behave (and think) in particular ways, a case of the majority influencing the individual (*majority influence*). But majorities can also be influenced by minorities (*minority influence*).

Is there anything that these different forms of social influence have in common? According to Turner (1991), the key idea in understanding what researchers mean by social influence is the concept of a *social norm*, 'a rule, value or standard shared by the members of a social group that prescribes appropriate, expected or desirable attitudes and conduct in matters relevant to the group …'.

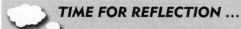

- Try to identify some of the social norms that operate in the different nursing situations you have experienced.

 From my diary (6): Year 1/Orthopaedic Ward

This incident occurred when I was working with Susan, a preceptee who, like me, was new on the ward. I noticed Emma (one of the HCAs), who was helping with a post-op patient's wash, quickly disconnect his heparin infusion and then re-connect it when she'd removed his theatre gown. I remarked to Susan that I thought HCAs weren't allowed to do that and she said that officially they weren't, but 'they all' (I assumed she meant the registered nurses) seemed to permit it. As she too will be registered soon I didn't like to question her further, but I felt uneasy about it. As the NMC code (NMC Guidance on Professional Conduct, revised 2011, page 13) states you should 'recognise and work within the limits of your competence', it seemed wrong.

Conformity

What is it?

Conformity has been defined in a number of ways. For Crutchfield (1954), it is 'yielding to group pressure'. Mann (1969) agrees with Crutchfield, but argues that it may take different forms and be based on motives other than group pressure. Zimbardo and Leippe (1991) define conformity as 'a change in belief or behaviour in response to real or imagined group pressure when there is no direct request to comply with the group nor any reason to justify the behaviour change'.

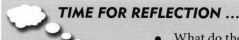

TIME FOR REFLECTION ...

- What do these definitions have in common?

Group pressure is the common denominator in definitions of conformity, although none of them specifies particular groups with particular beliefs or practices. Pressure is exerted by those groups that are important to the individual at a given time. Such groups may consist of 'significant others', such as family or peers (*membership groups*), or groups whose values a person admires or aspires to, but to which she/he does not actually belong (*reference groups*).

Conformity, then, does not imply adhering to any particular set of attitudes or values. Instead, it involves yielding to the real or imagined pressures of any group, whether it has majority or minority status (van Avermaet, 1996).

For Susan the registered nurses represent a membership group; for me they are still a reference group, although obviously one I aspire to join!

Experimental studies of conformity

A study by Jenness (1932) is sometimes cited as the very first experimental study of conformity. Jenness asked individual students to estimate the number of beans in a bottle and then had them discuss it to arrive at a group estimate. When they were asked individually to make a second estimate, there was a distinct shift towards the group's estimate. Sherif (1935) used a similar procedure in one of the classic conformity experiments (Key Study 8.1).

According to Sherif, participants used others' estimates as a frame of reference in what was an ambiguous situation. Note that

- Participants were not in any way instructed to agree with the others in the group (unlike the Jenness study), despite initially wide differences between individuals.
- When participants were tested again individually, their estimates closely resembled the group norm (rather than their original, individual estimates).

Susan knew the behaviour of the HCA wasn't officially correct but she was using the attitude of the registered staff as her 'frame of reference'.

KEY STUDY 8.1

If the light appears to move, it must be the Sherif

- Sherif used a visual illusion called the *autokinetic effect*: a stationary spot of light seen in an otherwise dark room appears to move.
- He told participants he was going to move the light, and their task was to say how far they thought the light moved.
- They were tested individually at first, being asked to estimate the extent of movement several times. The estimates fluctuated to begin with, but then 'settled down' and became quite consistent. However, there were wide differences between participants.
- They then heard the estimates of two other participants (the group condition). Under these conditions, the estimates of different participants *converged* (they became more *similar*). Thus, a *group norm* developed, which represented the average of the individual estimates.

Source: Sherif, M., Arch. Psychol., 27, 17–22, 1935.

An evaluation of Sherif's experiment

Despite its 'classic' status (Brown, 1996), Sherif's study seems to raise questions rather than provide answers:

- In what sense can Sherif's participants be described as a group?
- Can we speak of group norms without any direct interaction taking place or participants seeing themselves as engaged in some kind of joint activity?

In post-experimental interviews, participants all denied being influenced by others' judgements. They also claimed that they struggled to arrive at the 'correct' answers on their own. In other words, they did not consider themselves part of a group.

While Sherif believed he had demonstrated conformity, others, notably Asch, disagreed. According to Asch, the fact that the task used by Sherif was *ambiguous* (there was no right or wrong answer) made it difficult to draw any definite conclusions about conformity. A much stricter test of conformity would involve the individual's tendency to agree with other group members who unanimously give the *wrong answer* on a task where the solution is obvious or unambiguous. Asch devised a simple perceptual task that involved participants deciding which of three comparison lines of different lengths matched a standard line (Figure 8.1).

To ensure validity in research, we need to be sure we're measuring what we think we are measuring! But what were Sherif's participants demonstrating if not conformity?

Based on a pilot study, Asch concluded that the answers were obvious. Because his procedure for studying conformity can be adapted to investigate the effects of different variables on conformity, it is known as the *Asch paradigm*. This is described in Box 8.1.

Figure 8.1 Stimulus cards used in Asch's conformity experiments (1951, 1952, 1956).

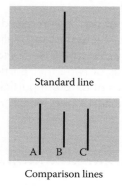

Standard line

Comparison lines

The important measure in the Asch paradigm is whether the naïve participant conforms and gives the same wrong answer as the unanimous stooges on the critical trials or remains independent and gives the obviously correct answer. Asch found a mean conformity rate of 32%; in other words, participants agreed with the incorrect majority answer in about one-third of the critical trials.

As van Avermaet (1996) has remarked, 'The results reveal the tremendous impact of an "obviously" incorrect but unanimous majority on the judgements of a lone individual.'

By ignoring the HCA's behaviour (which she thought was wrong) Susan conformed to the norms of what she obviously perceived as her membership group (two ward managers and four staff nurses).

Factors affecting conformity

Asch (1952, 1955) subsequently manipulated different variables to identify the crucial influences on conformity.

Size of the majority and unanimity

Where there were:

- one naïve participant and just one stooge, conformity was very low (about 3%), ('it's my word against yours').
- two stooges and one participant, conformity increased to 14%.
- three stooges, it reached the 32% that Asch originally reported. But beyond three, conformity did not continue to rise.

This suggests that it is the *unanimity* of the majority that is important (the stooges all agree with each other), rather than the actual size of the majority (the number of stooges).

This was demonstrated when one of the stooges (a *dissenter*) agreed with the naïve participant. With one 'supporter', conformity dropped from 32% to 5.5%. Significantly, a dissenter who disagrees with *both* the naïve participant and the majority has almost as much effect on reducing conformity as one who gives the correct answer (i.e. agrees with the naïve participant). In both cases, the majority is no longer unanimous.

Thus, just breaking the unanimity of the majority is sufficient to reduce conformity (Allen and Levine, 1971). According to Asch (1951), 'a unanimous majority of three is, under the given conditions, far more effective than a majority of eight containing one dissenter ...'. However, this reduction in conformity seems only to apply to unambiguous stimulus situations (like Asch's perceptual task) and not where opinions are being asked for (Allen and Levine, 1968).

Susan's remark that 'they all' seemed to permit the change in practice now seems highly significant; if just one had objected, it may well not have been allowed. (A research note to myself: the number of trained staff condoning the HCA's action are the **independent** variables. Whether Susan accepts the 'wrong' ward practice is the **dependent** variable.)

Task difficulty

When Asch made the comparison lines more similar in length (making the task more difficult), participants were more likely to yield to the incorrect majority answer. This was especially true when they felt confident that there was a right answer. When tasks are more ambiguous, as in expressing opinions or stating preferences (there is no objectively correct answer), conformity actually *decreases*.

Giving answers in private

Critics of Asch's experiment have pointed out that participants may conform because they are reluctant or embarrassed to expose their private views in face-to-face situations (as many of them indicated in post-experimental interviews). If so, the level of conformity should decrease if they are allowed to write down their answers, or where they remain anonymous in some other way. Deutsch and Gerard (1955) found evidence to support this hypothesis as did Asch himself: when the naïve participant was allowed to answer in writing (while the stooges still gave their answers publicly), conformity dropped to 12.5%.

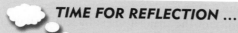 I can see how manipulating the independent variables allowed Asch to find out that a majority of three (in Susan's case, more) is enough to maximise conformity. Using interviews as well allowed him to find out **why** people conformed, which seems just as important.

Cross-cultural studies of conformity

As shown in Table 8.1, the vast majority of conformity studies using the Asch paradigm have been carried out in Britain and America. However, using meta-analysis (a 'study of studies'), Bond and Smith (1996) were able to compare the British and American studies with the small number carried out in other parts of the world. After all relevant factors have been taken into account, the studies can be compared in terms of an *averaged effect size* – in this case, the conformity rate.

TIME FOR REFLECTION ...

- Are there any patterns in the conformity rates (averaged effect size) in Table 8.1?
- For example, are those countries with the highest and lowest conformity geographically and/or culturally related?

According to Smith and Bond (1998), the countries represented in Table 8.1 can be described as *individualist* (such as the United States, the United Kingdom and other Western European countries) or *collectivist* (such as Japan, Fiji and the African countries). In individualist cultures, one's identity is defined by personal choices and achievements, while in collectivist cultures it

Table 8.1 Asch conformity studies by national culture

Nation	Number of studies	Averaged effect size
Asch's own U.S. studies	18	1.16
Other U.S. studies	79	0.90
Canada	1	1.37
United Kingdom	10	0.81
Belgium	4	0.91
France	2	0.56
Netherlands	1	0.74
Germany	1	0.92
Portugal	1	0.58
Japan	5	1.42
Brazil	3	1.60
Fiji	2	2.48
Hong Kong	1	1.93
Arab samples (Kuwait, Lebanon)	2	1.31
Africa (Zimbabwe, Republic of the Congo [Zaire], Ghana)	3	1.84

Source: Based on Bond, R.A., Smith, P.B., *Psychol. Bull.*, 119, 111–137, 1996; taken from Smith, P.B., Bond, R.A. *Social Psychology across Cultures: Analysis and Perspectives*, Prentice-Hall Europe, Hemel Hempstead, 1998.

is defined in terms of the collective group one belongs to (such as the family or religious group). As might be expected, the tendency is for more conformity in collectivist cultures (see Chapter 10).

Being brought up by Asian parents, I might be expected to be more, not less, conforming than Susan. However, she probably sees herself as a member of the trained staff 'collective'.

Majority or minority influence in Asch-type experiments?

Typically, the findings from experiments using the Asch paradigm have been interpreted as showing the impact of a (powerful) majority on the (vulnerable) individual (who is usually in a minority of one). While the stooges are, numerically, the majority, Asch himself was interested in the social and personal conditions that induce individuals to *resist* group pressure.

Spencer and Perrin (1998) ask if reports of Asch's experiments have overstated the power of the majority to force minority individuals to agree with obviously mistaken judgements. Indeed, Moscovici and Faucheux (1972) argued that it is more useful to think of the naïve participant as the majority (she/he embodies the 'conventional', self-evident 'truth') and the stooges as the minority (they reflect an unorthodox, unconventional, eccentric and even outrageous viewpoint). This corresponds to the distinction between the in-group and out-group respectively: Moscovici wanted to demonstrate the conditions under which people actually conform to the out-group. In Asch's experiments, this minority/out-group influenced the majority 32% of the time, and it is those participants remaining independent who are actually the conformists!

If the staff managers are 'breaking the rules' regarding the HCA, from Moscovici and Faucheux's (1972) point of view they are innovators/a minority out-group, rebelling against accepted practice. So Susan is identifying with the non-conformers – and, oh dear, I am, after all, the conforming one.

Is the majority always right?

Looked at from Moscovici and Faucheux's perspective, Asch-type experiments suggest how new ideas may come to be accepted (they explain *innovation*), rather than provide evidence about maintenance of the status quo. If groups always followed a majority decision rule ('the majority is always or probably right, so best go along with it'), or if social influence were about the inevitable conforming to the group, where would innovation come from (Spencer and Perrin, 1998)?

According to Moscovici (1976), there is a *conformity bias* in this area of research, such that all social influence is seen as serving the need to adapt to the status quo for the sake of uniformity and stability – the 'tyranny of the majority' (Martin and Hewstone, 2001; Wood, 2000). However, change is sometimes needed to adapt to changing circumstances, and this is very difficult to explain given the conformity bias. Without *active minorities*, social and scientific innovations would simply never happen (van Avermaet, 1996).

If the tendency to conform to the status quo had persisted, none of the nursing profession's adaptations to the changing demands of nursing care would have happened!

How do minorities exert an influence?

Moscovici (1976) re-analysed the data from one of Asch's (1955) experiments, in which he varied the proportion of neutral to critical trials (where stooges gave the right or wrong answers respectively). In the original experiment this proportion was 1:2 (see Box 8.1). When the proportion was 1:6, the conformity rate was 50%, but when it was 4:1 it dropped to 26.2%.

TIME FOR REFLECTION ...

- Try to account for these findings.
- Why should conformity rates *increase* as the ratio of neutral to critical trials *decreases*, but *decrease* when it *increases*?

Box 8.1 Asch paradigm

- Some of the participants who had taken part in the pilot study were asked to act as 'stooges' (or 'confederates' – accomplices of the experimenter). They were told they would be doing the task again, but this time in a group. The group would contain one person (a naïve participant) who was completely ignorant that they were stooges.
- On certain *critical* trials, which Asch would indicate by means of a secret signal, all the stooges were required to say out loud the same *wrong answer*. In Asch's original experiment, the stooges (usually seven to nine of them) and the naïve participant were seated either in a straight line or round a table. The situation was rigged so that the naïve participant was always the last or last but one to say the answer out loud (see Figure 8.2).
- On the first two trials (*neutral* trials), all the stooges gave the correct answers. But the next trial was a critical one (the stooges unanimously gave a wrong answer). This happened a further 11 times (making 12 critical trials in total), with 4 additional neutral trials (making 6 in total) between the critical trials.

Figure 8.2 A minority of one faces a unanimous majority. (Courtesy William Vandivert and *Scientific American*, November 1955.)

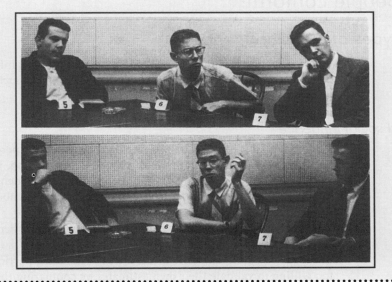

Moscovici interpreted these findings in terms of *consistency*. When there were more critical than neutral trials (the ratio *decreases*), the stooges (who embody the *minority* viewpoint) appear *more consistent* as a group, and this produces a higher conformity rate. They are more often agreeing with each other about something unconventional or novel, which makes it more likely that they will change the views of the majority (as represented by the naïve participant). Moscovici (1980) proposes that while majorities impose their views through directly requiring compliance (which often requires 'surveillance'), minorities use more *indirect* means to achieve a more lasting conversion.

Next day I asked Emma about the heparin and she explained there is no national definition of HCA's duties, it depended on the ward manager. This ward was always so busy that if she had to wait for a staff nurse to disconnect all the heparin infusions the washes would never get done! She also said that Sister had assessed her (she has an NVQ 3 qualification) as competent to do this task as long as a staff nurse checks the infusion rate immediately afterwards.

So, using Goodman's (1984) framework (see case study 2, page 230), in order to provide effective care for patients and fulfill efficiency requirements (level 1) the registered nurses (the minority group) have debated and changed accepted practice (level 2) which challenged the 'official' (majority) point of view.

According to Wood et al. (1994), minority influence most often occurs *privately* – that is, on measures that protect the converted majority individuals from appearing publicly to abandon their majority position. 'Thus, majorities can be converted by minorities, but majority individuals do not admit it to others, and perhaps not to themselves, thereby avoiding public identification with the unpopular minority position ...' (Fiske, 2004).

Why do people conform?

Different types of social influence

One very influential and widely accepted account of group influence is Deutsch and Gerard's (1955) distinction between *informational social influence* (ISI) and *normative social influence* (NSI).

Informational social influence

Underlying ISI is the need to be right, to have an accurate perception of reality. So when we are uncertain or face an ambiguous situation, we look to others to help us perceive the stimulus situation accurately (or define the situation). This involves a *social comparison* with other group members to reduce the uncertainty.

As we saw earlier, Sherif's experiment involves an inherently ambiguous situation: there is no actual movement of the light and so there cannot be any right or wrong answers. Under these conditions, participants were only too willing to validate their own estimates by comparing them with those of others. The results were consistent with Sherif's *social reality hypothesis*, which states that 'The less one can rely on one's own direct perception and behavioural contact with the physical world, the more susceptible one should be to influence from others ...' (Turner, 1991).

According to Festinger's (1954) *social comparison theory*, people have a basic need to evaluate their ideas and attitudes and, in turn, to confirm that they are correct. This can provide a reassuring sense of control over one's world and a satisfying sense of competence. In novel or ambiguous situations, social reality is defined by what others think and do. Significantly, Sherif's participants were relatively unaware of being influenced by the other judges.

As a student, I look to others all the time to ensure I'm doing the right thing, although reading this chapter is making me more wary of doing so!

Normative social influence

Underlying NSI is the need to be accepted by other people and to make a favourable impression on them. We conform to gain social approval and avoid rejection – we agree with others because of their power to reward, punish, accept or reject us.

Most of Asch's participants faced a *conflict* between two sources of information, which in unambiguous situations normally coincide – namely their own judgement (which they knew was correct) and that of others. If they chose their own judgement, they risked rejection and ridicule by the majority.

Susan needs to make a good impression on the ward managers as they will endorse her registration. As the role of the HCA could be said to be ambiguous, she's likely to conform to their judgement.

Internalisation and compliance

Related to ISI and NSI are two kinds of conformity.

1. *Internalisation* occurs when a private belief or opinion becomes consistent with a public belief or opinion. In other words, we say what we believe and believe what we say. Mann (1969) calls this *true conformity*, which can be thought of as a *conversion* to other people's points of view, especially in ambiguous situations.

2. *Compliance* occurs when the answers given publicly are not those that are privately believed (we say what we do not believe and what we believe we do not say). Compliance represents a compromise in situations where people face a conflict between what they privately believe and what others publicly say they believe.

So if Susan believes her colleagues' behaviour is right (internalisation) and supports them, it will be **true** conformity; if she just pretends to agree to it, believing its wrong, it's compliance.

TIME FOR REFLECTION …

- Which kind of conformity was most common in Sherif's and Asch's experiments?
- How are internalisation and compliance related to NSI and ISI?

In Sherif's experiment, participants were *internalising* others' judgements and making them their own. Faced with an ambiguous situation, participants were guided by what others believed to reduce their uncertainty. So, internalisation is related to ISI.

By contrast, most of Asch's participants knew that the majority answers on the critical trials were wrong, but often agreed with them publicly. They were *complying* with the majority to avoid ridicule or rejection. So, compliance is related to NSI.

I never discovered if Susan was internalising the 'minority' ward attitude – she was complying with it, for whatever reason.

Do we have to choose between ISI and NSI?

Remember that when Asch made the task more difficult by making the three comparison lines much more similar, conformity increased. Clearly, ISI was involved here. If we believe there is a correct answer and are uncertain what it is, it seems quite logical to expect that we would be more influenced by a unanimous majority. This is why having a supporter, or the presence of a dissenter, has the effect of reducing conformity. By breaking the group consensus, the participant is shown both that disagreement is possible and that the group is fallible. As Turner (1991) points out, both ISI and NSI can operate in conjunction with each other and should not be seen as opposed processes of influence (see Figure 8.3).

In an ambiguous situation, Susan deferred to the unanimous judgement of the group but was no doubt anxious for their approval, so both could have influenced her.

Conformity and group belongingness

The distinction between NSI and ISI has been called the *dual process dependency model* (DPDM) of social influence (e.g. Turner, 1991). But this model underestimates the role of group 'belongingness'. One important feature of conformity is that we are influenced by a group because, psychologically, we feel we belong to it. This is why a group's norms are relevant standards for our own attitudes and behaviour. The DPDM emphasises the *interpersonal* aspects of conformity experiments, which could just as easily occur between individuals as group members.

The *self-categorisation approach* suggests that – in Sherif's experiment, for example – participants assumed that the autokinetic effect was real and expected to agree with each other. In support of this, it is been shown that when participants discover that the autokinetic effect is an illusion, mutual influence and convergence cease – the need to agree at all is removed (Sperling, 1946). If, however, we believe that there *is* a correct answer, and we are uncertain what it is, then those whom we categorise as belonging to 'our' group will influence our judgements. As Brown (1988) has remarked, 'There is more to conformity than simply "defining social reality": it all depends on who is doing the defining' (Key Study 8.2).

Figure 8.3 The relationship between different kinds of influence and different kinds of conformity.

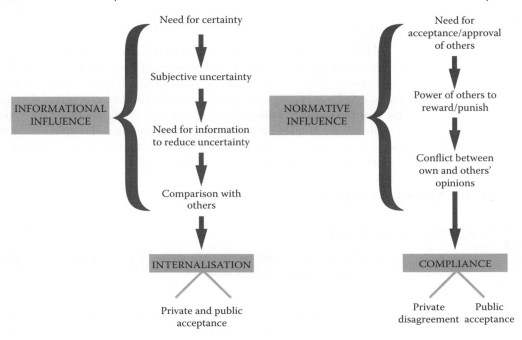

KEY STUDY 8.2

Knowing what to think by knowing who you are

- Abrams et al. replicated Sherif's experiment with psychology students, but manipulated categorisation: stooges were introduced as students at a nearby university, but were either fellow psychology students or students of ancient history.
- Convergence occurred only when others were categorised as being equivalent to self – that is, a member of the in-group (fellow psychology students). So self-categorisation may set limits on ISI.
- It should also set limits on NSI, since individuals will presumably have a stronger desire to receive rewards, approval and acceptance from those categorised in the same way as themselves than from those categorised differently.
- Using the Asch paradigm but again manipulating categorisation, Abrams et al. found that conformity exceeded the usual level of 32% in the in-group condition, but was greatly below this level in the out-group condition.

Source: Abrams, D. et al., *Br. J. Soc. Psychol.*, 29, 97–119, 1990.

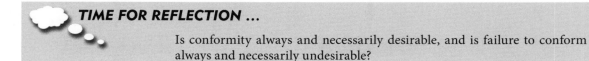

So Susan would value the point of view **and** the good opinion of her new membership group (the ward senior staff) more than that of another group (e.g. senior staff in general)?

Abrams et al. (1990) conclude that social influence occurs when we see ourselves as belonging to a group and possessing the same characteristics and reactions as other group members. This is what Turner (1991) calls *referent social influence*. What is important is not the validation of physical reality or the avoidance of social disapproval, but the upholding of a *group norm*: people are the source of information about the appropriate in-group norm. A social categorisation approach sees the NSI/ISI distinction as a false dichotomy since 'Information is intrinsically social ...' (Fiske, 2004).

Conformity: Good or bad?

TIME FOR REFLECTION ...

Is conformity always and necessarily desirable, and is failure to conform always and necessarily undesirable?

According to Zimbardo and Leippe (1991), in most circumstances, conformity serves a valuable social purpose in that it '... lubricates the machinery of social interaction [and] enables us to structure our social behaviour and predict the reactions of others'.

For most people, though, the word 'conformity' has a negative connotation. As a result, it is implicitly assumed that independence is 'good' and conformity is 'bad', a value judgement made explicit by Asch (1952). However, conformity can be highly functional, helping us to satisfy social and non-social needs, as well as being necessary (at least to a degree) for social life to proceed at all.

Since each of us has a limited (and often biased) store of information on which to make decisions, other people can often provide valuable additional information and expertise. Conforming with others under these circumstances may be a rational judgement. However, while conformity can help preserve harmony, 'There are obvious dangers to conformity. Failure to speak our minds against dangerous trends or attitudes (for example, racism) can easily be interpreted as support' (Krebs and Blackman, 1988).

The term 'conformity' is often used to convey undesirable behaviour. In laboratory research, it has most often been studied in terms of the 'conspiratorial group ... [being] shown to limit, constrain, and distort the individual's response ...' (Milgram, 1965). However, in the context of his famous studies of obedience, Milgram showed that the presence of two defiant peers significantly reduced the obedience rate among naïve participants, and he wrote an article (1965) called 'Liberating effects of group pressure' (see Chapter 9).

Also, whether conformity is considered good or bad is a matter of *culture*. In *individualist* cultures, people are often distressed by the possibility that others can influence their behaviour against their will: they prefer to believe they are in control of their destiny. So 'conformity', 'compliance', 'obedience' and other similar terms have negative connotations. But in *collectivist* cultures, adjusting one's behaviour to fit the requests and expectations of others is highly valued, and sometimes even a moral imperative (Fiske et al., 1998). In these cultures, conformity is seen as necessary for social functioning, rather than a sign of weakness (Nagayama Hall and Barongan, 2002).

Whether conformity is good or bad seems no more absolute than the role of the HCA!

Reflecting on this incident has made me aware that accepting the status quo may not always be desirable; the danger of conformity lies in the subtle way it operates and is based on a desire to belong and to 'fit in'.

Asch's classic experiments (1952, 1955) showed why a small group of staff agreeing a policy was enough to induce Susan's conformity; as a new member of staff, she would rely on her senior colleagues for information about appropriate 'in-group norms' (Turner, 1991).

Moscovici and Faucheux's (1972) view of Asch's experiment showed how the ward managers were an innovative minority; they saw the accepted practice was not achieving effectiveness and efficiency (Goodman level 1 criteria) and by challenging its underlying rationale of accountability were debating principles and goals (Goodman level 2 activity). Their non-conformity could result in changes to the 'official' role and improvement in the delivery of care which seems a good thing. However, as Zimbardo and Leippe (1991) argue, the conformists' tendency to compromise can sometimes be a positive quality, so deciding whether conformity is a good or bad thing in nursing must be judged (again) in its context and, crucially, its accountability. If Emma **had** been acting outside her role (as I thought) and compromising patient care, Susan's (and my) silence would be dangerous and unethical (Goodman level 3 consideration).

CHAPTER SUMMARY

- *Social influence* can be *active* or *deliberate*, as in persuasive communication and obedience, or *passive* or *non-deliberate*, as in social facilitation and conformity. A common feature of all social influence is the concept of a *social norm*.
- Definitions of *conformity* commonly refer to *group pressure*, whether the group is a *membership* or a *reference* group.
- In Sherif's experiment using the *autokinetic effect*, individual estimates *converged* to form a group norm. Asch criticised Sherif's use of an ambiguous task, and in his own experiments used a 'comparison of lines' task for which there was a correct answer.
- Asch found that the *unanimity/consensus of the majority* is crucial, not its size. The presence of a *supporter* or *dissenter* reduces conformity, because the majority is no longer unanimous.
- Conformity is increased when the task is made *more difficult* (more *ambiguous*) and reduced when participants give their answer *anonymously*.

- Replications of Asch's experiment have produced higher or lower rates of conformity according to when and where they were conducted. Both *socio-historical* and *cultural factors* seem to play a part.
- Asch's findings are usually interpreted as showing the impact of *majority influence*. But Moscovici believes that the stooge majority should be thought of as embodying unconventional, minority beliefs, and that conformity experiments show how new ideas come to be accepted (*innovation*).
- One way in which *minority influence* works is by displaying *consistency*.
- Two major *motives for conformity* are the need to be right Informational Social Influence (*ISI*) and the need to be accepted by others Normative Social Influence (*NSI*).
- ISI is related to Sherif's *social reality hypothesis* and Festinger's *social comparison theory* and is demonstrated through *internalisation/true conformity*. NSI is linked to *compliance*.

9

Obedience

Introduction and overview

Obedience is an active or deliberate form of social influence, which involves someone in authority requiring us to behave in a particular way in a particular situation. If we obey, we are said to be 'complying' with the authority figure's request or instruction. Compliance is a major kind of conformity, namely, one in which overt behaviour does not reflect private beliefs.

Compliance also occurs whenever we do what someone else 'asks' us to do, that is, whenever people make direct requests, such as when a friend asks us for a favour or a salesperson invites us to try a product or service. Many researchers believe that attempts to gain compliance through direct requests are the most common form of social influence (Hogg and Vaughan, 1995).

In the context of nursing, obedience can be seen to operate both within the profession (as when junior nurses comply with the wishes/requests of the charge nurse or ward sister) and between nursing staff and doctors. Although Florence Nightingale may well have been offended by doctors' definition of nurses as 'devoted and obedient', she must take the blame for starting the militaristic hierarchy that still survives (Heenan, 1990).

In the context of health psychology, compliance refers to the extent to which a patient's behaviour matches the advice or recommendations from their health professional (Horne et al., 2006; NICE, 2009a). In developed economies, the most common health intervention is the prescription of medication; not surprisingly, most research into compliance is concerned with the extent to which medication is taken as prescribed. However, there is growing awareness of the vital role of lifestyle factors (such as physical activity and diet) in managing chronic illnesses (Horne and Clatworthy, 2010).

Most researchers now prefer the term 'adherence', since this implies a more mutual relationship between the patient and the practitioner. Compliance implies that the practitioner is an authority figure, whereas the patient is a fairly passive recipient.

From my diary (7): Year 1/Orthopaedic Ward

I had a lesson in assertiveness today! I was helping Tameka (a Staff Nurse) settle 74-yr-old Mr Price, who had just come back from theatre having had a revision of total hip replacement. We did his observations and then looked at his drug chart and Tameka said at once, 'Oh, I don't think that's right.' She was familiar with IV Gentamycin being given prophylactically and thought the dose of 400mgs a bit high as she'd never given more than 320mgs before. Nigel, the F1, was at the nurses' station so we went over and Tameka told him that as she knew it was nephrotoxic she was worried it wasn't right. Nigel didn't even look at the chart but said dismissively, 'If that's what the consultant's written, that's what he wants,' and turned away. Tameka said very firmly, 'No, I'm not happy about giving that dose. I want to check it.' I felt uncomfortable as I could see Nigel was getting annoyed. He said, rather arrogantly I thought, that he'd no intention of questioning a consultant surgeon's prescription 'and it's not your job to either. Just give it!' and stalked off. Tameka muttered, 'Oh, yes it is,' picked up the phone and got through to Pharmacy. After asking Mr Price's weight (88kgs) age and condition (post–op with IV) the pharmacist said it would be all right to give it and apparently told her well done for checking. Tameka made a note of this and did so. A bit later, when the registrar came to the ward Tameka explained to him what happened and he said she was absolutely right to question anything she wasn't sure of.

Experimental studies of obedience

In the experiments of Sherif and Asch (see Chapter 8), participants showed conformity by giving a verbal response of some kind or pressing buttons representing answers on various tasks. In the most famous and controversial of all obedience experiments, Milgram's participants were required to kill another human being (see Box 9.1 and Figure 9.1).

Milgram's research

Milgram was attempting to test 'the "Germans are different" hypothesis'. This has been used by historians to explain the systematic destruction of millions of Jews, Poles and others by the Nazis during the 1930s and 1940s. It maintains that the Germans have a basic character defect, namely, a readiness to obey authority without question regardless of the acts demanded by the authority figure. It is this readiness to obey that provided Hitler with the cooperation he needed. After piloting his research in America Milgram planned to continue it in Germany, but his results showed this was unnecessary.

Participants

The participants in the original (1963) experiment were 20- to 50-year-old men from all walks of life. They answered advertisements asking for volunteers for a study of learning to be conducted at the Yale University, New Haven, Connecticut. It would take about 1 hour, and there would be a payment of $4.50.

Box 9.1 Milgram's basic experimental procedure

- When participants arrived at the Yale University psychology department, they were met by a young man in a grey laboratory coat, who introduced himself as Jack Williams, the experimenter. Also present was a Mr Wallace, who introduced himself as another participant. In fact, Mr Wallace was a stooge, and everything that happened after this was pre-planned, staged and scripted: everything, that is, except the degree to which the real participant obeyed the experimenter's instructions.

- The participants and Mr Wallace were told that the experiment was concerned with the effects of punishment on learning. They chose a piece of paper from a hat to (supposedly) determine who would be the teacher and who the learner; this was rigged so that a participant was always the teacher. They all went into an adjoining room, where Mr Wallace was strapped into a chair with his arms attached to electrodes, which would deliver a shock from the shock generator situated in an adjacent room (see Figure 9.1).

- The teacher was given a 45 V shock to convince him or her that it was real, for she was to operate the generator during the experiment. However, that was the only real shock that either the teacher or the learner was to receive throughout the entire experiment.

- The generator had a number of switches, each clearly marked with voltage levels and verbal descriptions, starting at 15 V and going up to 450 V in intervals of 15:

15–60	Slight shock
75–120	Moderate shock
135–180	Strong shock
195–240	Very strong shock
255–300	Intense shock
315–360	Intense to extreme shock
375–420	Danger: severe shock
435–450	XXX

- The learner had to perform a form of word association task and press one of four switches, which turned on a light on a panel in the generator room. Each time she made a mistake the teacher had to deliver a shock, and each successive mistake was punished by a shock 15 V higher than the one before.

Fourteen psychology students predicted that a few participants would break off early on, most would stop somewhere in the middle, and a few would continue right up to 450 V. Forty psychiatrists predicted that, on average, less than 1% would administer the highest voltage.

Figure 9.1 (a) Shock generator used in the experiments. Fifteen of the 30 switches have already been depressed. (b) Learner is strapped into chair and electrodes are attached to his wrist. Electrode paste is applied by the experimenter. (c) Subject receives sample shock from the generator. (d) Subject breaks off the experiment. (Copyright 1965 by Stanley Milgram from the film *Obedience*, distributed by the Pennsylvania State University, Audio Visual Services.) (From Milgram, S., *Obedience to Authority*, Harper & Row, New York, 1974.)

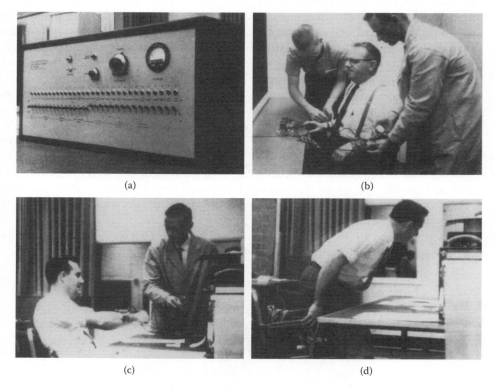

(a)　　　　　　　　　(b)

(c)　　　　　　　　　(d)

I'm feeling very uneasy at just the thought of this experiment. I don't think anybody would progress very far on such a scale, certainly not to the point of causing anyone harm or danger.

These estimates were based on what Milgram called the 'remote-victim condition', in which Mr Wallace was scripted to pound loudly on the wall at 300 V and after 315 V to stop pounding and give no further answers. In the second experiment (voice feedback), teachers heard a tape-recorded series of verbal responses, which they believed were the spontaneous reactions of Mr Wallace to the increasing shock levels. For example,

At 75, 90 and 105 V, he made a little grunt.
At 120 V, he shouted to the experimenter that the shocks were becoming painful.

At 150 V, he cried out, 'Experimenter, get me out of here! I won't be in the experiment any more! I refuse to go on!'; this continued with rising intensity until at 180 V he shouted, 'I can't stand the pain!'.

At 270 V, he let out an agonised scream (he continued to insist on being released).

After 330 V, there was ominous silence.

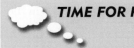

TIME FOR REFLECTION …

- If you had been one of Milgram's teacher participants, how far up the voltage scale would you have continued to punish wrong answers?

The teacher was instructed to treat no response as if it were an incorrect response, so the shocks could continue beyond 300 volts. In addition, the experimenter had a script prepared for whenever the teacher refused to continue or showed any resistance or reluctance to do so:

'Please continue' or 'please go on.'
'The experiment requires that you continue.'
'It's absolutely essential that you continue.'
'You have no other choice; you must go on.'

There were also special prods to reassure the participant that he or she was not doing the learner any permanent harm: 'Although the shocks may be painful there is no permanent tissue damage, so please go on.'

I think if I'd been in Tameka's position and another doctor, although a first Foundation Year one, was reinforcing the consultant's instructions to give the Gentamycin, I might have perceived him as being in charge and therefore responsible. But it's different of course as I wouldn't have been causing anyone pain.

Results

In the remote-victim experiment, every teacher shocked up to at least 300 V and 65% went all the way up to 450 V. In the voice-feedback condition, 62.5% of participants went on giving shocks up to 450 V.

Many displayed great anguish, attacked the experimenter verbally, twitched or laughed nervously. Many were observed to 'sweat, stutter, tremble, groan, bite their lips and dig their nails into their flesh'. Full-blown, uncontrollable seizures were observed for three participants (Milgram, 1974). Indeed, one experiment had to be stopped because the participant had a violently convulsive seizure.

I find it difficult to believe these results. The teachers' reactions indicate an immense degree of mental conflict yet two-thirds of them went on until they might have killed the learner!

To determine why the obedience levels were so high, Milgram conducted several variations using the voice-feedback condition as his baseline measure. In all, a further 16 variations were performed.

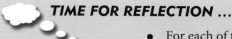

TIME FOR REFLECTION ...

- For each of the variations described in Key Study 9.1, estimate the rates of total obedience (those participants going all the way up to 450 V).
- Try to explain why it might have been higher or lower than 62.5% in the voice-feedback condition.

In variation 10, the obedience rate was 47.5 per cent. This still very high figure suggests that the institutional context played some part but wasn't a crucial factor.

In variation 3 the obedience rate dropped to 40 per cent, and in variation 4 it dropped further to 30 per cent. While it became much more uncomfortable for participants to see – as well as hear – the effects of their obedience, the figures are still very high.

In variation 7, obedience dropped to 20.5 per cent. Indeed, participants often pretended to deliver a shock or delivered one lower than they were asked to.

KEY STUDY 9.1

Some variations on Milgram's basic procedure

Institutional context (variation 10): In interviews following the first experiment, many participants said they continued delivering shocks because the research was being conducted at Yale University, a highly prestigious institution. So, Milgram transferred the experiment to a rundown office in downtown Bridgeport.

Proximity and touch proximity (variations 3 and 4): In the original procedure, the teacher and learner were in adjacent rooms and could not see one another. But in variation 3 they were in the same room (about 46 cm apart), and in variation 4 the teacher was required to force the learner's hand down on to the shock plate.

Remote authority (variation 7): The experimenter left the room (having first given the essential instructions) and gave subsequent instructions by telephone.

Two peers rebel (variation 17): The teacher was paired with two other (stooge) teachers. The stooge teachers read out the list of word pairs and informed the learner whether the response was correct. The naive participant delivered the shocks. At 150 V, the first stooge refused to continue and moved to another part of the room. At 210 V, the second stooge did the same. The experimenter ordered the real teacher to continue.

A peer administers the shocks (variation 18): The teacher was paired with another (stooge) teacher and had only to read out the word pairs (the shock being delivered by the stooge).

This suggests that they were trying to compromise between their conscience and the experimenter's instructions. In his absence, it was easier to follow their conscience.

In variation 17, there was only 10 per cent obedience. Most stopped obeying when the first or second stooge refused to continue. According to Milgram (1965), 'The effects of peer rebellion are most impressive in undercutting the experimenter's authority.' In other words, seeing other participants (our peers) disobey shows that it's possible to disobey, as well as how to disobey. Indeed, some participants said they didn't realise they could. This is a demonstration of the effects of conformity.

In variation 18, obedience rose to 92.5 per cent. This shows that it's easier for participants to shift responsibility from themselves to the person who actually 'throws the switch'.

All these external influences on behaviour are intriguing, especially the significant effect of 'peer rebellion' (like Tameka's). But most striking is the massive effect of not having to take responsibility for what you do.

Why do people obey?

According to Milgram (1974),

> The most fundamental lesson of our study is that ordinary people simply doing their jobs, without any particular hostility on their part, can become agents in a terrible destructive process.

Unless there is reason to believe that people who go all the way up to 450 V are unusually sadistic and/or obedient, explanations of obedience move away from personal characteristics to the characteristics of the social situation: most people facing that situation would probably act in a similar (obedient) way. What might some of these situational factors be?

Personal responsibility

Many participants raised the issue of responsibility for any harm to the learner. Although the experimenter did not always discuss this, when he did say 'I'm responsible for what goes on here' participants showed visible relief. Indeed, when participants are told they are responsible for what happens, obedience is sharply reduced (Hamilton, 1978).

Milgram saw this *diffusion of responsibility* to be crucial in understanding the atrocities committed by the Nazis and Eichmann's defence that he was 'just carrying out orders'. (Eichmann was in charge of the transportation of Jews and others to extermination camps and was eventually tried in Jerusalem in 1960. See Figure 9.2.)

Figure 9.2 Eichmann at his trial in Jerusalem, 1960.

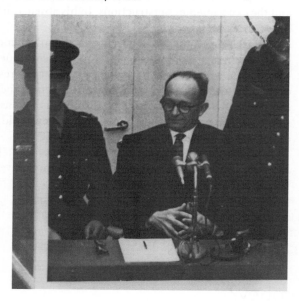

🔖 This is about accountability. When Tameka and I discussed the incident afterwards, she asked me if I would have given the Gentamycin if I knew I'd be held personally responsible for possible damage to Mr Price's ageing kidneys resulting in him needing dialysis – or worse. It scared me into changing my mind!

The distress and conflict displayed by many participants suggests that diffusion of responsibility cannot tell the whole story. The conflict seems to be between two opposing sets of demands: the external authority of the experimenter who says 'Shock' and the internal authority of the conscience, which says 'Don't shock'. The point at which conscience triumphs is, of course, where the participant (finally) stops obeying the experimenter, who, in a sense, ceases to be a legitimate authority in the eyes of the participant. In the original experiment, 35% reached that point somewhere before 450 V, and for many the crucial prod was when the experimenter said, 'You have no other choice, you must go on.' They were able to exercise the choice that, of course, they had from the start.

🔖 Interestingly enough, by telling Tameka that it wasn't her job to question the prescription, Nigel was – inadvertently – pointing out to her that it was.

The most common mental adjustment in the obedient participant is to see himself or herself as an agent of external authority (the *agentic state*). This represents the opposite of an *autonomous state* and is what makes it possible for us to function in a hierarchical social system. For a group to function as a whole, individuals must give up responsibility and defer to others of higher status in the social hierarchy. Legitimate authority thus replaces a person's own self-regulation (Turner, 1991). In Milgram's (1974) words,

> The essence of obedience consists in the fact that a person comes to view himself as the instrument for carrying out another person's wishes, and he, therefore, no longer regards himself as responsible for his actions. Once this critical shift of viewpoint has occurred in a person, all the essential features of obedience follow.

(For a critique of the agentic state explanation, see Gross [2012b].)

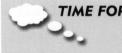 Although I'm very aware the nursing profession is fighting to establish its autonomy, I still perceived doctors' status as higher than ours and felt uncomfortable at the challenge to their orders. In contrast, Tameka certainly had no problem with refusing to be the traditional 'handmaiden'!

TIME FOR REFLECTION …

- What was it about Jack Williams, the experimenter, that conveyed to participants that he was 'in charge' in the experimental situation?

Authority figures often possess highly visible symbols of their power or status that make it difficult to refuse their commands. In Milgram's experiments, the experimenter always wore a grey laboratory coat to indicate his position as an authority figure. For Milgram (1974),

> A substantial proportion of people do what they are told to do, irrespective of the content of the act and without limitations of conscience, so long as they perceive that the command comes from a legitimate authority.

Another major study that demonstrates the impact of uniforms and other symbols of authority is Zimbardo et al.'s (1973) 'prison simulation experiment' (see Gross [2012b]).

Most of us in the health care team wear uniforms, or some indicator of our 'rank', which is significant. I've noticed the doctors' symbol of authority (their stethoscopes round their necks) is being adopted by some nurses. Is this another assertion of our bid for autonomy?

'Foot in the door' and not knowing how to disobey

According to Gilbert (1981), Milgram's participants may have been sucked in by the series of graduated demands. These began with the harmless advertisement for volunteers for a study of learning and memory, and ended with the instruction to deliver what appeared to be potentially lethal electric shocks to another person. Having begun the experiment, participants may have found it difficult to remove themselves from it.

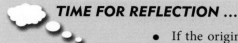

TIME FOR REFLECTION ...

- If the original advertisement had mentioned electric shocks (which it did not), do you think there would have been many volunteers?
- In what ways might such volunteers have constituted a more biased sample than those who participated in the actual experiments?

Presumably, fewer volunteers would have come forward. Those who did may well have been more sadistic than Milgram's sample (assuming that they believed they would be giving the electric shocks).

Socialisation

Despite our expressed ideal of independence, obedience is something we are socialised into from a very early age by significant others (including our parents and teachers). Obedience may be an ingrained habit that is difficult to resist (Brown, 1986).

Yes, and much of nursing work is carrying out doctors' instructions, which makes it more difficult to distinguish when it is, and isn't, legitimate to 'disobey'.

An evaluation of Milgram's research

In evaluating Milgram's experiments, *ethical issues* are usually more prominent than scientific ones (see Gross [2010]). However, Milgram asks whether the ethical criticisms are based as much on the nature of the (unexpected) results as on the procedure itself. Aronson (1988) asks whether we would question the ethics if none of the participants had gone beyond the 150 V level, which is the point at which most people were expected to stop (according to Milgram's students and the 40 psychiatrists he consulted). Aronson manipulated the results experimentally and found that the higher the percentage going right up to 450 V, the more harmful the effects of the experiment are judged to be.

Methodological issues

- Orne and Holland (1968) criticised Milgram's experiments for their lack of *mundane realism*, that is, the results do not extend beyond the particular laboratory setting in which they were collected. They base this claim on the further claim that cues in the experimental setting influenced the participants' perceptions of what was required of them. Obedience, then, might simply have been a response to the *demand characteristics* of the highly unusual experimental setting (see Chapter 1).
- Surveys (mostly conducted in the United States) have found that when presented with a hypothetical situation in which a doctor orders an excessive

dose of medication (Cunningham, 1983; Nursing, 1974; Rank and Jacobson, 1977), or an unsafe practice (Raven and Haley, 1980; Redfearn, 1982), the vast majority believe they would refuse to carry out the order. Nurses with advanced degrees (Nursing, 1974) and more assertive nurses (Redfearn, 1982) are even less likely to see themselves as compliant.

- Surveys like these provide interesting data regarding nurses' self-perceptions (Krackow and Blass, 1995). However, when we are asked to predict our own behaviour, we usually present ourselves favourably (Redfearn, 1982).

- Two field (naturalistic) experiments were conducted to determine what nurses would actually do when faced with the conflict between (i) carrying out an order, which could potentially harm the patient, and (ii) refusing to carry out the order, which might bring the doctor's wrath on the nurse's head. Hofling et al.'s (1966) study is described in Key Study 9.2 and the study by Rank and Jacobson (1977) in Key Study 9.3.

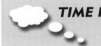

TIME FOR REFLECTION ...

- What do you think you'd have done if you'd been one of the nurses?

- In interviews, 22 graduate nurses who had not participated in the actual experiment were presented with the same situation as an issue to discuss; all said they would not have given the drug without written authorisation, especially as it exceeded the maximum daily dose.

KEY STUDY 9.2

A naturalistic study of nurses

- Twenty-two nurses working in various American hospitals received telephone calls from a stooge 'Dr Smith of the psychiatric department', instructing them to give Mr Jones (Dr Smith's patient) 20 mg of a drug called Astrofen.
- Dr Smith said that he was in a desperate hurry and would sign the drug authorisation form when he came to see the patient in 10 minutes' time.
- The label on the box containing the Astrofen (which was actually a harmless sugar pill) clearly stated that the maximum daily dose was 10 mg.
- So, if the nurse obeyed Dr Smith's instructions, he would be exceeding the maximum daily dose. Also, he would be breaking the rules requiring written authorisation before any drug is given and that a nurse be absolutely sure that Dr Smith is a genuine doctor.

Source: Hofling, K.C. et al., *Journal of Nervous & Mental Disorders, 143,* 171–180, 1966.

KEY STUDY 9.3

A replication of Hofling et al.'s experiment

- Rank and Jacobson (1977) repeated the experiment, but with two important changes:
  - They recorded any checking that the nurses did.
  - They changed the prescription to 30 mg of Valium, a real drug with which they were familiar.
- They also pointed out that Hofling et al.'s participants were working the night shift, when there are few resources available if a nurse chooses to question an order.
- Rank and Jacobson hypothesised that if nurses, familiar with a drug, were ordered to give an overdose and if they were allowed normal contact with other nurses and reference materials, they would not carry out the order.
- Under these conditions, only 2 out of 18 nurses prepared to administer the drug without any checking; 10 prepared the drug but then tried to recontact the doctor, pharmacy or a supervisor; and 6 tried to check the order before preparing the drug.

Source: Rank, S.G. and Jacobson, C.K., *Journal of Health & Social Behaviour*, 18, 188–193, 1977.

- In the experiment, a real doctor was posted nearby, unseen by the nurses, who observed what the nurses did following the telephone call; 21 out of the 22 nurses complied without hesitation, and 11 later said they had not noticed the dosage discrepancy.
- However, could the unfamiliarity of Astrofen (a dummy drug, invented for the purposes of the experiment) have influenced the nurses' responses? Also, Hofling et al. failed to report what proportion of nurses actually tried to check the instruction with fellow nurses or superiors; they reported only the number of nurses who (eventually) complied.

This is fascinating as the issue is still relevant today. The study results seem to reflect the increasing autonomy in the nursing profession. Nearly all the 1966 night duty nurses acted with 'blind obedience'; only 2 of the 18 1977 nurses didn't check the drug at all. The night duty argument shouldn't apply surely? I think that now, day or night, everyone would check the drug and its side effects and question it if they were uncertain. Although … after reading about the Milgram experiment can I be sure of that?

- According to Krackow and Blass (1995), these two studies provide some evidence of nurses' compliance with inappropriate orders. However, both studies were conducted some years ago, at a time when individuals in our society were perhaps more likely to comply with authority. Their own study was designed to provide a more contemporary perspective on the extent to which nurses actually follow doctors' orders that they believe may have harmful consequences for the patient. More specifically, it aimed at identifying the factors – demographic, situational and atributional – that would distinguish between instances of nurses' obedience to and defiance of doctors' inappropriate orders. This study is described in Key Study 9.4.

KEY STUDY 9.4

When nurses obey or defy doctors' inappropriate orders

- The participants were 500 registered nurses, a representative sample of all registered nurses in the U.S. state of Maryland. Their mean age was 38.8 (ranging from 23 to 64 years). They had 1–35 years of nursing experience (a mean of 13 years).

- Participants were randomly assigned to receive one of two versions of a questionnaire. One version asked the respondent to 'recall the most recent time you carried out a physician's order that you felt could have harmful consequences to the patient …'. The other version asked the nurse to recall when he refused to carry out such an order. The rest of the questions were identical in both versions.

- The compliant and non-compliant nurses did not differ significantly with respect to age, gender, nursing qualifications, years of experience, work setting or job title/ status.

- There was also no significant difference based on the type of order given (e.g., relating to medication or some other matter), time of day when the order was given, how the order was given (verbal/written/telephone), the gender of the doctor or the doctor's position and status.

- Compliance also did not differ as a function of the years in which the incident took place (1950s to 1992).

- Nurses, overall, attributed most of the responsibility to the doctor, less to themselves, and least to the patient. Compliant nurses assigned more responsibility to the doctor than to themselves, but among non-compliant nurses responsibility was more evenly split between themselves and the doctors.

- Regardless of whether they were compliant or non-compliant, nurses rated a statement reflecting doctor power as legitimate authority ('The physician had the right to provide the overall direction for patient care') as being the most accurate. Next most accurate was a statement reflecting the doctor's expert power. ('By virtue of his or her many years of medical training, and/or information about the patient, I trusted that the physician had the expertise to make sound decisions'). The lowest accuracy rating was given to the statement reflecting informational power ('The physician shared information with me which led me to understand the rationale for carrying out the prescribed treatment').

Source: Krackow, A. and Blass, T., *Journal of Social Behaviour and Personality, 10*(3), 585–594, 1995.

(Research note to myself!) So the tendency to comply (the dependent variable) hasn't changed, but the factors that affect it (the independent variables) have. Of them the strongest influence was the perception of the doctors as the accepted authority, then as being the experts. The weakest influence on compliance was when they shared information and explanations with nurses, which seems more like the doctor–nurse relationship now. Nigel, however, still seems to think we should see the consultant (and him?) as the expert to be obeyed.

Krackow and Blass conclude that their findings, as indicated earlier by Hofling et al. and Rank and Jacobson, 'provide contemporary evidence that Milgram's work may still be generalisable to the nurse/physician relationship'. Their study indicates that the nurse perceives the doctor primarily as a legitimate authority (consistent with Milgram's explanation; see earlier). Again,

> The fact that one-half of the respondents in this study carried out inappropriate orders indicates that in spite of societal changes in the perception and acceptance of authority, the obedience paradigm is still relevant … (Krackow and Blass, 1995).

Although all nurses attributed greater responsibility for (potential) harmful consequences to the doctor than to themselves, those who were obedient accepted less responsibility themselves than those who were defiant. This is consistent with Milgram's (1974) finding that obedient participants accepted less responsibility for delivering electric shocks compared with defiant participants; this, in turn, is consistent with his agentic state explanation. However, all Milgram's participants assigned the same amount of responsibility to the experimenter, whereas the obedient shifted more responsibility to the learner than did the disobedient. In Krackow and Blass's study, both compliant and non-compliant nurses assigned minimal and equal amounts of responsibility to the patient. The patient is only passively involved in this situation, while the stooge learner in Milgram's experiments was perceived as a volunteer and an active participant.

So, the most significant influence after all was the perception of how responsible we are for our actions. Non-compliance seems to be linked to awareness of accountability. Tameka asking me if I'd have given the Gentamycin made me remember that as a student I'm responsible for not doing what I'm not trained to do. The NMC Code (2002) states, 'You must possess the knowledge, skills and abilities required for lawful, safe and effective practice without direct supervision' (Tschudin, 2003: 99). This means that Tameka is accountable for her own safe practice and therefore obliged to question what she thinks is unsafe.

TIME FOR REFLECTION …

- How do you see the relationship between nursing and medical staff?
- Who has more power/authority, and who perceives themselves as having greater power/authority?
- What forms does this greater power/authority take?
- How do these power/authority differences affect patient care? (See Critical Discussion 9.1.)

CRITICAL DISCUSSION 9.1

Nurse–doctor relationship

- Thirty years ago, at least, the stereotypical roles associated with doctors and nurses were very much in place (Robotham, 1999). Stein (1967) described a definite doctor–nurse 'game' being played out in wards across U.S. hospitals where power was weighted in favour of the medical staff. Nurses were able to suggest courses of action to doctors in such a way as to enable doctors to restate these as their own, so maintaining their superior public image. The system was undeniably hierarchical. This appears to have been replicated in U.K. hospitals.

- According to Stein et al. (1990), 'The game is dead … one of the players (the nurse) has unilaterally decided to stop playing the game and instead is consciously and actively attempting to change both nursing and how nurses relate to other health professionals.' However, Tellis-Nyak and Tellis-Nyak (1984) and Porter (1995) believe the model still applies.

- While doctors have a lot of respect for nurses, it is often subverted by problems and the issue of responsibility. Quite often, a task is transferred to the nurse but the responsibility stays with the doctor.

- In an interview study of general practitioners (GPs) and district nurses, Rowe (1999) found that nurses were keen to expand their roles and it was acknowledged by all participants that district nurses had become experts in certain areas, such as wound care and palliative care. But both groups agreed that the doctors had a continuing responsibility for their registered patients, which made the GPs cautious when delegating care to nursing colleagues. This, in turn, made nurses feel they needed to earn the GPs' trust to be able to expand their areas of work. But this sits rather uneasily with the claim that nursing is controlling its own agenda and with the United Kingdom Central Council's *Code of Professional Conduct*, which states, 'As a registered nurse, midwife or health visitor you are personally accountable for your practice'. GPs felt threatened by nurses taking over areas of work traditionally seen as theirs, making it difficult for them to share responsibility with nurses.

- However, nurses as a whole might look towards midwifery to see which path the nurse–doctor relationship could take. Midwives have been used to working officially with professional accountability and responsibility for some time now (Rowe, 1999) (see Key Study 9.4).

- According to Brooking (1991), while nurses are no longer subservient to the more powerful medical profession, medicine retains much of its power in relation to nursing for reasons such as the following:
  - Doctors usually have legal responsibility for admission, discharge, diagnosis and prescription and see themselves as having overall responsibility for all aspects of care and treatment.
  - Nurses are required (in part of their role at least) to carry out medically prescribed treatment, but the converse is not true.
  - Nurses may feel accountable to doctors even for nursing treatments; nurses, in contrast, are unlikely to comment to doctors on matters of diagnosis and prescription.

(Continued)

CRITICAL DISCUSSION 9.1 *(Continued)*

- Doctors have greater knowledge of disease and its treatment as a result of their longer and more intense education.
- Nursing is still a predominantly female profession, whereas most senior doctors are male.
- None of these differences would matter if nurses were not clearly dissatisfied with their relationships with doctors (and vice versa) (Brooking, 1991). But why should this matter? Brooking argues,

    … If we can agree that teamwork in health care is essential, it should also be self-evident that teams will function most effectively when their various members understand and respect each other's roles and perspectives …

Having responsibility means 'to know the boundaries clearly and to be accountable, especially if any limits are overstepped' (Tschudin 2003: 99). Nigel obviously regarded the doctor's prescriptive role as absolute and considered Tameka had overstepped hers!

Issues of generalisation

As we noted earlier, Orne and Holland (1968) argued that Milgram's experiments lack mundane realism (or *external* or *ecological validity*). But Milgram (1974) maintains that the process of complying with the demands of an authority figure is essentially the same, whether the setting is the artificial one of the psychological laboratory or a naturally occurring one in the outside world. While there are, of course, differences between laboratory studies of obedience and the obedience observed in Nazi Germany, 'differences in scale, numbers and political context may turn out to be relatively unimportant as long as certain essential features are retained'. The essential features that Milgram refers to is the agentic state – seeing yourself as the instrument of someone else's will (see pages 194 and 195).

What do Milgram's studies tell us about ourselves?

Perhaps one of the reasons Milgram's research has been so heavily criticised is that it paints an unacceptable picture of human beings. Thus, it is far easier for us to believe that a war criminal like Eichmann was an inhuman monster than that 'ordinary people' can be destructively obedient (what Arendt [1965] called the 'banality of evil').

Power of social situations

Social roles provide models of power and powerlessness, as in parent–child, teacher–student and employer–employee relationships. Rather than asking what makes some people more obedient than others, or how we would have reacted if we had been one of Milgram's participants, we could instead ask how we would behave if put into a position of authority ourselves. How easily could we assume the role and use the power that goes with it?

Zimbardo's research

As we noted earlier, Zimbardo et al.'s (1973) prison simulation experiment illustrates the impact of uniforms and other visible symbols of authority, and for this reason it is usually discussed in relation to obedience. However, it is also relevant to certain aspects of conformity and, like Milgram's obedience studies, it demonstrates the power of social situations to make people act in uncharacteristic ways. A brutalising atmosphere (like a prison) can induce brutality in people who are not usually brutal (see Gross [2010, 2012b]).

Patient compliance: Doing what you are told

TIME FOR REFLECTION ...

- Have you ever been non-compliant? For example, have you ever failed to complete a course of antibiotics?
- Why did not you comply?
- Why do you think it is important to understand non-compliance?

Concepts of compliance and adherence

As we noted in the *Introduction and overview*, the term compliance implies that the patient is passively obeying the requests of the more powerful health professional. Not surprisingly, the traditional concept of compliance is becoming increasingly unsuitable in modern patient-centred nursing. As Marland (1998) puts it, 'The value judgements inherent in the label of non-compliance serve only to scupper any attempts to involve patients as partners in care'.

The traditional definition implies a paternalistic view of the nurse–patient relationship, where the nurse is the expert and the patient is in a dependent, childlike role. (This mirrors the view of the doctor–nurse–patient triad, as father–mother–child, respectively.) If the patient is not yielding and acquiescent, the label non-compliant may cause the patient to be viewed as troublesome (Holm, 1993). The non-compliant patient may be seen as failing in a moral duty towards the nurse ('letting me down'). Hence, the term adherence will be used in the rest of this section.

 Are nurses to patients as doctors are to nurses? The role of both the 'passive nurse' and the role of the 'passive patient' are changing, and patient empowerment is described by the RCN (2003) as a central function in nursing. But Hewitt (2002) suggests that nurses' deference to medical staff leaves the patients with the perception that nurses are powerless, so they're not likely to be seen as facilitators of patients' empowerment (Christensen and Hewitt-Taylor, 2006). Obviously not so in Tameka's case.

Operationalising adherence/non-adherence

There are numerous ways in which patients' behaviour can deviate from recommendations, with varying implications for clinical outcomes (Horne and Clatworthy, 2010). For example, a patient could

- Take all the required medication but not at the correct time.
- Miss occasional doses.
- Take 'drug holidays' (i.e., miss 3 or more days' doses).
- Take lower or fewer doses than prescribed.
- Never take the medication.
- Take larger or more frequent doses than prescribed.

According to Horne and Clatworthy (2010), there is no universally accepted way of measuring adherence/non-adherence that distinguishes 'adherers' from 'non-adherers'. However, the method used can impact the resulting adherence rates. Table 9.1 describes some common methods used to measure adherence to medication.

None of these methods represents a 'gold standard'. At first sight, it may appear that direct measures, such as biological assays, would be the best methods. However, the amount of a drug/drug metabolite in a biological fluid is determined not only by the amount taken but also by individual variation in pharmacokinetic processes (e.g., the absorption, distribution, metabolism and elimination of the medicine). These measures can, therefore, indicate whether someone has taken any of the medicine but is unlikely to be sensitive to dose or timing variations (i.e., they are qualitative but not quantitative measures of adherence) (Horne and Clatworthy, 2010).

Indirect, behavioural measures of adherence (such as electronic monitoring of medication containers) may provide objective measures of adherence. However, they are subject to the Hawthorne effect: people may change their behaviour because they know they are being monitored. In this way, they may in themselves act as adherence interventions, rather than giving an accurate estimation of adherence levels (Horne and Clatworthy, 2010).

Self-report measures are often criticised for being subjective and prone to response bias (e.g., people overestimate their adherence). However, they are the only means of finding out why the person was non-adherent (e.g., was it intentional or unintentional?).

So the direct/indirect methods (i.e., all but the 'self-report measures') are to find out whether or not adherence occurs, not why it doesn't. It's not always lack of information given to patients. On two occasions I've heard staff nurses explaining to pre-op patients who were smokers how not smoking prior to the operation would help them cope with the anaesthetic better. Both ignored their advice and as soon as they were able went outside to smoke. One, pushed in a wheelchair by his helpful partner, was taken ill outside and had to be brought back and given oxygen.

Table 9.1 Methods of measuring medication adherence

Direct	
Observation	Adherence assessment is made by directly observing patients taking their medication. Widely used in the treatment of tuberculosis, but as an intervention to improve adherence rather than as a means of measuring adherence.
Biological assays	Usually blood or urine samples are taken and analysed to detect levels of the drug/ drug metabolites.
Indirect	
Pill count	Patients are asked to bring all their medication containers to their appointment. The remaining tablets are counted and the percentage of prescribed doses taken is calculated.
Self-report	Patients are asked to describe their adherence either in an interview or through completion of a questionnaire or diary.
Repeat prescription/pharmacy refill records	Records of when the patients collect or fill prescriptions are monitored. Actual collect/fill date is compared with the date medication would have been needed if all doses had been taken as prescribed.
Electronic monitor	Caps of medication bottles contain a computer chip and record each time the container is opened. Caps are scanned and the data downloaded onto a computer.

Source: Horne, R. and Clatworthy, J., *Health Psychology* (2nd edn.), BPS Blackwell, Oxford, 2010.

TIME FOR REFLECTION ...

- What might be some of the advantages and disadvantages of these different methods?

Problem of non-adherence

As more and more people are being treated with medicines to manage the effects of chronic disease, the issue of adherence is of pressing importance to nursing. It is an important area of research primarily because following health professionals' recommendations is considered essential to patient recovery.

According to Ekerling and Kohrs (1984), about 50% of patients with enduring health problems do not comply with medical regimes, regardless of diagnosis. This suggests that their non-adherence is not simply explained in terms of particular symptoms. According to the World Health Organisation (2003), approximately a third to a half of all medication prescribed for long-term conditions are not taken as directed; rates vary widely between 5% and 100% (DiMatteo, 2004). One reason for this variation relates to differences in methods of assessment (see Table 9.1).

Wouldn't some of these, like self-report, be extremely suspect, especially if they wanted to give an impression of complying? And doesn't wanting to present an impression of compliance suggest an 'obedient' attitude? That doesn't seem to fit the idea of autonomous patients.

Impact of non-adherence

The implicit assumption behind adherence research is that adherence improves patient outcomes. DiMatteo et al. (2002) reviewed 63 studies investigating the relationship between adherence to medical advice (including prescribed medication, diet modification, physical activity and eye patching) and outcomes (including survival, reported pain, blood pressure control, visual acuity, cholesterol levels and organ rejection). Overall, the odds of having good treatment outcomes were three times higher among high adherers than low adherers.

Focusing specifically on medication adherence and using an objective outcome measure, a review of 21 studies found that the odds of dying among those with high adherence were almost half those of low adherers (Simpson et al., 2006).

So the 'motivation' element works both ways – if you believe in the treatment you will adhere, if you adhere you get better.

The impact of adherence varies across conditions, ranging from minor effects on outcomes in some conditions to making the difference between life and death in others. Non-adherence cannot be explained by the type or severity of disease, with rates of 25%–30% noted across 17 disease conditions (DiMatteo, 2004). A key priority for adherence research and the development of adherence interventions is, therefore, to focus on the conditions where adherence matters most, that is,

- Where there is strong evidence supporting the benefits of medication
- Where high levels of adherence to treatment are essential to ensure efficacy or prevent problems, such as treatment resistance in HIV, transplantation and moderate to severe asthma (Horne et al., 2006)

A different kind of impact of non-adherence is the financial burden it places on the National Health Service NHS. NICE (2009b) estimated that hospital admissions resulting from medication non-adherence costs the NHS up to £196 million annually. In addition, up to £4 billion per year is wasted on prescribed medication that is not taken as directed.

 This is a socio-economic and political issue which is becoming more and more relevant in the NHS now.

Explaining non-adherence

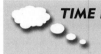 **TIME FOR REFLECTION ...**

- Which models of health behaviour do the five factors listed in Box 9.2 derive from (see Chapter 10)?

 It seems to me that Diana (an obese patient – see case study 2, page 234) only managed partial adherence to her 'treatment'. She seemed to understand the severity and risks of her weight and smoking (1 and 2) and did take her BP medication faithfully but lacked the confidence and motivation to believe she could maintain the behaviour (dieting and giving up smoking) that would reduce the threat (3,4 and 5).

A more general factor that might help explain adherence is that patients who are highly adherent to medications are more likely to engage in other health-promoting behaviours (Horne and Clatworthy, 2010).

According to Marland (1998), chronic illness often involves a close nurse–patient relationship. The nurse may learn why the patient chooses not to follow

---

Box 9.2 What makes patients adhere?

According to Damrosch (1995), there is theoretical agreement regarding the importance of five factors that make patients most likely to comply:

1. They perceive the high severity of the disorder (*serious consequences*). For example, Brewer et al. (2002) examined the relationship between illness cognitions (see Chapter 10) and adherence to medication and cholesterol control in patients with hypercholesterolaemia (very high cholesterol). A belief that the illness has serious consequences was related to medication adherence.
2. They believe the probability of getting the disorder is also high (*personal susceptibility*).
3. They have confidence in their ability to perform the behaviour prescribed to reduce the threat (*self-efficacy*).
4. They are also confident the prescribed regimen will overcome the threat (*response efficacy*).
5. They have the intention to perform the behaviour (*behavioural intention*).

Damrosch refers to these five points as the *double high/double efficacy/behavioural intention* model.

the advice of health professionals, which may help the nurse gain a deeper understanding of the patient's decision-making processes. This may, in turn, result in interventions that ensure a match between the patient's wishes and therapeutic effectiveness. When patients fail to discuss their medication-taking behaviour openly, they may decide their own level of dose, which may be sub-therapeutic. The prescriber may then decide to increase the dose, as the patient seems not to be responding. If the patient then decides to take the prescribed dose, there may be side-effects or even toxicity. As Marland says, 'It is essential … to find ways to establish an open and honest therapeutic alliance. The traditional concept of compliance is a barrier to such a relationship.'

Cheesman (2006) says the term 'compliance' has been replaced by the term 'concordance' – where prescribing and medicine taking are based on partnership and increasing patient empowerment. However, as in the nurse–doctor relationship, doesn't increased autonomy mean patients are expected to take increased responsibility and accountability for non-adherence?

Variables that do not seem to influence adherence rates

Knowing how is not enough, as demonstrated by the following:

- While providing the patient with clear information is essential, it is not sufficient to guarantee adherence (Horne and Clatworthy, 2010).
- Information-based interventions do not tend to improve adherence to long-term treatments (Kripalani et al., 2007).

There is also little evidence that adherence behaviours can be explained in terms of

- Personality characteristics
- Socio-demographic variables (such as gender and age)

The notion of the non-adherent patient is a myth: most of us are non-adherent some of the time. Non-adherence is a *variable behaviour*, not a trait characteristic. Personality traits and socio-demographic variables are *fixed* variables; they can help identify groups that are 'at risk' for non-adherence but can do little to inform the type or content of these interventions. For this, we need to identify potentially *modifiable* causes of non-adherence (Horne and Clatworthy, 2010).

Perceptions and practicalities approach

As with most other behaviours relating to health and illness, the many causes of non-adherence can be classified as intentional/volitional and unintentional/non-volitional. The recognition that human behaviour can be understood as a combination of both types of factors is fundamental to modern psychology (Horne and Clatworthy, 2010). This distinction forms the basis of the *perceptions and practicalities approach* (Horne, 2001) for understanding non-adherence and developing interventions to support optimal adherence (see Figure 9.3).

Figure 9.3 Perceptions and practicalities approach. (From Horne, R. and Clatworthy, J., *Health Psychology* (2nd edn.), BPS Blackwell, Oxford, 2010.)

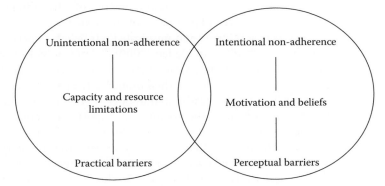

Unintentional non-adherence occurs when limitations in the patient's resources (including abilities) thwart his or her intentions to adhere; these resources include the following:

- Poor recall or comprehension of instructions
- Difficulties in administering the treatment
- Financial costs of the treatment
- Simply forgetting to take it

Intentional non-adherence occurs when the patient decides not to follow the treatment recommendations; this reflects the following:

- The beliefs (and other cognitions) and preferences or emotions influencing the person's motivation to begin and continue with a treatment; these cognitive and motivational factors can produce perceptual barriers to intentional non-adherence.

Perceptual and practical barriers need to be addressed by different types of interventions. For example, perceptual barriers might be addressed by cognitive behavioural techniques (see Chapters 2 and 3) or motivational interviewing; by contrast, practical barriers might be overcome by interventions that increase capacity or improve ability (such as reminder systems to reduce forgetting).

Each individual will have a unique mix of perceptual and practical barriers to adherence, affected by socio-demographic, cultural and economic factors, as well as personality traits. Interventions should be tailored to meet the needs of individuals.

This again seems relevant to Diana (case study 2, page 240), but it also sounds very complicated and some require specialist skills; I wonder how practical it would be for a community nurse like Sally to deliver?

Practitioner variables and doctor–patient communication

Doctors' sensitivity to patients' non-verbal expression of feelings (such as tone of voice) is a good predictor of adherence. For example, Dimatteo et al. (1993)

conducted a 2-year longitudinal study of over 1800 patients with diabetes, heart disease or hypertension and 186 doctors. The doctors' job satisfaction, willingness to answer questions and practice of scheduling follow-up appointments were all powerful predictors of adherence.

The way practitioners communicate their beliefs to patients also influences adherence. According to Ogden (2000), '… not only do health professionals hold their own subjective views, but … these views may be communicated to the patient in a way that may then influence the patient's choice of treatment.'

According to the traditional model of doctor–patient communication (the *education model*), the doctor is an expert who communicates his or her knowledge to a naive patient. The doctor is an authority figure, who instructs or directs the patient. Research has suggested that the communication process may be improved if a sharing, more interactive (two-way), *patient-centred* consulting style is used. This may produce greater patient commitment to any advice given, potentially higher levels of adherence and greater patient satisfaction.

However, a field experimental study by Savage and Armstrong (1990) of patients attending a group practice in an inner-city area of London found a preference for the education model. Patients (aged 16–75, without serious illnesses) seemed to prefer an authority figure, who offered a formal diagnosis, to a 'sharing' doctor who asked for their views.

On my community placement, I went with a diabetic patient to the diabetes clinic. I met one young patient who'd researched her condition on the Internet and knew all about the cause and complications. She asked lots of questions and was very much in control of her diet and health regime. My elderly patient was the opposite; she answered but didn't ask any questions and kept emphasising she'd stuck faithfully to the doctor's instructions. She seemed very anxious for the doctor's approval.

Patient and regimen variables

Adherence is likely to decrease over time. It's also more problematic for conditions with no obvious symptoms, especially if treatment produces unpleasant side-effects, such as reduced sex drive. Also, the more complex the regimen, the lower the adherence. For example, home monitoring of blood sugar up to 10 times per day and multiple insulin injections have been shown to greatly reduce or eliminate adherence. But this is a lifelong practice, which is probably daunting to many patients (Damrosch, 1995).

According to Ley's (1981, 1989) *cognitive hypothesis model*, compliance can be predicted by a combination of the following:

- Satisfaction with the process of consultation (see earlier)
- Understanding of the information given
- Recall of this information

Ley's model has been influential in promoting research into communication between health professionals and patients. But it is consistent with the education model of doctor–patient communication and so is subject to the same criticisms (see the study by Ogden [2004]).

Preferring a more interactive approach, Ogden et al. (1999) investigated (1) the level of agreement between patient and health professional and (2) the impact of this agreement on patient outcome. It is important to understand the extent to which the two individuals 'speak the same language', share the same beliefs, and agree about the desired content and outcome of any consultation. This is especially relevant to general practice, where patient and health professional perspectives are most likely to coincide.

Once a treatment is prescribed, the patient is often left to his or her own devices. Adherence then depends on his or her interpretation of the illness, treatment and symptoms. Siegel et al. (1999) studied middle-aged and older HIV-positive people and their drug adherence. Once taking the drugs, they would question their efficacy and safety if they noticed any unusual symptoms. If they perceived these as side-effects of the drugs, or if the drugs seemed to be having no effect, the conditions were ripe for non-adherence. But according to Forshaw (2002),

- because a drug seems to be doing nothing that doesn't mean it is, and unpleasant symptoms that appear after taking the drug aren't necessarily caused by the drug;
- drugs can sometimes take a while to start working, but people often expect immediate results. Also, we often think that if a problem seems to have cleared up, then it has. People commonly stop taking their antibiotics when the symptoms have eased – but these often recur because they're just the final stage of unseen bodily processes.

Forshaw (2002) believes that

> Careful education of patients as to exactly what to expect from a treatment can improve adherence, especially in cases where non-adherence stems from lack of knowledge rather than rebelliousness ...

So we are back to the 'knowledge' argument again; the fact it keeps recurring is surely significant in spite of the knowledgeable smokers' rebellion!

Adherence and the placebo effect

Evidence suggests that simply adhering to medical recommendations to take pills may benefit patients recovering from a heart attack, regardless of whether the pills taken are active drugs or inert placebos (see Chapter 3 and Gross [2012b]). This has implications for understanding the mind–body relationship ('I believe I've taken my medication' is related to actually getting better) and the central role of beliefs and expectations in health and illness (Ogden, 2000).

Ogden cites data suggesting that the best predictor of mortality in men who had survived a heart attack was not taking the lipid-lowering drug compared with a placebo but adherence to taking any drug at all (active or placebo).

Adherers had lower mortality after 5 years than non-adherers in both experimental and placebo groups. Ogden concludes by saying '… "doing as the doctor suggests" appears to be beneficial to health, but not for the traditional reasons ("the drugs are good for you") but perhaps because by taking medication, the patient expects to get better …'.

But I wonder … would the ones who took the medication faithfully be more likely to adhere to a healthy diet and exercise etc.?

In Simpson et al.'s (2006) review of 21 studies (see page 206), those who adhered to medication were significantly less likely to die than those who adhered to a placebo (as we would expect). However, there was also an 'adherence effect' in the placebo group: the odds of dying among high adherers to the placebo were approximately half those of low placebo adherers.

The incident with Tameka makes me aware of how power and accountability affect our relationships in relation to obedience and adherence. Being autonomous professionals means accepting responsibility for what we do as opposed to being in an 'agentic state'. Florence Nightingale did advocate intelligent obedience, but said also that blind obedience 'might … do for a horse' but it was 'a very poor thing for a nurse' (Kuhse 1997, page 26). My feelings of discomfort when Tameka challenged a doctor's authority must indicate that I still lack conviction in the idea of nurse–doctor equality. However, the example of Tameka asserting her own authority will give me confidence in future to question instructions that worry me. Even as a student, I'm accountable; all health professionals are equally responsible within our very different roles. However, nurses provide care, psychological support and advocacy on a continuous basis, so they should not have to be subservient to any other health care professional (doctor or otherwise).

Considering all these role relationships has helped me understand why 'concordance', where autonomous patients see themselves as responsible partners in their own care, is more likely to produce adherence to therapeutic behaviour. Milgram's and other studies have helped explain some significant behaviour during one small incident at work which led to much wider issues. And again Goodman's (1984) third level of reflection (see case study 2, page 230) helps me link ethical and socio-economic influences to the way we think and behave.

CHAPTER SUMMARY

- *Compliance* is a factor in different kinds of social influence, including conformity, obedience and our responses to other people's direct requests.
- While both conformity and obedience involve the abdication of personal responsibility, *obedience* involves orders from someone in higher authority with influence being in one direction only.

- Milgram's series of 18 obedience experiments involves a basic procedure (*remote victim/voice feedback*) and variations on this, involving the manipulation of critical variables.
- Increasing the proximity to the victim (proximity and touch proximity: variations 3 and 4); reducing the proximity of the experimenter (remote authority: variation 7) and having the social support of rebel fellow teachers (two peers rebel: variation 17) all reduced obedience, while having someone else actually deliver the shock increased it (a peer administers the shocks: variation 18).
- According to Milgram, two related variables that are crucial for understanding obedience are *acceptance/denial of responsibility* and the *agentic state*. The latter represents the opposite of the *autonomous state* and is what makes it possible to function in a hierarchical social system.
- The wearing of uniform and other such symbols of authority are also important, as demonstrated in Zimbardo et al.'s prison simulation experiment.
- Milgram's experiments have caused great ethical controversy but have also been criticised on scientific grounds.
- The *mundane realism* of Milgram's procedure is supported by Hofling et al.'s naturalistic experiment involving nurses, and Milgram believes that obedience is essentially the same process regardless of the particular context.
- Hofling et al.'s experiment also showed that what nurses say they would do if given potentially dangerous orders by a doctor and what they actually do are two different things: social situations are very powerful influences over individuals' behaviour. However, Rank and Jacobson's replication challenged the findings of the original study.
- Krackow and Blass's more recent replication found that nurses perceive the doctor primarily as a legitimate authority; this is consistent with Milgram's agentic state account of obedience and shows that his work is still valid.
- Patient *non-adherence* is very common, although this varies depending on the particular disorder. It applies to both chronic and acute conditions, and even to organ transplant patients.
- Adherence/non-adherence can be measured in various ways, both direct (observation and biological assays) and indirect (pill count, self-report, repeat prescription/pharmacy refill records and electronic monitor).
- The *double high/double efficacy/behavioural intention model* identifies the five factors that make adherence most likely: serious consequences, personal susceptibility, self-efficacy, response efficacy and behavioural intention.
- Adherence is unaffected by access to information, personality characteristics or socio-demographic variables (such as gender and age).

- The distinction between *unintentional* and *intentional non-adherence* has important implications for interventions, which must first identify the individual's specific barriers; appropriate techniques are then selected for each barrier.
- Adherence is affected by both *practitioner* and *patient/regimen variables*. The former include how doctors communicate their beliefs to patients, and the latter include patients' satisfaction with the consultation and their understanding/recall of the information given.
- Simply adhering to medical recommendations to take pills may benefit patients recovering from a heart attack regardless of whether the pills taken are active drugs or inert placebos.

10 Social cognition and health behaviour

Introduction and overview

According to the biomedical model, *disease* is a deviation from a measurable biological norm. This view, which still dominates medical thinking and practice, is based on several invalid assumptions. Most importantly, the *specificity assumption* maintains that understanding of an illness is greater if it can be defined at a more-specific biochemical level. According to Maes and van Elderen (1998), traditional medicine is more focused on disease than on health: 'It would be more appropriate to call our health care systems "disease care systems", as the primary aim is to treat or cure people with various diseases rather than to promote health or prevent disease'.

By contrast with the biomedical model's *reactive* attitude towards *illness*, the biopsychosocial (BPS) model underlying Health Psychology adopts a more *proactive* attitude towards *health*. Many definitions of health have been proposed since the 1940s, mostly in terms of the *absence* of disease, dysfunction, pain, suffering, and discomfort. Also, in opposition to the biomedical model's reductionist view, the BPS model adopts a *holistic* approach – that is, the *person as a whole* needs to be taken into account. It maintains that both *'micro-level'* (small-scale causes, such as chemical imbalances) and *'macro-level'* (large-scale causes, such as the extent of available social support) processes interact to determine someone's health status.

Health beliefs (HBs) are important determinants of health behaviour. Understanding why people do or do not practise behaviours to protect their health can be assisted by the study of *models/theories of health behaviour*, such as,

- The Health Belief Model (HBM)
- The Theory of Reasoned Action (TRA)
- The Theory of Planned Behaviour (TPB)
- The Protection Motivation Theory (PMT)
- The Health Action Process Approach (HAPA)

According to Ogden (2004), these various models/theories are often referred to, collectively, as *social cognition models*, because they regard cognitions as being shared by individuals within the same society (see Chapter 2). But Ogden prefers to distinguish between

- Social cognition models (such as TRA and TPB), which aim to account for social behaviour in general and are much broader than health models
- Cognition models (such as HBM, PMT and HAPA), which are specifically *health models*

 From my diary (2): Year 1/Community/District Nurse

Today Sally, my community nurse mentor, and I visited Diana who is 42, morbidly obese (her BMI is 46.5), with a pressure sore that needs dressing. Sally went through Diana's medical history for my benefit: medications, diet, etc. and explained that she lives alone following her divorce some years ago and is a smoker; she is hypertensive and has had several attacks of bronchitis. She's had a shower room and a bariatric toilet installed, has a bariatric reclining chair and wheelchair but was in bed when we arrived.

According to Bulman and Schutz (2008, page 35) a good reflective description should include 'what you were thinking at the time; how you were feeling at the time.' And my first reaction when I saw Diana (although I'd tried to prepare myself) was shock. Sally's attitude was matter-of-fact, which helped; she showed me how to take Diana's blood pressure (BP) and I was pleased I got the same reading as Sally at my second attempt. As she attended to the small sore on Diana's hip I chatted to her, trying hard not to let my feelings (a mixture of bewilderment and disapproval) show. Eventually (perhaps reflecting what was on my mind) I asked how her diet was going and she confessed she'd eaten a whole packet of chocolate biscuits the evening before which a (well-meaning) friend had brought. She said she knew she was 'hopeless' and looked so downcast that I felt sorry for her then, but later when Sally was discussing Diana's chesty cough with her I was off again – thinking, well, it's all her own fault for smoking.

Defining health and illness

Health beliefs

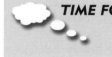
TIME FOR REFLECTION ...

- What do you understand by the terms 'health' and 'illness'?
- Are you healthy if you're not ill, or is health a more positive state than this?

According to Holland and Hogg (2001), the concept of health is broad and complex, with a wide range of meanings. HBs are ideas or conceptualisations about health and illness derived from the prevailing worldview and, like the culture which determines that worldview, they may change over time. For example, despite the link with skin cancer, sunbathing/suntans are still associated with health and well-being (Holland and Hogg, 2001). Like health behaviour, HBs may be *health damaging* as well as *health promoting* (sunbathing again).

Box 10.1 Defining health and illness

- According to the World Health Organization (WHO, 1947), *health* is 'a complete state of physical, mental, and social well-being and not merely the absence of disease or infirmity'. Including 'social well-being' in the definition opened the way to conceptualising the individual as a social being, part of a bigger entity than his/her own body (Uskul, 2010). Later, WHO (1982) referred to the importance of sociocultural factors by claiming that if actions are to be effective in the prevention of diseases and in the promotion of health and well-being, they must be based on an understanding of culture, tradition, beliefs and patterns of family interaction.
- *Disease* is a 'state of the body characterised by deviations from the norm or measurable biological or somatic variables' (Maes and van Elderen, 1998).
- *Illness* is 'the state of being ill, implying that illness is a more psychological concept, which is closely related to one's own perception of a health problem (e.g. pain)' (Maes and van Elderen, 1998). Subjective psychological symptoms, such as anxiety, also play a substantial role in the construction of illness. Similarly, although illness is usually associated with evidence of medical abnormality, 'it also incorporates aspects of the individual's wider functioning, self-perceptions and behaviours, and requires consideration of social context and societal norms' (Turpin and Slade, 1998).
- The concepts of health and illness incorporate physical, psychological and social aspects, reflecting the BPS model.

Diana's weight and BP deviate from the norm, she has mobility problems, hypertension, intermittent bronchitis, a chronic cough and a bedsore, yet she didn't seem to consider herself ill. However, I certainly don't consider her healthy.

According to Ogden (2004), most people define health *positively* (not just as the absence of illness). Lau (1995) found that young, healthy adults described 'being healthy' in terms of several dimensions:

- *Physiological/physical* (e.g. good condition/has energy)
- *Psychological* (happy, energetic, feeling good)
- *Behavioural* (eating and sleeping properly)
- *Future consequences* (live longer)
- *The absence of* (not sick, no disease, no symptoms)

Diana doesn't meet any of these criteria, which is sad. She could be healthy if she changed her lifestyle, but this would mean changing her health beliefs and behaviour.

Health beliefs in nursing practice

According to Holland and Hogg (2001), conflicting HBs can leave both nurses and patients feeling frustrated and failing to understand each other. Ultimately, this may cause the patient to abandon or ignore health care services (see Chapter 13).

Nurses enter the profession with ideas about health and illness that are unique and that have been shaped by their ethnic and cultural background. They then bring those beliefs to the health arena, hospital wards, community and therapeutic settings, influencing nursing practice in the prevention and treatment of illness. These beliefs may change as nurses integrate with their professional colleagues and absorb the beliefs, values and attitudes of the nursing culture. This is reflected in nursing language, such as 'doing the obs', 'off duty', 'doing the cares', 'doing the backs' and 'handover'. As with all cultures, the nursing culture may become 'hidden', because nursing practices become the norm ('second nature'). Unless nurses are aware of this, a gap may develop between the nurse/other health care providers and the recipient (Holland and Hogg, 2001; see Chapter 13).

Box 10.2 Three categories/systems of health beliefs (Holland and Hogg, 2001)

1. *HBs based on biomedicine*: This corresponds to the biomedical model, which was developed in and dominates the health systems of North America and Western Europe. It has been exported all over the world. Diseases are caused by *pathogens* (bacteria/viruses) entering the body or by biochemical changes in the body due to conditions or events (such as wear and tear, accidents, nutritional deficiencies, the ageing process, injury, stress, smoking and alcohol). The body is a complex machine, whose various parts function together to ensure health. Health practitioners are highly educated, powerful and respected specialists, whose position and power are upheld by the law. In general, they concentrate on treating just the diseased/injured body part, with mind and body being seen as two separate entities (see Chapter 3): 'Biomedicine may be regarded as an attacking force, and militaristic terminology such as "battling cancer", "fighting disease", or "winning the war against germs" is commonly used …'.

2. *HBs based on personality (or magico-religious) systems*: Illness is caused by (1) the active intervention of a sensate agent, possibly a supernatural force (such as God or some other deity); (2) non-humans (such as ghosts, ancestors or evil spirits) or (3) human beings, witches or sorcerers. These are all forces beyond the individual's control, but illness may be punishment for some misdeed. The 'evil eye' as a cause of illness or distress is accepted in Europe, the Middle East, North Africa, Central and South America. An Indian Muslim woman who, according to a biomedical perspective, might have been diagnosed with post-natal depression and treated with antidepressants, believed that her low mood, insomnia and leg pains were caused by the 'Jinns' (malevolent spirits that cause ill health). The Imam at her local mosque performed the appropriate ceremony and she returned to 'normal' health.

3. *HBs in naturalistic systems*: Naturalism (or *holism*) dates back to the ancient civilisations of Greece, India and China. They explain illness in personal and systemic terms. Health is the balance between elements (such as heat and cold) in the body. Human life is only one aspect of nature and is part of the natural cosmos. Any disturbance or imbalance causes illness, disease or misfortune. These beliefs form the basis of traditional health practices in many Asian countries (including China, Japan, Singapore, Taiwan and Korea), as well as South America, the Philippines, Iran and Pakistan.

Health beliefs also change over time within the same culture; nursing culture has changed radically since the inception of Project 2000. For instance, 'doing the backs' reflects a task-based approach that is out of date; my own beliefs are already being challenged by knowledge of the biopsychosocial model in nursing. However, reflecting with Sally on our visit, I confessed I found it difficult to feel sympathetic towards Diana as I felt her condition was self-inflicted. She agreed that Diana's behaviour was frustrating sometimes, but we must care for her as she is, not as we think she ought to be.

Although our National Health Service was based on a biomedical model, the nursing profession no longer accepts the 'mind–body split'; the BPS model is fundamental to nursing practice.

Culture and health

Traditionally, medical anthropologists have been interested in the role of sociolcultural factors in health and illness. They have extensively examined how illness is conceptualised and treated differently across cultures (Helman, 1994; Kleinman, 1980). Medical sociologists have studied the effects of larger societal structures or institutions, such as medical delivery systems, on health and illness (Bird et al., 2000). Now, psychologists are asking research questions that incorporate sociocultural variables into health and illness, investigating them in groups from different sociocultural backgrounds (Uskul, 2010).

As Box 10.2 shows, HBs differ between cultures. Culture represents one of the 'macro-level' processes referred to above (see Boxes 10.3 and 10.5). *Cross-cultural health psychology* (Berry, 1994) involves two related domains:

1. The earlier, more established study of how cultural factors influence various aspects of health. Cross-cultural research can help researchers test their theories and assumptions in different cultural environments; practitioners

---

Box 10.3 Health, disease and illness as cultural concepts

- Many studies have shown that the very concepts of health and disease are defined differently across cultures. While 'disease' may be rooted in pathological biological processes (common to all), 'illness' is now widely recognised as a culturally influenced subjective experience of suffering and discomfort (Berry, 1998) (see Box 10.1).
- Recognising certain conditions as either healthy or a disease is also linked to culture. For example, trance is seen as an important curing (health-seeking) mechanism in some cultures, but may be classified as a sign of psychiatric disorder in others. Similarly, how a condition is expressed is also linked to cultural norms, as in the tendency to express psychological problems *somatically* (in the form of bodily symptoms) in some cultures (e.g. Chinese) more than in others.
- Disease and disability are highly variable. Cultural factors (such as diet, substance abuse and social relationships within the family) contribute to the prevalence of diseases including heart disease, cancer and schizophrenia (Berry, 1998).

in the field can be equipped with the knowledge to interact with individuals from different cultural backgrounds (Uskul, 2010).

2. The more recent and very active study of the health of individuals and groups as they settle into and adapt to new cultural circumstances, through migration, and of their persistence over generations as ethnic groups.

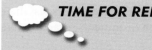 At this time, in Western culture, obesity is well defined as contributing to disease; Diana is showing clear signs of the damage it is doing to her health.

Acculturation

Cross-cultural psychologists believe that there's a complex pattern of continuity and change in how people who have developed in one cultural context behave when they move to and live in a new cultural context. This process of adaptation to the new ('host') culture is called *acculturation*. With increasing acculturation (the longer immigrants live in the host country), health status 'migrates' to the national norm (Berry, 1998).

For example, coronary heart disease (CHD) among Polish immigrants to Canada increased, while for immigrants from Australia and New Zealand, the reverse was true. Immigrants from 26 out of 29 countries shifted their rates towards those of the Canadian-born population. Similar patterns have been found for stomach and intestinal cancer among immigrants to the United States (Berry, 1998).

TIME FOR REFLECTION ...

- How could you explain such findings?
- What is it about living in a different cultural situation that can increase or decrease your chances of developing life-threatening diseases?

One possibility is exposure to widely shared risk factors in the physical environment (e.g. climate, pollution, pathogens), over which there's little choice. Alternatively, it could be due to choosing to pursue assimilation (or possible integration) as the way to acculturate. This may expose immigrants to *cultural* risk factors, such as diet, lifestyle and substance abuse. This 'behavioural shift' interpretation would be supported if health status both improved *and* declined relative to national norms. However, the main evidence points to a *decline*, supporting the 'acculturative stress' (or even 'psychopathology') interpretation – the very process of acculturation may involve risk factors that can reduce health status. This explanation is supported by evidence that stress can lower resistance to disease, such as hypertension and diabetes (Berry, 1998) (see also Chapter 5).

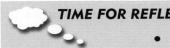 My Asian parents must have experienced 'acculturative stress', but they still maintain their (healthy) vegetarian diet whereas I've adopted a more Western (though still healthy!) one.

Culture and the experience of different medical conditions

According to Uskul (2010):

> Our sociocultural environments shape our psychology regarding health and illness – that is, how we think of, feel about and act upon our physical states. Perhaps more striking is that individuals' (reported) physical experiences seem to also be shaped by their sociocultural environments

TIME FOR REFLECTION ...

- How does this view of the impact of sociocultural environments relate to the BPS model of health and illness?

Two examples of the impact of sociocultural influences are menopause and pain.

Menopause

The experience of menopause illustrates how previously universally defined physical signs of a certain stage of the life cycle may actually vary, depending on cultural characteristics. For example, Lock (1986) observed that Japanese women view menopause as a natural life-cycle transition; the biological marker of cessation of menstruation is not considered to be of any great importance. Japanese women also reported different (and fewer) symptoms from those in the West. For example, the former experienced hot flushes or sudden perspiration very infrequently, while these were among the most commonly reported by Western women.

Pain

In Poland, labour pains are both expected and accepted by women giving birth, while in the United States, they are not accepted and analgesia is commonly demanded (Zborowski, 1952). Zborowski claims that this illustrates how a cultural group's expectations and acceptance of pain as a 'normal' part of life will determine whether it is seen as a clinical problem requiring a clinical solution.

How one reacts to pain killers may also differ between cultures and not all cultures are equally willing to use 'pain-killing' medication (Uskul, 2010). Poliakoff (1993) suggested that many Chinese people fear that such medication will make them feel that they are out of control; this makes them reluctant to use them. Similarly, Hindus who believe that they are close to death may wish to do so 'clear-headed' rather than sedated; they may also believe that pain (and other negative feelings) are the result of wrongs they have committed in the past (Poliakoff, 1993).

Culture and health care seeking

Uskul (2010) cites evidence that people from different sociocultural backgrounds tend to differ in the extent to which they delay seeking medical help. For example, being a member of an ethnic minority group can add to delay. Black women tend to have a more advanced breast cancer when detected and, as a consequence, have poorer survival rates than white women once the cancer is detected. Hispanic women also have later-staged tumours and decreased survival rates. Gentleman and Lee (1997) found that Canadian women are less likely to have mammograms if they are single, have less education, are unemployed and are immigrants from South America, Central America, the Caribbean, Africa or Asia.

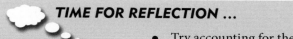

TIME FOR REFLECTION ...

- Try accounting for these differences.

Cultural differences in delay in health care seeking have been attributed to a diverse set of factors, ranging from knowledge and beliefs regarding causes of the disease, associated symptoms, curability and consequences to trust in doctors (Uskul, 2010). Factors of a more sociocultural nature have also been considered. For example, in the context of breast cancer again, women's place in their society can shape their help-seeking behaviour by influencing their priorities. Chinese women indicate concern about potential or actual disruptions in performing their duties in the event of breast cancer symptoms (Facione et al., 2000; Mo, 1992). Similarly, South Asian societies focus on how women should act, how they should fulfil their family responsibilities and how they should maintain their proper place in the community; these all involve putting others first and may result in delaying engagement in health care behaviours (Bhakta et al., 1995; Bottorf et al., 1998).

Maisie (see case study 1, page 50) delayed seeing a doctor about her pain through fear: she knew cancer caused her husband's death, believed she had the same condition and assumed the outcome would be the same. (However, this could well be cross-cultural.)

Culture and doctor–patient relationships

Some cultural norms heavily regulate gender relationships even in health care settings such as hospitals. Female members of certain cultural groups may be reluctant to be examined by male doctors; even the anticipation of this happening may contribute to delays in – or complete avoidance of – seeking health care (Facione et al., 2000; Uskul and Ahmad, 2003). Some Asian women, despite having lived in North America for a while and speaking English, indicated that they may choose to access traditional Chinese medicine: the traditional Chinese doctor examines the patient without asking her to take her clothes off (Facione et al., 2000).

Yes, my own mother, although considerably anglicised, will go to great lengths to see a female rather than a male doctor. She would feel even more strongly about male nurses.

Individualism–collectivism, health and illness

Psychologists have identified a number of *cultural syndromes* as a way of accounting for observed cultural differences and similarities in human psychology. Some examples include the following: *tight versus loose* (Triandis, 1995); *masculine versus feminine* (Hofstede, 1980) and *high versus low power distance* (Hofstede, 1980). The most commonly used cultural syndrome is *individualism–collectivism* (Hofstede, 1980; Triandis, 1995). This is described in Box 10.4.

My own divorce was very much disapproved of by my Asian grandmother; less so by my anglicised parents.

Box 10.4 Individualism–collectivism

- *Individualism–collectivism* refers to whether one's identity is defined by personal choices and achievements (the autonomous individual: *individualism*) or by characteristics of the collective group to which one is more or less permanently attached, such as the family, tribal or religious group, or country (*collectivism*).
- In *individualistic* cultures (such as the United States and the United Kingdom), the self is seen as *independent*: people are agentic and, therefore, responsible for their own decisions and actions. There is a focus on the positive outcomes one hopes to approach rather than the negative outcomes one hopes to avoid. Relationships are regarded as freely chosen and easy to both enter and exit.
- In *collectivist* cultures (such as many East Asian countries), the self is seen as *interdependent*, embedded within the social context and defined by social relations and membership in groups. People are seen as relational or communal and their decisions and actions as heavily influenced by social, mutual obligations and the fulfillment of in-group expectations. Individuals tend to be motivated to fit in with their group and maintain social harmony; they focus on their responsibilities and obligations while trying to avoid behaviour that might cause social disruption or disappoint significant others. Relationships are seen as less voluntary and more difficult to leave.

Source: Based on Smith, P.B. & Bond, M.H. *Social Psychology Across Cultures* (2nd edn.). Hemel Hempstead, UK: Prentice-Hall Europe, 1998; Marcus, H.R. and Kitayama, S. *Psychological Review*, 98, 224–253, 1991; Triandis, H., Theoretical concepts that are applicable to the analysis of ethnocentrism. In R.W. Brislin (ed.), *Applied Cross-Cultural Psychology*, Newbury Park, CA: Sage, 1990; *Culture and Social Behaviour*, New York, McGraw-Hill, 1994; *Individualism and Collectivism*, Boulder, CO, Westview Press, 1995.

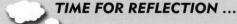

TIME FOR REFLECTION ...

- How do you think such cultural differences in how the self and relationships are perceived might impact on how health and illness are experienced and acted upon?

Individualism is likely to make individuals focus on the physical body and wellness: having a healthy body can be characterised as a goal in its own right. Both Rose (1996) and Lock (1999) link the American cultural focus on wellness, avoidance of illness and improvement of health to the American cultural focus on self-actualisation and personal responsibility (see Chapter 2). Similarly, Americans' desire to maintain health has been linked to their wish to be autonomous individuals (Baumeister, 1997; Crawford, 1984).

By contrast, *collectivism* is likely to regard illness as a to-be-avoided breakdown in one's abilities to carry out one's duties and obligations (Uskul and Hynie, 2007; Uskul and Oyserman, 2010). Having a healthy body is a resource that facilitates fitting into the social order. Collectivists, therefore, will experience a strong desire to avoid the negative social obligation consequences of ill-health.

Illness cognitions/representations

In the same study described above (see page 217), Lau (1995) asked participants 'What does it mean to be sick?' Responses revealed several dimensions:

- *Not feeling normal* ('I don't feel right')
- *Consequences of illness* ('I can't do what I normally do')
- *Timeline* (how long the symptoms last)
- *Absence of health* (not being healthy)

These dimensions have been described within the context of *illness cognitions* (illness beliefs or representations), a patient's own implicit common-sense beliefs about their illness (Leventhal et al., 1980, 1997). These provide patients with a framework for coping with and understanding their illness, telling them what to look out for if they're becoming ill. Based on interviews with adults who were chronically ill, recently diagnosed with cancer or healthy, Leventhal et al. identified five cognitive dimensions of these beliefs (overlapping with those found by Lau: see above).

1. *Identity:* the label given to the illness (medical diagnosis) and the symptoms experienced.
2. *Perceived cause:* may be biological (virus/lesion) or psychosocial (stress/health-related behaviour).
3. *Timeline:* beliefs about how long the illness will last (acute/short term or chronic/long term).
4. *Consequences:* may be physical (pain/lack of mobility), emotional (loss of social contact/loneliness), or some combination of these.
5. *Curability and controllability:* can it be treated/cured? How controllable is it – either by themselves or powerful others (e.g. doctors)?

Health locus of control (HLoC) refers to an individual's belief as to whether their health

- Is controllable by them (e.g. 'I'm directly responsible for my health')
- Is in the hands of fate (e.g. 'Whether I'm well or not is a matter of luck')
- Is under the control of powerful others (e.g. 'I can only do what my doctor tells me to do')

The first example describes someone with an *internal* HLoC, while the second and third describe an *external* HLoC (see Chapter 5).

Diana has developed identifiable 'diseases': hypertension and bronchitis. Although she 'knows' that over-eating and smoking contributes to both I'm not sure she perceives them as a cause. She watches a great deal of TV and doesn't go out as, apart from her reduced mobility, she gets upset if people stare at her. She seems to accept her obesity as her fate, something she 'can't help' and, although she felt guilty at 'breaking her diet', felt 'hopeless' at controlling her behaviour. She's clearly an external HLoC person.

Box 10.5 Culture and illness cognitions/representations

- A small number of studies have shown that illness cognitions/representations are closely linked to a culture's philosophical and spiritual orientations that shape individuals' connectedness with other people and the physical world.
- In *individualistic* cultures, physiological aspects of illness are given greater weight and are typically seen as separate from the social and physical environments in which individuals are embedded.
- In *collectivist* cultures, physiological aspects of illness are given lesser weight and illness beliefs are shaped by holistic worldviews connecting relational, collective and physical forces. For example, Maori in New Zealand identify spiritual, mental, physical and family well-being as interrelated dimensions of health: a breakdown in one dimension is likely to cause illness (Durie, 1994).
- In India, belief in Karma, God and spirits are understood to be important determinants of many events in one's life, including illness and suffering (Kohli and Dalal, 1998). Karma holds that good and bad deeds accumulate through a series of lives and people face the consequences: physical suffering is typically attributed to one's misdeeds in this and/or previous lives. God is an external agent who controls reward and punishment, not always according to what one deserves. The belief in fate implies that one can do little to change the course of events.
- In studies with Indian patients, Kohli and Dalal (1998) found that belief in fate and God's will are negatively correlated with perceived controllability, that is patients who attribute their illness to fate and God's will perceive little control over the course of their illness. However, patients who believe God's will to be the cause of their illness show *greater* perceived recovery.
- As we saw above (page 224), collectivism is associated with an interpretation of ill-health in terms of social responsibility and a desire to avoid the failure to fulfil social obligations. For example, Uskul and Hynie (2007) found that patients in collectivist cultures are more likely to report shame and embarrassment about their illness.

According to Uskul (2010):

> ...the health-care process is likely to be facilitated if attention is paid to patients' culturally shaped appraisals of their symptoms, the assumptions they make about the causes and how responses to medical advice are conditioned by the culturally shaped theories they use to understand their bodily responses. Understanding the illness theories used by patients offers the potential for improved communication, better treatment and enhanced adherence to medical advice.

Although part of an individualistic culture, Diana seems to blame the fact she 'puts on weight easily' (a physiological cause) for her obesity and that she 'can't help' smoking to reduce the undoubted stress she feels. As this is at odds with treatment, it isn't likely she will be able to adhere to professional advice.

Illness and Health Psychology

According to the BPS model:

- Individuals are not just passive victims, but are responsible for taking their medication, changing their beliefs and behaviour
- Health and illness exist on a continuum – people are not *either* healthy *or* ill, but progress along the continuum, in both directions
- Psychological factors contribute to the *aetiology* (causation) of illness – they are not just consequences of illness.

According to Ogden (2000, 2004), health psychology aims to

- *Evaluate* the role of behaviour in the aetiology of illness, such as the link between smoking, CHD, cholesterol level, lack of exercise, high blood pressure and stress (see Chapter 5)
- *Predict* unhealthy behaviours – for example, smoking, alcohol consumption and high-fat diets are related to beliefs, and beliefs about health and illness can be used to predict behaviour (see Chapter 12)

TIME FOR REFLECTION ...

- Can you think of examples of where your being ill was (partly) caused by psychological factors and where your illness affected you psychologically?

- *Understand* the role of psychological factors in the experience of illness – for example, understanding the psychological consequences of illness could help to alleviate pain, nausea, vomiting, anxiety and depression (see Chapter 3)
- *Evaluate* the role of psychological factors in the treatment of illness (see Chapter 3)

These aims are put into practice by

- *Promoting* health behaviour, such as changing beliefs and behaviour (see Chapter 6)
- *Preventing* illness – for example, by training health professionals to improve communication skills and to carry out interventions that may help prevent illness (see Chapter 9)

All these factors relate to Diana. She is progressing towards worse illness, but, according to this model, could reverse that direction by changing her health beliefs. But in this case, conflicting beliefs of the professional and patient (see Holland and Hogg, 2001) are leaving us all frustrated. So far, Sally said, the nurses, doctor, physiotherapist, dietician, occupational therapist and social services have all failed to change Diana's beliefs and behaviour!

Health behaviour

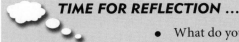

TIME FOR REFLECTION ...

- What do you understand by the term 'health behaviour'?
- Can you identify different types – and examples – of health behaviour?

Steptoe et al. (2010) distinguish between two broad types of health behaviour: those that increase risk and those that promote health (see Table 10.1).

- They define risk behaviour as *'any activity undertaken by people with a frequency or intensity that increases risk of disease or injury'* (their emphasis). This indicates that the amount or 'dose' of the behaviour may be important: while cigarette smoking is not qualified in terms of how much (implying that *any* cigarette smoking is risky), it is *excessive* alcohol consumption that is risky. Indeed, they cite evidence that moderate consumption is associated with *more favourable* health outcomes than either heavy drinking or complete abstinence.
- Positive health behaviours are *'activities that may help to prevent disease, detect disease and disability at an early stage, promote and enhance health, or protect from risk of injury'* (their emphasis).

The definitions above show that the concept of health behaviour is fluid: activities that are included can and do change as medical knowledge advances. For example, it's only in the past 25 years or so that using a condom as a precautionary

Table 10.1 Common risk-increasing and health-promoting behaviours

Risk increasing	Health promoting
Cigarette smoking	Regular physical exercise
Taking narcotic drugs	Eating fruit and vegetables
Excessive alcohol consumption	Using sunscreen
Eating large amounts of high-fat foods	Wearing a seatbelt
Some sexual behaviours	Driving sensibly
Drink driving	Taking advantage of medical and dental screening opportunities (such as cancer screening)

Source: Steptoe, A. et al., The role of behaviour in health. In D. French, K. Vedhara, A.A. Kaptein and J. Weinman (eds.), *Health Psychology* (2nd edn.), Oxford, BPS Blackwell, 2010.

measure when having sex with someone whose sexual history is unknown to us has become common practice (as opposed to a form of contraception).

Steptoe et al.'s definitions also recognise that certain health-relevant activities may be performed for non-health reasons. For example, tooth-brushing and eating a low-fat diet may be driven by non-health motives such as wishing to look good. For this reason, 'Health psychologists need to view behaviour in a broad context, and recognise that health motivations and cognitions are part of a wider set of influences on health behaviour' (Steptoe et al., 2010).

Diana's behaviour is definitely risk-taking. Interestingly, the fact that healthy behaviour need not be health-motivated may be a clue to helping her.

Determinants of health behaviour

According to Steptoe et al., appreciating this wider set of influences on health behaviour is important for three major reasons:

1. Recognising the broader social and cultural context provides a fuller understanding of individual behaviour.
2. Non-psychological (i.e. non-individual) factors may limit the impact that interventions can have on changing behaviour.
3. The broader determinants remind us that most people do not engage in positive health activities or risky behaviours primarily for health reasons, or often even for conscious reasons at all.

Steptoe et al. identify several different kinds of factors that can affect health behaviour (see Figure 10.1):

1. *Sociocultural and national factors*, including national, cultural and religious *tradition* regarding food and cooking, alcohol and smoking and sexual behaviour.

2. *Legislative factors*, such as laws regarding tobacco and alcohol and other drugs (see Chapter 12).
3. *Macroeconomics*, including the overall state of the national economy and the availability of individuals' disposable income.
4. *Systems of provision and services*, such as manufacturers making readily available palatable low-fat foods, the availability of sport and leisure facilities, and the provision of smoke-free environments.
5. *Health-service provision*, including the availability of appropriate health services (such as cancer screening, immunisation programmes and health checks for markers like blood pressure and cholesterol level).
6. *Sociodemographic factors*: age, gender, and socioeconomic status.
7. *Health status*: the ability to perform many health behaviours is affected by personal health, while illness may provide additional motivation for behaviour change. For example, many people with disabilities or chronic lung disease are limited in the physical exercise they are capable of. Diagnosis with a condition such as CHD or non-insulin-dependent diabetes may provide the stimulus for weight reduction through dietary change and physical exercise.

Figure 10.1 Summary of determinants of health behaviour. (Based on Steptoe, A. et al., The role of behaviour in health. In D. French, K. Vedhara, A.A. Kaptein and J. Weinman (eds.), *Health Psychology* (2nd edn.), Oxford, BPS Blackwell, 2010.)

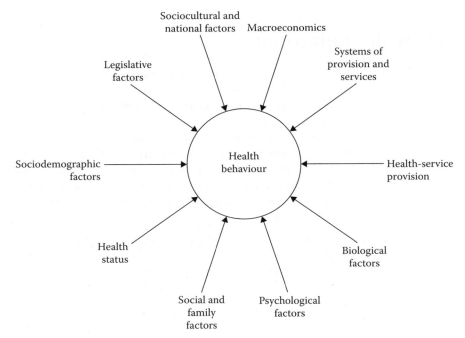

8. *Social and family factors*: family habits have a strong impact on food choice, cigarette smoking, alcohol consumption and physical exercise habits. Health behaviours have been successfully modified through social support interventions, as in studies of supportive lay health advisors to encourage breast cancer screening among rural African American women (Earp et al., 2002).

9. *Psychological factors*, which are largely (but not exclusively) cognitive. (These are discussed further in relation to models of health behaviour: see pages 231 through 241).

10. *Biological factors*: dietary choice may be influenced partly by the metabolic or psychological effects of particular nutrients, while alcohol has an important reciprocal relationship with biological stress responses (Sayette, 1993) (see Chapter 4). There is also increasing interest in investigating the impact of genetic factors on health-related behaviours; twin studies have found evidence for a heritable component to smoking initiation and nicotine addiction, as well as to body weight and obesity (Plomin et al., 2000) (see Chapters 2 and 11).

Goodman's (1984) model of Reflective Practice is helpful in analysing all the above factors. The first-level reflection is concerned with 'what works' (in terms of accepted accountability, efficiency and effectiveness); level two reflection assesses the consequences of actions and beliefs as well as their rationale which introduces debate on principles and practice. The third level incorporates much wider ethical and political concerns that affect health behaviour and links the 'setting of everyday practice and the broader social structure and forces' (Bulman in Bulman and Schutz, 2008, page 233).

Models of health behaviour

As we saw in the *Introduction and Overview*, Ogden (2004) distinguishes between cognition models, which are specifically *health* models, and social cognition models, which are general accounts of cognitions shared by individuals within a particular society.

A fundamentally important question for health psychology is why people adopt – or do not adopt – particular health-related behaviours. Models of health behaviour try to answer this question, and most of those discussed below belong to the family of *expectancy-value models* (Stroebe, 2000). These assume that decisions between different courses of action are based on two types of cognition:

1. *Subjective probabilities* that a given action will produce a set of expected outcomes
2. *Evaluation* of action outcomes

So, considering the consequences for Diana, she might think, a) I will lose weight and therefore be healthier if I change my diet and lifestyle and b) as a result I'll feel healthier, be more attractive – but will forever be 'on a diet'.

Individuals will choose from among various alternative courses of action the one most likely to produce positive consequences and avoid negative ones. Different models differ in terms of the *types* of beliefs and attitudes that should be used in predicting a particular class of behaviour. They are *rational reasoning models*, which assume that individuals consciously deliberate about the likely consequences of behavioural alternatives available to them before engaging in action.

Theory of Reasoned Action

This has been used extensively to examine predictions of behaviour and was central to the debate within social psychology regarding the relationship between attitudes and behaviour (see Chapter 6). TRA assumes that behaviour is a function of the *intention* to perform that behaviour (Ajzen and Fishbein, 1970; Fishbein, 1967; Fishbein and Ajzen, 1975). A behavioural intention is determined by

- A person's *attitude* to the behaviour, which is determined by (1) beliefs about the outcome of the behaviour, and (2) evaluation of the expected outcome
- *Subjective norms* – a person's beliefs about the desirability of carrying out a certain health behaviour in the social group, society and culture s/he belongs to (see Figure 10.2).

Figure 10.2 Main components of the theory of reasoned action. (Adapted from Penny, G., Health psychology. In H. Coolican (ed.), *Applied Psychology*, London, Hodder & Stoughton, 1996; Maes, S. and van Elderen, T., Health psychology and stress. In M.W. Eysenck (ed.), *Psychology: An Integrated Approach*, London, Longman, 1998.)

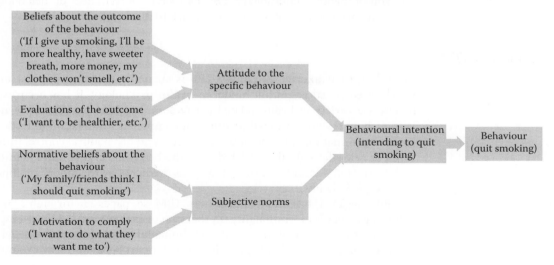

An attitude is comprised of what we think/believe, feel and do about certain things (Chapter 6, pages 128 and 129). I concluded from Diana that she did believe sticking to her diet would make her healthier, felt she **should** do it and so was guilty and depressed that she'd 'failed again'.

Evaluation of TRA

TRA has successfully predicted a wide range of behaviours, including blood donation, smoking marijuana, dental hygiene and family planning. However, attitudes and behaviour are only *weakly* related: people do not always do what they say they intend to (see Chapter 6). The model does not consider people's past behaviour, despite evidence that this is a good predictor of future behaviour. Nor does it account for people's irrational decisions (Penny, 1996). Similarly, Maes and Elderen (1998) argue that 'The assumption that behaviour is a function of intentions … limits the applicability … of the model to volitional behaviour, that is, to behaviours that are perceived to be under personal control'

A purely cognitive approach like TRA doesn't help us understand **why** Diana, for instance, eats biscuits on impulse i.e. what comes between her intention and 'giving in'.

Theory of Planned Behaviour

This represents a modification of TRA. It reflects the influence of Bandura's (1977, 1986) concept of *self-efficacy* – our belief that we can act effectively and exercise some control over events that influence our lives. Ajzen (1991) added the concept of self-efficacy to TRA, claiming that control beliefs are important determinants of *perceived behavioural control* (PBC). This is crucial for understanding motivation: if, for example, you think you are unable to quit smoking, you probably would not try. PBC can have a *direct* effect on behaviour, bypassing behavioural intentions (see Figure 10.3).

Evaluation of TPB

According to Walker et al. (2004), TPB is currently the most popular and widely used social cognition model in health psychology. It has been used to assess a variety of health-related behaviours. For example, Brubaker and Wickersham (1990) examined its different components in relation to testicular self-examination: attitude, subjective norm and behavioural control (measured as self-efficacy) all correlated with the behavioural intention. Schifter and Ajzen (1985) found that weight loss was predicted by the model's components, especially PBC.

TPB (like TRA) has the advantage over HBM (see pages 233 through 235) of including a degree of irrationality (in the form of evaluations), and it attempts to address the problem of social and environmental factors (normative beliefs). The extra 'ingredient' of PBC provides a role for past behaviour. For example,

Figure 10.3 Main components of the theory of Planned Behaviour. (Adapted from Ogden, J., *Health Psychology: A Textbook* (3rd edn.), Maidenhead, UK, Open University Press/McGraw-Hill Education, 2004.)

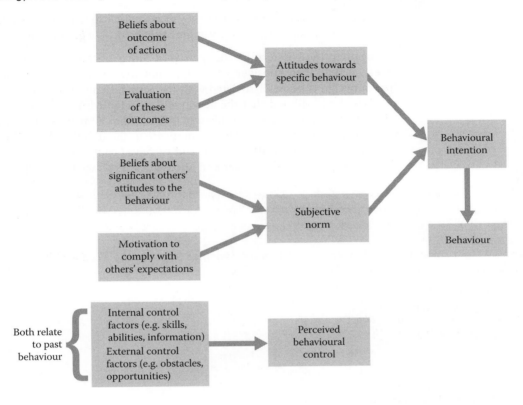

if you've tried several times in the past to quit smoking, you're less likely to believe you can do so successfully in the future and, therefore, you're less likely to intend to try (Ogden, 2000; Penny, 1996).

This sounds more realistic, if more complicated. It shows Diana needs to believe in her ability to succeed (self-efficacy), which her past failures to diet and give up smoking undermine. But it still doesn't explain *why* she fails each time – or how we can help her change.

Health Belief Model

This was originally developed by social psychologists working in the U.S. Public Health Service (Becker, 1974; Janz and Becker, 1984). They wanted to understand why people failed to make use of disease prevention and screening tests for early detection of diseases not associated with clear-cut symptoms (at least in the early stages). It was later also applied to patients' responses to symptoms and adherence to prescribed medication among acutely and chronically ill patients. More recently, it has been used to predict a wide range of health-related behaviours (Ogden, 2004).

HBM assumes that the likelihood that people will engage in a particular health behaviour is a function of

- The extent to which they believe they're *susceptible* to the associated disease
- Their perception of the *severity of the consequences* of getting the disease

Together, these determine the *perceived threat* of the disease. Given the threat, people then consider whether or not the action will bring benefits that outweigh the costs associated with the action. In addition, *cues to action* increase the likelihood that the action will be adopted; these might include advice from others, a health problem or mass-media campaigns. Other important concepts include *general health motivation* (the individual's readiness to be concerned about health matters) and *perceived control* (e.g. 'I'm confident I can give up smoking' – Becker and Rosenstock, 1987, see Figure 10.4).

I think the idea of cost is important. In Diana's case, she may well consider food and cigarettes the most (or only) pleasurable things in her life and her motivation would have to be very high to give them up. Seeing herself as 'hopeless' indicates her perceived behavioural control isn't high, either.

Figure 10.4 Main Components of the Health Belief Model. (Adapted from Stroebe, W., *Social Psychology and Health* (2nd edn.), Buckingham, Open University Press, 2000.)

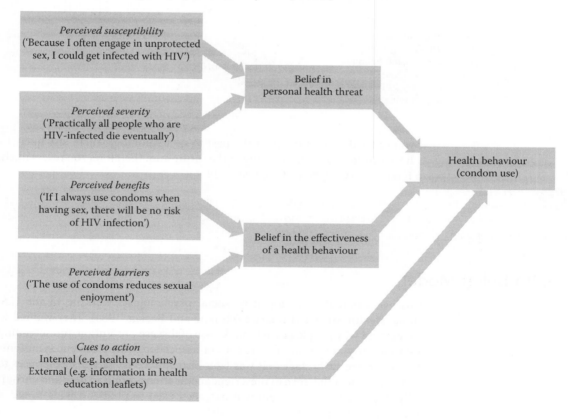

Perceived susceptibility
('Because I often engage in unprotected sex, I could get infected with HIV')

Perceived severity
('Practically all people who are HIV-infected die eventually')

Perceived benefits
('If I always use condoms when having sex, there will be no risk of HIV infection')

Perceived barriers
('The use of condoms reduces sexual enjoyment')

Cues to action
Internal (e.g. health problems)
External (e.g. information in health education leaflets)

Belief in personal health threat

Belief in the effectiveness of a health behaviour

Health behaviour (condom use)

Evaluation of HBM

- It allows for demographic variables – such as age and gender – and psychological characteristics – such as ways of coping with stress and locus of control (see Chapter 5) – that might affect HBs (Forshaw, 2002). For example, young women are likely to engage in dieting behaviour. So 'the HBM covers most, if not all, of the factors which, on the face of it, should be relevant in determining if a person engages in a particular behaviour' (Forshaw, 2002).
- There is considerable evidence supporting the HBM's predictions, in relation to a wide range of behaviours. Dietary compliance, safe sex, having vaccinations, having regular dental checks, participation in regular exercise programmes – all are related to people's perception of their susceptibility to the related health problem, their belief that the problem is severe and their perception that the benefits of preventative action outweigh the costs (Becker, 1974; Becker and Rosenstock, 1984; Becker et al., 1977).
- However, there is also conflicting evidence. For example, Janz and Becker (1984) found that healthy behavioural intentions are related to *low* perceived seriousness (not high as the model predicts). Also, several studies have suggested an association between *low* susceptibility (not high) and healthy behaviour (Ogden, 2004).
- HBM has also been criticised for assuming that people's behaviour is governed by rational decision-making processes, ignoring emotional factors, such as fear and anxiety, and overemphasising the individual. A factor that may explain the persistence of unhealthy behaviours is people's inaccurate perceptions of risk and susceptibility.

So this model has partial success; perhaps the complexity of human behaviour makes it unrealistic to expect one model to deal with all aspects of it?

Perceptions of invulnerability

According to Ogden (2000), one of the most consistent findings to emerge from the research is the perception of personal invulnerability to HIV, in both heterosexual and homosexual populations. For example, Woodcock et al. (1992) interviewed 125 16–25 year olds about their sexual behaviour and examined how they evaluated their personal risk. Even though most acknowledged some degree of risk, some managed to dismiss it by claiming, 'it would show by now', 'it was in the past', 'AIDS wasn't around in those days', 'it's been blown out of proportion' and 'AIDS is a risk you take in living'. The themes of being run over by a bus and 'it couldn't happen to me' were also quite common. These are classic examples of people *rationalising* behaviour that conflicts with important aspects of self-concept [see Festinger's (1957) *cognitive dissonance theory* in Chapter 6]. Most commonly, people denied that they had ever put themselves at risk.

While most models, such as HBM, TRA and TPB, emphasise people's rational decision-making, including their assessment of personal susceptibility to/being at risk from HIV:

> ...many people do not appear to believe that they are themselves at risk, which is perhaps why they do not engage in self-protective behaviour, and even when some acknowledgement of risk is made, this is often dismissed and does not appear to relate to behaviour change (Ogden, 2000).

Unrealistic optimism – the compelling sense that we are somehow less vulnerable to the kinds of problems others face ('it only happens to other people') – can be very hard to break down, thus undermining the extent to which we adopt health precautions (see Box 10.6). AIDS fits perfectly the profile of a risk for which most people tend to manifest unrealistic optimism (Harris and Middleton, 1995).

As Diana's hypertension is at present being treated by medication and although Sally has explained its association with heart attack and stroke, she probably doesn't perceive it as a threat.

Unlike TRA and TPB, there is no explicit reference in HBM to behavioural *intention*. Instead, central beliefs and perceptions act directly on the likelihood of behaviour. But it has been shown that adding intention to HBM increases its level of predictability, so it is now typically added when testing it. However, this blurs the distinction between HBM and other models. According to Harris

---

Box 10.6 Are we unrealistic optimists?

- Weinstein (1983, 1984) asked participants to examine a list of health problems and to state, 'Compared with other people of your age and sex, are your chances of getting [the problem] greater than, about the same, or less than theirs?' Most believed they were *less* likely, displaying what Weinstein called *unrealistic optimism*: not everyone can be less likely! Weinstein identified four cognitive factors contributing to unrealistic optimism:
  - Lack of personal experience with the problem
  - Belief that the problem is preventable by individual action
  - Belief that, if the problem has not yet appeared, it would not appear in the future
  - Belief that the problem is uncommon
- This suggests that perception of one's own risk *is not* a rational process. People show *selective focus*, ignoring their own risk-taking behaviour (e.g. the times they have not used a condom) and concentrating primarily on their risk-reducing behaviour (the times they have).
- This is compounded by the tendency to ignore others' risk-reducing, and emphasise their own risk-taking, behaviour. These tendencies produce unrealistic optimism.

and Middleton (1995), the trend is towards the development of generic models of health behaviour that incorporate the best 'bits' of other models. HAPA is a good example of such a generic model (see pages 239 through 241).

Protection Motivation Theory

PMT (Rogers, 1975, 1985; Rogers and Prentice-Dunn, 1997; Schwarzer, 1992) is an extension of HBM that includes *fear* as a motivating factor. Like HBM, it is a cognitive model, but unlike it, it proposes a motivation to protect oneself from danger (*protection motivation*). Once aroused, fear acts to promote, sustain and direct self-protective activity. Neither threat (HBM) nor fear (PMT) plays any role in TRA or TPB (Harris and Middleton, 1995).

Protection motivation arises as a result of combining two cognitive appraisals:

- *Threat appraisal* considers the current risky behaviour (e.g. smoking).
- *Perceived vulnerability* is defined as the perceived likelihood of the adverse outcome occurring and is conditional upon continuing the risky behaviour.

Perceived severity refers to the perceived extent of harm likely if the adverse outcome occurs. *Perceived rewards* of the risky behaviour increase the likelihood of its performance. *Fear* has only an *indirect* influence on protection motivation: fear arousal influences the appraisal of the threat's severity (threats that arouse more fear are seen as more severe). According to Rogers and Prentice-Dunn (1997):

Overall threat appraisal = (perceived severity + vulnerability)

− (rewards of the maladapative behaviour).

For example, a smoker would have a high threat appraisal if she believed she was very likely to develop CHD if she continued to smoke, that CHD is a life-threatening condition and that there were few benefits of continuing to smoke (Wright, 2010).

The severity of a heart attack is irrelevant if you believe it won't happen to you (unrealistic optimism). Diana believes smoking calms her, stops her eating so much and is of course addicted to nicotine.

Other components of PMT include the following:

- *Coping appraisal* considers the risk-reducing behaviour (e.g. quitting smoking).
- *Response efficacy* refers to the perceived effectiveness of the risk-reducing behaviour at reducing the threat.
- *Self-efficacy*.
- Beliefs about any physical or psychological costs (*response costs*) of the risk-reducing behaviour reduce its likelihood.

- Overall coping appraisal = (response efficacy + self-efficacy) – (perceived costs of the risk-reducing behaviour). For example, smokers might believe that quitting smoking would be an effective way to reduce their risk of CHD, feel fairly confident in their ability to quit, but be concerned that quitting may cause weight gain (Wright, 2010).

Threat and coping appraisals interact to influence motivation for risk-reducing behaviour: the impact of our threat appraisal on motivation depends on the level of our efficacy appraisal. According to Rogers and Prentice-Dunn (1997), if people believe they can cope with the threat (i.e. have high efficacy appraisals), then the greater the perceived threat, the greater their intentions for the risk-reducing behaviour. However, if people have low efficacy, then as perceived threat increases, their intentions to perform risk-reducing behaviour will decrease. (These two situations represent *positive* and *negative correlations*, respectively.)

It follows (according to PMT) that interventions aimed at increasing perceived threat will be counterproductive in individuals who have low efficacy for the risk-reducing behaviour. Ruiter and Kok (2006) argue that most smokers would have low self-efficacy, due to having already made several unsuccessful attempts to quit: their intentions to quit would decrease when faced with warning labels that increase their threat appraisals.

Yes, this is exactly relevant to Diana's case. The message 'Smoking Kills!' on every pack of cigarettes probably makes Diana more anxious – for which her remedy is smoking!

An evaluation of PMT

- PMT has been applied to a wide range of health threats and behaviours (Wright, 2010). Wright summarises the conclusions from two major meta-analytic studies (a 'study of studies' which measures the influence of/relationship between variables in terms of *effect size*) conducted by Milne et al. (2000) and Witte and Allen (2000).
- Together, these two meta-analyses suggest that variables specified by PMT have small to moderate relationships with intentions for, and actual, risk-reducing behaviour. Milne et al., focusing on health-related behaviours, found that PMT constructs predicted intentions more strongly than behaviour. Witte and Allen reviewed a broader range of behaviours and found a similar strength of prediction for intentions and behaviour (Wright, 2010).
- Milne et al. found stronger relationships between self-efficacy and response efficacy and intentions/behaviour than between threat variables and intentions/behaviour. This implies that reinforcing these beliefs may be an optimal strategy for increasing protective behaviours (Wright, 2010). Witte and Allen reported small, but very similar, effect sizes for these two sets of relationships.
- Most experimental manipulations of PMT variables have relied on written messages, which may be less suited for increasing self-efficacy than other PMT constructs (Wright, 2010). According to Bandura (1997), verbal

persuasion is a weaker influence on self-efficacy than *enactive mastery* experiences (e.g. successfully going a day without smoking) or *vicarious mastery* experiences (e.g. seeing someone similar to oneself successfully quitting).

So if Diana believed in her ability to succeed it would be more effective than any threat of illness. Vicarious mastery is used by slimming clubs where there is face to face encouragement, support and peer example. But what chance of this for Diana?

Health action process approach

Schwarzer (1992) criticised TPB for its lack of a *temporal* element – it does not describe either the order of the different beliefs or any direction of causality. Schwarzer attempted to address this issue in his HAPA. This explicitly brought together elements from TRA, TPB and HBM to form a generic model (see Figure 10.5).

The *decision-making/motivational stage* is an attempt to identify the key general processes involved when people make up their minds about whether or not to adopt health precautions. The *action/maintenance stage* tries to identify the factors that determine how hard they try and how long they persist. This is lacking in the other models (Harris and Middleton, 1995).

Figure 10.5 Major components of the Health Action Process Approach. (Based on Harris, P. and Middleton, W., Social cognition and health behaviour. In D. Messer and C. Meldrum (eds.), *Psychology for Nurses and Health Care Professionals*. Hemel Hempstead, UK, Prentice Hall/Harvester Wheatsheaf, 1995; Schwarzer, R., Self-efficacy in the adoption and maintenance of health behaviours: theoretical approaches and a new model. In R. Schwarzer (ed.), *Self Efficacy: Thought Control of Action*. Washington, DC, Hemisphere, 1992.)

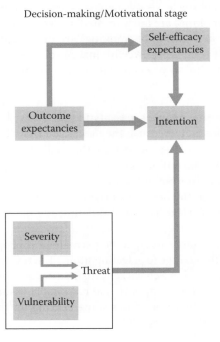

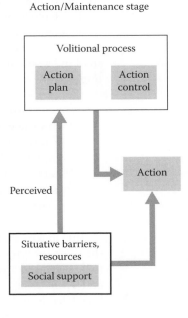

So the HAPA helps analyse Diana's lifestyle and attitude, her thoughts, feelings and the different stages of changing health behaviour. The barriers and support elements are also important; Diana's sister who smokes with her and the 'friend' who brought chocolate biscuits are barriers, not supports and a wider social influence, Diana's TV, serves up tempting food advertisements! However, political awareness of the economic cost of obesity has stimulated food labelling which may help to educate people about adverse consequences of some foods.

According to Schwarzer, self-efficacy is the most important factor, followed by outcome expectancy and threat. Consistent with this, he suggests that they (especially threat) may exert most of their impact on intention indirectly. So, perceiving yourself as at risk of lung cancer may be more influential in producing your intention to give up smoking if it prompts you to think of ways in which you might increase your self-efficacy for quitting. It will be less influential if it contributes to an intention to quit that you feel will be difficult to carry through.

So if Diana decided to try nicotine patches and ban smoking in the house, it would increase her self-efficacy; but if she decided simply to save her cigarette money for a holiday as soon as she'd got to her target weight (a long-term reward), that wouldn't?

Evaluation of HAPA

Perhaps more than the other models, HAPA addresses the key issue of *behaviour change*. This represents one of the central difficulties people face when adopting healthier regimes. According to Schwarzer, the key to successful *action control* (the amount of effort invested and the degree to which people will persevere in the face of obstacles) is *self-reinforcement*. The rewards associated with old habits (e.g. smoking) are fairly immediate (see Chapter 12), while those associated with the new ones (not smoking) are more remote and less tangible – and in the short term less powerful. Just as you cannot be sure the smoking would have killed you, so you can quit and die of something equally unpleasant:

> As a consequence, some people are ready to take risks with their health precisely because they construe this in terms of a gamble – they hope that they will be among the lucky few who will not get ill or believe that there are many other risks out of their control and that they might as well reap the benefits of their unhealthy habits in the meantime (Harris and Middleton, 1995).

This means that change is more likely to be permanent if people focus on the short-term rewards of the change (e.g. feeling fitter). The rewards that have to be sacrificed are often *social*, but Schwarzer's distinction between *perceived* and *actual* social support is consistent with the reasonable assumption that how friends and family actually respond has some bearing on the final outcome ('action') (Harris and Middleton, 1995).

Schwarzer's claim that self-efficacy is consistently the best predictor of behavioural intentions and change for a variety of behaviours is supported by studies of the effective use of contraception, addicts' intention to use clean needles, breast self-examination, quitting smoking, losing weight and exercising (Ogden, 2004). However, HAPA is subject to many of the limitations of all the models.

How effective are health belief models that do not facilitate behaviour change? HAPA includes planning strategies to maintain changed behaviour. And that – back to behaviourism – includes rewarding oneself to compensate for loss of pleasure (balancing cost by benefit). But does it address the underlying causes of negative health behaviour – the reason why Diana's health-damaging behaviour began and is so resistant to change?

An evaluation of models of health behaviour

A limitation shared by all the models is their failure to consistently predict behavioural intentions. Most seriously of all, they are unable to predict actual behaviour (the *intention–behaviour gap*). One response to these criticisms has been the concept of *implementation intentions* (Gollwitzer, 1993). Carrying out an intention involves the development of specific plans about what to do given a specific set of environmental conditions. These plans describe the 'what' and 'when' of a particular behaviour. There is some evidence that encouraging people to make implementation intentions can actually increase the correlation between intentions and behaviour for taking vitamin pills and performing breast self-examination (Ogden, 2000). Overall, current models are relatively poor predictors of actual behaviour (Turpin and Slade, 1998).

Implementation intentions can also allow a person to rehearse positive health behaviour, e.g. where children practise saying 'no' to drugs or sexual advances.

The models are all very general, covering all kinds of health-related behaviours; it may simply be invalid to apply the same model to a whole range of behaviours and illnesses. It may be necessary to model specific behaviour, such as in response to the threat of AIDS (as in Catania et al.'s AIDS risk-reduction model, 1990).

To date, most models of health behaviour are designed and tested in a Western cultural context and are therefore likely to be biased; they are *culturally relative* and we cannot just assume that they apply universally (Forshaw, 2002; Uskul, 2010). For example Sissons Joshi's (1995) study of causal beliefs about insulin-dependent diabetes in England and India found that far more Indian diabetics believed that eating too much sweet food caused their diabetes (38 per cent compared with 6 per cent of the English sample).

According to Uskul (2010), the incorporation of sociocultural factors into existing health models can contribute to a comprehensive understanding of the moderating factors that determine how illness cognitions are shaped or when behaviour is likely to change:

> It is time to collate the vast amount of knowledge accumulated in the hitherto disconnected subfields of cultural and health psychology and to explore the degree to which theories and models developed in the West can be used to understand health and illness-related psychological experiences elsewhere (Uskul, 2010).

Identifying 'causal belief' is part of understanding 'where patients are coming from', whatever their culture. The theory of each health model helped me understand how many factors are involved in changing health behaviour, but the HAPA model is most useful in day-to-day nursing, as it provides a practical (what works) framework 'to promote health and healing', which is firmly encompassed in the nursing role. (RCNONLINE www.rcn.org.uk/direct. Published: 2003-04-14)

Applications of models of health behaviour

Eating behaviour

Some studies have used the TRA and the TPB to explore the cognitive predictors of actual behaviour. For example, Shepherd and Stockley (1985) used the TRA to predict fat intake, and reported that it was more strongly predicted by attitude than by subjective norms. Similarly, attitude has also been found to be the best predictor of table salt use (Shepherd and Farleigh, 1986), eating in fast-food restaurants (Axelson et al., 1983), the frequency of consuming low-fat milk (Shepherd, 1988), and healthy eating defined as high levels of fibre and fruit and vegetables and low levels of fat (Povey et al., 2000). The social norms component of these models has consistently failed to predict eating behaviour (Ogden, 2010a).

Some studies have explored the impact of adding extra variables to the standard framework of the social cognition models. For example, Shepherd and Stockley (1987) examined the predictors of fat intake and included a measure of nutritional knowledge; they found that this was associated with neither their measure of attitudes nor their participants' behaviour. Povey et al. (2000) included additional measures of descriptive norms (e.g. 'To what extent do you think the following groups eat a healthy diet?') and of perceived social support (e.g. 'To what extent do you think the following groups would be supportive if you tried to eat a healthy diet?'); these variables did not add anything to the core cognitions of the TPB.

Other studies have explored the role of *ambivalence* in relation to food choice. Central to different definitions of ambivalence is the simultaneous presence of both positive and negative values, which seems particularly pertinent to food choice (e.g. 'tasty', 'healthy', 'a treat' versus 'fattening') (Ogden, 2010a).

KEY STUDY 10.1

Does ambivalence affect how much meat or chocolate we eat?

- Sparks et al. (2001) incorporated the concept of ambivalence into the TPB and assessed whether it predicted meat or chocolate consumption.
- 325 participants completed a questionnaire that included a measure of ambivalence assessed in terms of the mean of both positive and negative evaluations (e.g. 'How positive is chocolate?' and 'How negative is chocolate'?), then subtracting this mean from the *absolute* difference between the two evaluations (total positive minus total negative). This computation provides a score that reflects the balance between positive and negative feelings.
- In line with previous TPB studies, the results showed that attitudes *per se* were the best predictor of the intention to eat both meat and chocolate.
- However, the results also showed that the relationship between attitude and intention was weaker in those participants with higher ambivalence; that is holding both positive and negative attitudes to food makes it less likely that the overall attitude will be translated into an intention to eat it.

Source: Sparks, P. et al., *British Journal of Health Psychology*, 6, 53–68, 2001.

Consistent with research using social cognition models in other health-related areas, research into eating behaviour has also added *implementation intentions* as a means of changing eating behaviour which relate to the specific 'where' and 'when' a particular behaviour will occur (Ogden, 2010a).

For example, Armitage (2004) asked 264 participants recruited from a workplace in the north of England to rate their motivation to eat a low-fat diet; they were then randomly allocated to either the implementation or the control condition. Those in the implementation condition were asked to describe a plan for eating a low-fat diet for the next month and to formulate their plans in as much detail as possible. Their food intake was measured using a food questionnaire after 1 month. The results showed that this simple intervention produced a significant decrease in the proportion of energy derived from fat; this decrease could not be explained by baseline differences in motivations. The implementation intention had changed subsequent behaviour.

These studies seem to indicate that a **positive** attitude towards foods is a better predictor to eating behaviour than subjective or social norms, nutritional knowledge or support groups. However, again, providing a practical way to implement the changed behaviour is more use in helping patients like Diana.

Control and weight loss

Although all the evidence indicates that most people regain any weight they might lose, a minority do succeed; Ogden (2010b) has been trying to determine what makes these people different. One way of doing this was to explore the psychological impact of obesity surgery.

Surgery is generally regarded as the most effective form of weight loss (by reducing the size of the stomach and, thereby reducing the amount of food that can be consumed). However, just as critically, after surgery, most (not all) participants reported feeling less hungry and less preoccupied with food (Ogden et al., 2006). As they could not eat as much, they simply stopped thinking about it. They also reported feeling much more in control of their eating and spoke about a 'rebirth' and being liberated. Paradoxically, by having control imposed over how much they ate, participants felt *more*, not less, in control of their eating behaviour.

Ogden's previous research on dieting had shown that trying to control what you eat can lead to *loss* of control; surgery, however, which takes control away from the patient, actually made him/her feel more in control. Ogden (2010b) calls this the 'paradox of control'. This resonated with several other areas of successful behaviour change interventions, such as seat belt laws, smoking bans and the removal of fizzy drink machines from schools: relying on willpower and self-control can have a rebound effect, but imposing control can be liberating (Ogden, 2010b).

The final 'paradox of control' suggests that battling against both subjective and social norms can overwhelm some people and only an imposed control by surgical intervention will help. However, this implies the failure of all health behaviour models and in many cultures is not an option. It also, I think, reverts to a biomedical model of health care that is at odds with the biopsychosocial nature of the condition. Level 3 of Goodman's 1984 model for reflective analysis prompts consideration of the social, economic, political and ethical issues so evident in health behaviour and education. Discovering the different factors involved in health promotion has made me re-consider my attitude to Diana and her problems; I realise my initial (judgmental) feelings about her were vastly uninformed and shall try to remember this in similar situations!

CHAPTER SUMMARY

- The *biomedical model* adopts a reactive and reductionist approach to *disease*, while the *BPS model* adopts a more proactive and holistic approach towards *health* and underpins *health psychology*.
- Health beliefs (*HBs*) are important determinants of health behaviour and can be *health damaging* as well as *health promoting*. For most Western people, being healthy is the norm and is defined in positive terms.
- While the concept of *disease* reflects the biomedical model, *illness* (like the concept of health) incorporates physical, psychological and social aspects, reflecting the BPS model.
- HBs vary across cultures, which represent *macro-level* influences on people's health status. Conflicting HBs can leave both nurses and patients feeling frustrated and failing to understand one another.
- HBs *based on biomedicine* dominate the health systems of North America and Western Europe. Others are based on *personality (or magico-religious) systems* and *naturalistic systems* (holism).

- The migration of immigrants' health status to the host nation's norm through *acculturation* is best explained in terms of risk factors associated with adapting to the new culture ('acculturative stress').
- Two examples of the impact of *sociocultural influences* on individuals' experience of bodily states are *menopause* and *pain*.
- Sociocultural factors also influence the extent to which individuals delay seeking medical help and social support, the doctor–patient relationship and basic understanding of what illness means.
- The most commonly cited *cultural syndrome* in the context of individual understanding of health and illness is *individualism–collectivism*.
- *Illness cognitions* provide patients with a framework/schema for coping with and understanding their illness. Five associated dimensions are *identity, perceived cause, timeline, consequences,* and *curability and controllability*.
- An important distinction is made between *risk-increasing* and *health-promoting behaviours*, but what is included within each category changes over time.
- Health behaviour is determined by sociocultural and national factors, legislative factors, macroeconomics, systems of provision and services, health-service provision, sociodemographic, social and family factors, health status, psychological and biological factors.
- *Social cognition models* can be divided into those that are specifically *health models* (HBM, PMT, HAPA) and *cognition models* (TRA and TPB, PMT).
- Both types of model try to explain why people adopt/do not adopt particular health-related behaviours. These *expectancy–value models* assume that people choose between alternative courses of action, based on *subjective probabilities* and *evaluation* of action outcomes.
- All models fail to predict actual behaviour (the *intention–behaviour gap*) and they are also *culturally relative*.
- Most models emphasise people's rational decision-making and underestimate their *perception of personal invulnerability/unrealistic optimism*.
- These models have been applied to a range of health behaviours, such as eating behaviour; adding *implementation intentions* to these models provides a means of changing behaviour by specifying where and when a particular behaviour will occur.

Neuropsychological and genetic aspects of illness

Introduction and overview

Neuropsychologists are concerned with the relationship between the structure and function of the brain and cognitive or physiological processes; like clinical psychologists (see Chapter 1), they may also help to assess and rehabilitate brain-injured people and those with neurobiological disorders (including dementia, strokes and tumours).

Recalling information from long-term memory is an ability that appears to decline with age (see Chapter 19); significant memory deficits are also a feature of *dementia* (mental frailty), one of the two most common forms of cognitive impairment. Dementia is usually of insidious onset (i.e., quite gradual but dangerous); its diagnosis requires the presence of progressive decline in two or more domains of cognition, giving rise to significant impairment of activities of daily living (Zeman and Torrens, 2010).

While the layperson may associate dementia in general and Alzheimer's disease (AD) in particular, with old age, there are, in fact, several causes of dementia. AD is a form of *primary degeneration*, a disease process that is more likely to affect us as we get older (Smith, 1998). Other causes include head injury, hypothyroidism, excessive use of alcohol, anticholinergics, hypnotics and genetics (Zeman and Torrens, 2010). Clearly, these latter causes are not age-related.

A stroke refers to any acute and persistent neurological deficit of vascular origin, whether caused by cerebral ischaemia or intracerebral haemorrhage (Garrard, 2010). A major cause of strokes is high blood pressure (BP). While both high BP and strokes are much more common in older people, it is becoming increasingly common for people under 30 to suffer strokes after taking drugs such as cocaine (Laurance, 2000; see Chapter 12). Especially severe strokes can cause coma, in which there is an absence of both wakefulness and awareness; these represent two key components of *consciousness* (Laureys, 2005). The presence or absence of these two components can be used to distinguish (at least theoretically) between different normal and abnormal states/conditions, including a comatose patient, a patient under general anaesthetic, and a patient in a *vegetative state* (VS) (Monti and Owen, 2010).

According to the biopsychosocial model of health (Engel, 1977; see Chapter 3), we need to understand disease in terms of the complex interrelationships between biological, psychological and social variables. However, an increasingly important role in the biological part of the equation is being played by discoveries within genetics; according to Hamilton-West (2011), these discoveries lead us to ask a number of questions, including the following:

- To what extent are individual differences in the risk of developing specific diseases genetically determined and to what extent might they be shaped by environmental factors (including the psychosocial environment)?
- To what extent are health-related behaviours, such as smoking and drinking alcohol, genetically determined?
- To what extent may health outcomes (and behavioural predictors of health outcomes) be amenable to psychological intervention (see Chapter 10)?
- How will advances in genetic research change the way we diagnose and treat disease?

 From my diary (15): Year 3/Elderly Care Ward

An interesting day. Back from days off and at lunch time I was trying to get Phyllis, a very confused, 70-year-old patient with Alzheimer's disease (AD), to eat her lunch. She was admitted two days ago with a urinary tract infection and was doubly incontinent so no urine specimen was obtained. She was being treated with IV fluids and a 48 hr course of Gentamycin which reduced her pyrexia. She was also dehydrated and malnourished so is on a Feed Chart and food supplements arranged by the dietician.

She's still confused; she pushed the plate away, saying she'd had her breakfast and then started searching in the locker drawer saying something about money. As it pulled on her IV line I tried to distract her but she suddenly became aggressive and agitated and kept repeating, 'you took it'. So I just concentrated on keeping the IV line intact until she gave up.

When her daughter arrived that evening I found it was Janet, an ex-patient who I remembered as being very upset following her abortion last year (case study 10, page 128). She said Phyllis had been ill for 'some time' and although she worked full-time Janet had visited daily and with the neighbours 'keeping an eye on her' they'd managed. Recently, however, Phyllis has got much worse, 'wetting and messing everywhere' so she's just had a DST (Decision Support Tool) assessment by a Community Nurse and is waiting for a bed in a nursing home. I asked Janet if she'd been caring for Phyllis when she'd had her operation last year and she looked embarrassed and said, 'Yes, trying to.' It added another perspective to her decision to terminate her pregnancy.

Dementia and Alzheimer's disease

Dementia

Until about 200 years ago, people died young and relatively quickly – mainly from infections. During the twentieth century, average life expectancy in the world doubled, and people in developed countries now tend to die old and slowly – from degenerative diseases brought on by ageing ('the expansion of morbidity'), in particular cancer, and vascular and neurodegenerative disease: these are the price we pay in Western society for living longer (Brown, 2007). The increased lifespan has not been matched by an extension of health: the years we gain are mostly spent with disability, disease and dementia. Between 1991 and 2001, life expectancy in the United Kingdom increased by 2.2 years, but healthy life expectancy increased by only 0.6 years: people experienced ill health for an extra 1.6 years of their lives. This is because we have not been able to slow the ageing process (Brown, 2007).

However, severe dementia affects only a minority of elderly people, in contrast with physical frailty (see Chapter 19); sometimes, they coincide, as in late-onset Parkinson's disease (Coleman and O'Hanlon, 2004). The sudden onset of physical disability (as in a stroke) or more gradually (as with osteoarthritis) represents one form of pathway into later life. Dementia represents a very different pathway:

> ... The many disabling consequences arising from mental frailty make dementia the major health problem of later life in modern western society. It is the most age-related of all the disabling conditions affecting older people ... (Coleman and O'Hanlon, 2004).

? RESEARCH QUESTION ...

- What do you think Coleman and O'Hanlon mean when they say that dementia is the most age-related condition affecting older people?
- What are the implications for current and future health care provision for these people?

Epidemiology

The rate of dementia changes with age in a strikingly consistent way. The average rate is 5.6% at age 75–79, 10.5% at 80–84 and 39% at 90–95 (Black et al., 1990). According to McVeigh (2009), almost 80% of people who live to 95 already suffer some form of mild to severe dementia. It is unclear whether the rate continues to increase in centenarians. According to Benjamin and Burns (2010), the prevalence of dementia doubles with every 5-year increase across the entire age range, from 30 to 95 years and over. But with so many more people surviving into their 90s, overall prevalence is increasing. Indeed, a report by the King's Fund health care charity predicts that the number of people in the United Kingdom with dementia will increase by 61% – to more than 1.1 million people – by 2026.

The increase in longevity and its accelerating rate has enormous implications for health and social service requirements of older adults in the coming years (Kroger, 2007).

 Many of our older patients have dementia to complicate their physical illnesses, but thankfully, it's not inevitable; last week we had a woman in who is 91, very mentally alert and still driving!

Causes and varieties of dementia

Dementia is a clinical syndrome characterised by multiple cognitive deficits; behavioural and psychological symptoms and neurological difficulties may also be present. These deficits impair the ability to function at work, socially, and in everyday activities, but the level of consciousness usually remains intact (Benjamin and Burns, 2010). Table 11.1 shows the wide range of causes of dementia.

Phyllis could have been confused as a result of her UTI and dehydration as well but if so it should have lessened now.

For diagnostic purposes, a broad distinction is made between *cortical* and *subcortical* dementia (Zeman and Torrens, 2010):

- *Cortical dementias* such as AD produce the classic neuropsychological deficit syndromes of amnesia (loss of memory), aphasia (or dysphasia: loss of language function), agnosia (loss of perceptual – predominantly visual – function), and apraxia (loss of simple motor skills).
- *Subcortical dementias* include those of multiple sclerosis, Huntington's disease and subcortical cerebrovascular disease and are characterised by slowing of cognition, often associated with altered behaviour and personality. Another feature of subcortical dementias is dysexecutive syndrome, in which the executive (decision-making) network that directs attention is impaired. Table 11.2 shows a comparison between cortical (e.g., AD) and subcortical (e.g., Huntington's disease) dementia.

When I gave Phyllis her spoon at lunch time she looked at it as if she didn't know what it was or what to do with it; she didn't attempt to use it. Phyllis has become atypically aggressive which indicates frontal lobe involvement.

Table 11.1 Causes of dementia

Cause	Example
Degenerative	Alzheimer's disease; Lewy body disease; frontotemporal dementias Parkinson's disease; Huntington's disease
Vascular	Single infarct; multi-infarct; diffuse white matter ischaemia
Endocrine	Hypothyroidism; hyperparathyroidism; Cushing's disease; Addison's disease
Metabolic	Hypercalcaemia; uraemia; hepatic encephalopathy
Infectious	Creutzfeldt–Jacob disease; human immunodeficiency virus/HIV; syphilis
Vitamin deficiency	B12; folate
Toxins	Alcohol; heavy metals
Other	Normal pressure hydrocephalus; subdural haematoma; tumours
Source: Benjamin, B. and Burns, A., Old-age psychiatry. In B.K. Puri and I. Treasaden (eds.), *Psychiatry: An Evidence-Based Text*, Hodder Arnold, London, 2010.	

Table 11.2 Features of cortical versus subcortical dementia

Function	Cortical (e.g., Alzheimer's (disease)	Subcortical (e.g., Huntington's disease)
Alertness	Normal	'Slowed up'
Attention	Normal early	Impaired
Executive function	Normal early	Impaired
Episodic memory	Amnesia	Forgetfulness
Language	Aphasic	Reduced output
Praxis	Apraxia	Relatively normal
Perception	Impaired	Impaired
Personality	Preserved (unless frontal type)[a]	Apathetic, inert

Source: Zeman, A. and Torrens, L., Cognitive assessment. In B.K. Puri and I. Treasaden (eds.), *Psychiatry: An Evidence-Based Text*, Hodder Arnold, London, 2010.

[a] This refers to the frontal lobe of the brain, believed to control personality.

Clinical features

As we have seen, dementia involves a number of cognitive deficits (see Table 11.2).

- *Aphasia* Language difficulties (aphasia) may present as a decrease in the quality of speech, and there may be difficulties understanding written and spoken language. In the late stages of dementia, speech may become incomprehensible or the patient may be mute.
- *Apraxia* may present as difficulties in getting dressed and using cutlery, despite intact motor and sensory abilities and comprehension of the task.
- *Agnosia* involves difficulties in recognising objects or familiar people despite no impairment in visual function.
- Impaired *executive functioning* involves loss of the ability to plan activities and think in abstract terms (especially in frontal lobe dementia).
- Common *behavioural and psychological symptoms of dementia* (BPSD) include depression, a variety of psychotic symptoms (including paranoid ideation, delusions and hallucinations), aggression, wandering and changes in sleep and eating patterns. Personality changes can be very distressing for relatives and are a prominent feature of frontal lobe dementias. The person may lose interest in friends and family as a result of apathy and neglect household tasks. Neglect of self-care tasks (such as eating, personal hygiene and toilet activities) makes it difficult or impossible for the person to live independently in the community.
- *Neurological features* may be evident early depending on the type of dementia. Some common examples are parkinsonism in Lewy body disease, focal neurological signs in vascular dementia and primitive reflexes in the frontotemporal dementias. All dementias involve a progressive loss of motor function in the end stages.

Phyllis had been neglecting eating and personal hygiene for months which Janet had coped with but when Phyllis became doubly incontinent, caring for her at home was impossible. She was also considered to be a potential danger to herself and others as she kept leaving the lighted gas rings on.

Dementia and emotion

- Compared with their cognitive abilities, the emotions of people with dementia remain intact longer, and these help us to continue making contact (Coleman and O'Hanlon, 2004). As Coleman and O'Hanlon observe, 'Dementia care is much more about responding to emotions and maintaining a sense of well-being than it is about preserving cognitive function'.

  > Precisely because the world to a confused person is likely to appear less certain, one would expect people suffering from a dementing condition to be more emotional. Unexpected things will happen more often. There will be sadness over losing things, anger at being frustrated in achieving aims, and fear and anxiety because of uncertainty over what might happen … There will also be more expressions of joy as problems are solved and familiar faces recognised. It is also probable that emotions will be expressed more extremely, and that resulting moods will be more prolonged ….

- Anxiety and nervousness are major problems and tend to persist, which is why staff often have recourse to sedative medication. While some of this can be attributed to changes in the brain, much may arise from real feelings of loss and tension; for example, even severely demented people remain sensitive to the moods of others around them.
- Feelings may become dissociated from the event that induced them. For example, reassuring someone who is sad and worried about losing something that it has since been found may have little effect: the feelings persist because the person cannot now remember that something was lost in the first place.

When Phyllis started scrabbling in the drawer again, Janet said reassuringly, 'Don't worry, Mum, I paid the cleaner', which seemed to quieten her. Janet's explanation that Phyllis kept cash for this in a kitchen drawer made sense of her behaviour.

Alzheimer's disease

AD was first described by Alois Alzheimer in 1906. Based on the autopsy of Auguste D., Alzheimer identified abnormalities in the cellular structure of her cerebral cortex, consisting of the loss of intact cells and the accumulation of pathological material. Alzheimer's observations represent an important identification of a biological basis of cognitive change.

AD is the most common form of dementia, accounting for 50%–70% of all cases; one in eight people over 65 in the United Kingdom and almost half of people over 85 have AD (Benjamin and Burns, 2010). However, even very late in life, cortical neurons seem capable of responding to enriched conditions by forming new functional connections with other neurons. This is supported by the finding that those who keep mentally active maintain their cognitive abilities (Rogers et al., 1990). Similarly, education, an active mind and enriched experience seem to go some way towards preventing dementia (Ott et al., 1995).

AD is one of the most debilitating and dreaded of the common diseases of ageing: 417,000 people in the United Kingdom were estimated to have AD in 2007 (Benjamin and Burns, 2010) and this figure was expected to have risen to over 1 million in 2010. While AD used to be described more generally as 'senile dementia', it is now referred to as 'senile dementia of the Alzheimer's type'. People at the height of their intellectual powers can be struck down with it, a classic example being Iris Murdoch (see Figure 11.1) (Rose, 2003).

More ordinarily, Phyllis can no longer do her daily crossword, or read her library books. Janet brought her magazines with lots of pictures which she does seem to enjoy.

Figure 11.1 Judi Dench as Iris Murdoch, the gifted more list and academic, in *Iris* (2001). She died from AD. (Based on Toates, F., *Biological Psychology: An Integrative Approach*, Pearson Education Ltd, Harlow, 2001.)

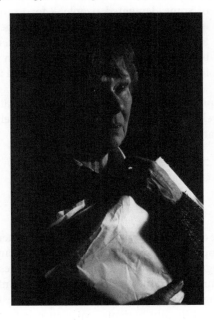

Brain disease or behavioural syndrome?

Patients experience a frightening loss of sense of their own identity and access to their store of personal (episodic) memories. Their brains shrink, and the neurons themselves change appearance – they develop 'tangles and plaques' (Rose, 2003). ('Plaques' refer to clumps of protein fragment called amyloid: Coleman and O'Hanlon, 2004.)

AD is selective to brain regions and types of cell within regions (Damasio et al., 1990). Most atrophy (loss of brain tissue) takes place in temporal lobe structures (e.g., the hippocampus and entorhinal cortex, a region of the cortex linked to the hippocampus; see Chapter 2). There is a particularly marked reduction in cerebral blood flow and glucose metabolism in the temporal lobe, indicating loss of neurons or lower activity in remaining neurons – or both (Morris, 1996a). A spread of pathology from the temporal lobes to parietal and frontal lobes can be correlated with a disruption of attention as well as an initial memory impairment (Perry and Hodges, 1999).

Phyllis often just sits and stares, not attending to what is said to her or happening which indicates the disease progression. She has recently started on Aricept (which boosts cholinergic functioning and slows the progression) but it's too soon to see if it works for her.

However, Coleman and O'Hanlon (2004) point out that AD, unlike heart disease, cancer and other physical diseases, is not, strictly speaking, a disease but a *behavioural syndrome*: we cannot yet define its severity in terms of brain pathology. Indeed,

> ... post-mortem studies show that the states of the brains of some demented people – for example, the number of plaques – are well within the range of those of mentally well-preserved individuals, whereas some people become demented with comparatively little accompanying neuropathology ... (Coleman and O'Hanlon, 2004).

Improved understanding of the disease at the biochemical and physiological levels may, in time, provide a better correlation between biological markers (indicators) and actual impairment.

This immediately questions the biological markers as diagnostic of the disease; does it perhaps suggest the possibility of an environmental influence on its development?

Clinical features

- The onset of the disease is insidious, and memory loss is the characteristic early symptom. Although memory loss for recent events occurs first, as the disease progresses long-term memory also becomes affected. Disorientation in time is common, and the patient may get lost in unfamiliar places.
- Language is also commonly affected in the early stages. The most common difficulty patients experience is finding words (*nominal dysphasia*):

they may describe the function of an object without being able to name it (e.g., 'a thing you write with' for 'pen'). The second most common language problem is *fluent dysphasia*: fluent speech with little understandable content.

- Other cognitive, behavioural and psychiatric features described in pages 251 and 252 in relation to dementia also develop (see pages x). Impairment of judgement is an important symptom that may put the patient at risk and cause concern for relatives (Benjamin and Burns, 2010).

- For some patients, perception of individual items and appreciation of their semantic significance remains intact only if they are presented in a simple context; other items disrupt perception of target items (Saffran et al., 1990). This is demonstrated by the 'table-cloth experiment': people are asked to close their eyes, an item is placed on the table and they are then asked to open their eyes and 'pick up the thing on the table'. Patterns on the table-cloth make the task more difficult. The integration needed to perform the task successfully seems to involve connections between cortical areas that are compromised in AD (Toates, 2001).

- There are large individual differences in cognitive loss (Funnell, 1996; Morris, 1996b).

📋 Phyllis has 'fluent dysphasia' as she talks to herself but it often doesn't make sense to us. However, the example of the money may mean it makes sense to her.

Is AD a disease process or a part of normal ageing?

Some researchers claim that AD is an *accelerated form* of normal changes in the ageing brain, so that we would all get the disease if we lived long enough. The opposing view is that cognitive decline is not an inevitable part of ageing, but rather it reflects a *disease process* that is more likely to affect us as get older (Smith, 1998).

Work by the Oxford Project to Investigate Memory and Ageing (OPTIMA) has used X-ray computerised tomography (CT) to examine the *medial temporal lobe* (MTL). While this tiny area comprises only 2% of the volume of the entire cerebral cortex, it includes the *hippocampus*, known to be crucial for memory. Also, the neurons of the MTL connect with almost all other parts of the cortex, so that any damage to this part of the brain is likely to have consequences for the functioning of the rest of the cortex.

X-ray CT images show that the MTL is markedly smaller in people with dementia who eventually die of AD than in age-matched controls without cognitive deficit. Repeated CT scans over periods of several years found that shrinkage is slow in control participants (about 1%–1.5% per year), compared with an alarming rate of some 15% in Alzheimer's patients (Smith, 1998) (see Figure 11.2).

📋 Janet told me that her mother has 'gone down quickly recently'. She added sadly that Phyllis was scared of 'losing her mind' and intended to make a living will (or Advance Decision form) to avoid prolonging suffering but she'd deteriorated so quickly it was now too late.

These, and other supportive data, led the OPTIMA researchers to conclude that AD is distinct from normal ageing and that it cannot simply be

Figure 11.2 CT scan of the brain of an Alzheimer's patient (left) and of a normal person (right).

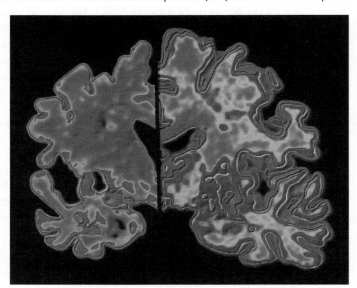

an acceleration of normal ageing. Although cognitive decline does appear to increase with age for the population as a whole, if we rigorously exclude those with pathological changes (such as early AD), then a majority may not show any significant decline. According to Smith (1998), 'We must abandon the fatalistic view that mental decline is an inevitable accompaniment of ageing'. Consistent with this conclusion is the belief that negative cultural stereotypes of ageing can actually cause memory decline in elderly people (see Chapter 19).

Is AD a psychological rather than a neuropathological condition?

Coleman and O'Hanlon (2004) believe that, at present, AD is more appropriately defined as an acquired progressive global deterioration of mental functioning. While the clinical features described earlier include behavioural and psychological changes as well as cognitive ones, missing from the list is *personality change*; patients' tendency to behave in ways uncharacteristic of their former selves was something emphasised by Alzheimer when first describing the condition. In practice, it can be very difficult to distinguish personality from cognition.

Because even very healthy people sometimes complain of some of the memory and language impairments included in the list of clinical features mentioned earlier, a more helpful criterion than memory loss is the loss of *automatic intelligence* – the ability to apply the intelligence the individual has acquired during life in an automatic way. Normally, we do not have to think about who we are, where we are, what we are doing and what we are going to do next: we operate automatically. When we decide to do something, we simply activate strategies and procedures (e.g., for driving a car, or having a shower) that reflect earlier learning.

... Even well-learned procedures are lost by persons in advanced states of dementia. As a result they can also lose a sense of where they are in the world and what they are doing. It is the loss of the past self that most sharply distinguishes dementia from other severe memory disorders resulting from neurological injury, where a person loses the ability to learn new information, but retains earlier memories ... (Coleman and O'Hanlon, 2004).

Coleman and O'Hanlon go on to describe other forms of memory impairment involved in AD, which really represent parts of the self that we normally just take for granted. For example,

- Failure of *schematic memory*, which automatically allows us to make sense of new experiences and to recognise and put new objects and experiences in the right categories. An early sign of AD may involve forgetting that you can now buy milk in plastic bottles at most general stores/supermarkets/garages – and not just in glass bottles from the dairy (a *reference schema*).
- Related to schematic memory is the distinction between *automatic* and *effortful* memory (Hasher and Zacks, 1979) or automatic encoding versus purposeful learning. In AD, there is a breakdown in the automatic encoding of information (not having to consciously try to remember certain things); this is disruptive because a greater proportion of our life (and, consequently, our sense of self) relies on automatic coding than purposeful learning.

From all the distinguishing features (above) of AD such as rapid shrinking of the MTL and deterioration of the connections between cortical areas, the most difficult consequence for carers must be personality change and loss of self which Coleman and O'Hanlon (2004) say most sharply distinguishes AD from other memory disorders. I know Janet finds her mother's atypical aggression very upsetting.

Experience of dementia

For any person involved in dementia care, it is important to try to appreciate what it is like to be demented. While closing our eyes gives us some, limited, insight into the experience of blindness, trying to put ourselves in the place of someone with AD requires a huge effort of imagination and empathy.

According to Sabat (2001) and Sabat and Harre (1992), when we refer to loss of self in AD, it is principally the *social* (as opposed to the *personal*) self that we have in mind. While loss of the social self is greatly influenced by others' behaviour towards the person with AD (including two-way communication), the personal self is usually preserved until the late stages and is demonstrated by the use of 'I' and 'my'. Indeed, close observation and discussion with people in the early stages of AD show that they have some insight and awareness of what is happening to them (Froggatt, 1988).

One problem is people's failure to understand the increasingly fragmented and fragile cues the AD sufferer expresses; this can result in misunderstanding the meaning of the latter's behaviour. In short, the fundamental cause of loss of the social self is found in the nature of the social interactions and the interpretations that occur as a result of communication difficulties: 'The ultimate result of such a situation is the fencing off of the sufferer so that no adequate self can be constructed' (Sabat, 2001).

Janet said she'll bring us a copy of the 'This is me' form, which she downloaded from the Alzheimer's website in preparation for the nursing home. Apparently it provides a detailed history of Phyllis's likes and dislikes, habits and characteristics; it will help us pick up cues so we can understand and care for her better.

Stroke

According to Coleman and O'Hanlon (2004), a major stroke (or *cerebrovascular accident* [CVA]) can mark entry into what is increasingly referred to as the 'fourth age', when issues of disability and frailty come to predominate the lives of older people.

> … This is 'old age' proper, the time of life when many people finally do ascribe the adjective 'old' to themselves. It is what many have been waiting for all along, expecting it with varying degrees of apprehension ….

Causes

As we noted in the '*Introduction and overview*', a stroke refers to any acute and persistent neurological deficit of vascular origin, whether caused by cerebral *ischaemia* (lack of blood flow) or *intracerebral haemorrhage*. Figure 11.3 summarises the major causes of strokes and the factors that contribute to these causes.

Neurological deficits

The neurological deficit that follows an ischaemic stroke depends on the distribution and extent of the lesion (actual tissue damage or abnormal tissue): the middle vertebral artery is implicated in a majority of cases, producing

- A *contralateral hemiparesis* (muscle weakness on the opposite side of the body to the lesion, usually affecting the face, arm or leg but worse in the arm).
- *Homonymous quadrantanopia* or *quadrantanopsia* (loss of vision in the same quadrant of the visual field in both eyes).
- *Isolated anterior cerebral artery territory infarction* (an area of tissue death due to a local lack of oxygen): this is rare but is associated primarily with contralateral leg weakness and personality change (disinhibition).

Epidemiology

Strokes are remarkably common – especially in individuals over the age of 65. In the United Kingdom, an estimated 130,000 people suffer a stroke every year, including about 1,000 under 30 years of age (see page 260) (Davey, 2008).

Figure 11.3 Major causes of strokes and factors contributing to these causes. (Based on Davey, G., *Psychopathology: Research, Assessment and Treatment in Clinical Psychology*, BPS Blackwell, Chichester, 2008.)

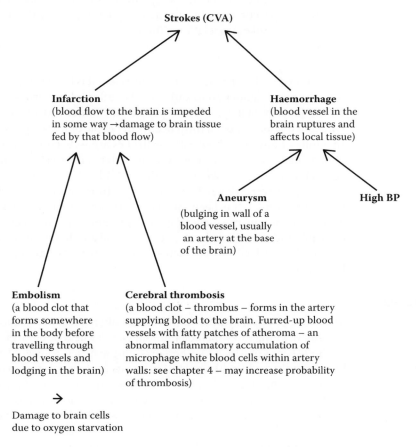

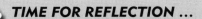

Damage to brain cells
due to oxygen starvation

TIME FOR REFLECTION …

- What do you understand by 'disinhibition' in relation to personality change?

The individual's behaviour becomes less controlled and constrained, more antisocial, more extreme, compared with how it was before the stroke.

Posterior cerebral artery stroke typically gives rise to brainstem-related and cerebellar signs (e.g., lack of coordination, poor balance, general clumsiness and unsteadiness – often mistaken for being drunk – and difficulty with stabilising eye movements) or *homonymous hemianopia* (or *hemianopsia*) (reduced vision affecting half of the visual field of one or both eyes).

About a third of stroke victims will die as a direct result of their stroke (Stroke Association, 2009). Strokes are the third most common cause of death in the United Kingdom and the single most common cause of disability: over 250,000 people currently live in the United Kingdom with a disability caused by a stroke (Stroke Association, 2006).

Stroke in younger adults

As we noted in the *Introduction and overview*, it is becoming increasingly common for people under 30 to suffer strokes after taking drugs, such as cocaine. Of the (approximately) 150,000 people who suffer a stroke every year in the United Kingdom, about a third occurs in people of working age (i.e., below 65). In adults of any age, about 80% of strokes are ischaemic, with the remaining 20% being haemorrhagic; however, the latter is relatively common in younger adults (40%–50%) (Stroke Association, 2011d).

Using any recreational drug makes it 6.5 times more likely that an individual will have a stroke. It is been estimated that 14% of strokes in 18–44-year-olds are caused by drug use including ecstasy (methylenedioxymethamphetamine), cannabis and stimulants (such as cocaine and amphetamines) (see Chapter 12). Other lifestyle factors that increase the chances of having a stroke include binge drinking.

Clinical features

The overt, physical symptoms of a stroke often occur very suddenly and without any warning; they include numbness, weakness or paralysis on one side of the body (signs of which may be a drooping arm, leg, a lowered eyelid or a dribbling mouth), sudden blurred vision or loss of sight, confusion or unsteadiness and a severe headache. Paralysis usually occurs in just one limb or just one side of the body because a CVA usually damages tissue in just one hemisphere of the brain: the paralysis is on the opposite side to the affected hemisphere (i.e., *contralateral*).

The type and severity of symptoms will depend entirely on the brain area affected by the CVA. One of the most common forms of stroke is thrombosis in the left middle cerebral artery, affecting the left hemisphere: this causes disability to the right-hand side of the body and significant impairment in language ability, since, at least for most right-handed people, the left hemisphere is dominant for language production and comprehension (see Chapter 2 and Gross, 2010).

Many individuals have 'silent strokes', which occur in parts of the brain involved in minor functions; these do not produce any obvious cognitive or physical impairment. The prevalence of 'silent strokes' in 55–64-year-olds has been estimated at 11%, but this rises to 40% in 80–85-year-olds (Davey, 2008).

I have experience of two people who suffered recently from very different 'strokes'. One is Carrie, who is 83 and has been on the ward for a week with right hemiparesis and aphasia. She collapsed in a supermarket, was unable to move her right arm or leg and couldn't speak. She was sent by ambulance to A and E immediately, had a CT scan which showed a left middle cerebral thrombus and she was admitted.

Halim, a 54-year-old is a friend of my father's who, a few weeks ago, had a Transient Ischaemic Attack (TIA) the morning after flying home from a holiday. Halim's a Muslim and as far as I know *doesn't* drink, smoke or take drugs! His symptoms were mild; tingling in his left arm and leg with slight loss of function and the left side of his mouth felt numb. His wife drove him to A and E; he wasn't admitted but had bloods taken (including fasting lipids), an ECG, a CT scan and later a 2-hr BP monitor. He's recovering at home on an APAI (antiplatelet inhibitor) to prevent further clotting.

Communication problems

- *Aphasia* (or *dysphasia*) is the most common language disorder caused by stroke; problems may relate mainly to understanding what is being said by others (*receptive aphasia*) or to expressing what you want to say (*expressive aphasia*). Where there is a combination of problems that changes all or most aspects of the person's communication and she/he is described as having *mixed* (or *global*) *aphasia* (Stroke Association, 2011a).

- *Dysarthria* refers to weakness of the muscles involved in speech; this may affect the muscles used in moving the tongue, lips or mouth, those that control breathing or those that produce vocal sound. Consequently, the person's voice may sound different, she/he may have difficulty speaking clearly; some find their speech sounds slurred, strained, quiet or slow. All of these effects may make it difficult for others to understand what is being said (Stroke Association, 2011a).

- *Dyspraxia* of speech involves the inability to move muscles in the correct order to make the sounds needed for clear speech (even in the absence of dysarthria or paralysis). This may prevent the person from pronouncing words clearly, especially when *asked* to say or repeat them. These difficulties can be frightening and distressing, adding to the depression that is commonly experienced. If the ability to read is affected, everyday activities (e.g., choosing from a menu or reading signs or prescriptions) can become problematical (Stroke Association, 2011a).

Mary can say only two words and one of them is a swear word! But her almost total 'expressive aphasia' is expressive – she says them quite clearly and differently in response to things said to her.

Cognitive problems

- *Visual memory* (e.g., for faces and pictures) is usually more affected after a stroke in the *right* hemisphere, while *verbal* (or *language*) *memory* (e.g., for names, stories or conversations) tends to be affected following a *left* hemisphere stroke (Stroke Association, 2010).

- *Short-term memory* problems are the most common following a stroke, with *anterograde* amnesia/forgetting (i.e., the ability to store new memories) also commonly affected (Stroke Association, 2010). While dementia is defined partly in terms of memory deficits, having memory deficits does not, of course, equal dementia. However, dementia does sometimes occur following a stroke.

- Following a stroke, the person's *selective attention* may be affected; this can take the form of becoming easily distracted, a feeling of 'switching off' from ongoing conversations or events. The person's ability to *multi-task* (i.e., do two or more things at the same time) may also be affected, as in needing to concentrate on driving and avoid talking (Stroke Association, 2010); strictly, this demonstrates *divided* (as opposed to selective or focused) *attention* (see Chapter 1).

- People who have suffered a right-hemisphere stroke involving the parietal lobe (see Chapter 2) may completely ignore stimuli occurring on the left side. For example, they may fail to eat food from the left side of their plate and be unaware of their body on that side. The fascinating thing about this *unilateral visual neglect* is that these effects occur even though the pathways from the sense receptors (the rods and cones in the retina of the eye) to the brain's occipital lobe (through the optic nerve) remain intact (Figure 11.4).

Mary seems to enjoy her limited communication with us and then her attention seems good. But sometimes she looks anxious and confused; so, as I do with Phyllis, I try to talk to her in simple sentences, one thought at a time.

- Other cognitive problems include impairment of (1) *executive functioning* (such as decision-making, planning and making judgements), which becomes slower and, generally, less effective and (2) *social cognition*, such as seeing things from another person's point of view and trying to appreciate his/her motives and intentions (see Chapter 1).

Depression and other affective problems

- Strokes can sometimes cause subtle changes to *emotional aspects* of speech; for example, the person's tone of voice may sound 'flat' or his/her facial expression may not vary. Understanding humour may also become a

Figure 11.4 An example of left-sided unilateral visual neglect.

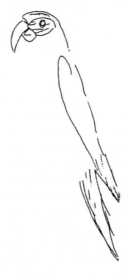

problem, as can knowing when to take turns in a conversation. All of these can be misinterpreted as signs of depression, which is the most common psychological change following stroke: an estimated 50% of stroke survivors suffer significant depression in the first year following their stroke (Stroke Association, 2011b).

- Levels of depression are correlated with the severity of both physical and cognitive deficits (Kauhanen et al., 1999). Recovery from physical and cognitive impairments is significantly delayed in those with depression, and mortality rate 1 year following the stroke is significantly higher in those with depression compared with those without (Morris et al., 1993; Robinson et al., 1986). According to Davey (2008), there seems to be a *bidirectional* (two-way) link between stroke and depression, with some studies indicating that depression may even be a risk factor for strokes.

- Similarly, treating post-stroke depression with antidepressant medication also has the effect of significantly decreasing mortality rates over a 9-year period (Robinson et al., 2000). Together, all these findings suggest that depression is an important feature of disability caused by strokes; clinical psychologists could help to manage depression in attempts to improve recovery rates and reduce mortality rates (Davey, 2008) (see Chapter 1).

- Depression is closely related to *anxiety*, that is, they are often found to coexist (they are *co-morbid*); anxiety is also one of the 'stress emotions' (see Chapter 4).

- *Emotionalism* is common and refers to how the person becomes more emotional than before the stroke and/or has difficulty controlling his/her emotions. Emotional reactions to everyday things become very intense and emotions are very close to the surface; from the point of view of other people, it takes very little to upset the person. She/he may start to cry for no apparent reason, laugh inappropriately or even swing from one to the other quite suddenly (Stroke Association, 2011c).

- *Anger* may become more common and less controlled for many stroke victims, who may direct it at relatives and carers – including nurses and other health professionals. This can be explained, at least partly, by the frustration, embarrassment and bewilderment produced by the communication and cognitive changes described in page 261.

- Some commonly reported *personality changes* include becoming impatient and irritable, withdrawn and introspective; showing a loss of inhibition (as in swearing or making inappropriate comments); becoming aggressive (verbally or physically) and impulsive; showing a loss of interest in activities that were previously enjoyed and showing more stress, anger, and depression (Stress Association, 2011c).

Yes, Mary does cry and seems frustrated at times, but isn't aggressive; she has a sweet personality. She tries so hard to co-operate – I keep telling her she'll be better when she's had more speech therapy and physiotherapy.

Dementia

Vascular dementia is the second most common type of dementia in the United Kingdom after AD (see Table 11.2). The two main types of vascular dementia related to stroke are *multi-infarct dementia* (MID) and *single-infarct dementia* (SID) (Stroke Association, 2009).

Consciousness and the vegetative state

As we saw in the *Introduction and overview*, consciousness can be conceptualised as comprising two key components (Laureys, 2005): (1) *level* (i.e., wakefulness) and (2) *content* (i.e., awareness).   shows how these two components are typically present or absent in different normal and abnormal states/conditions.

Note that in Table 11.3, in between the healthy (awake) individual and comatose patient (which are at opposite ends of the spectrum), wakefulness and awareness typically appear to vary together (both very low during general anaesthesia, jointly returning as we progress from deep sedation/sleep to wakefulness). However, in VS, they seem to dissociate; VS patients appear to be awake but they are not aware. The reverse dissociation occurs naturally during rapid eye movement (REM) sleep and especially during oneiric (dream-related) experiences, where a subjective feeling of awareness is often present despite the individual not being awake.

Some VS patients will never make any significant recovery and will be diagnosed as in *permanent* VS (in the United Kingdom, such a diagnosis is made after at least 6 months – for non-traumatic brain injury – and 12 months (for traumatic ones: Monti and Owen, 2010). But other patients do regain some (transient) level of awareness, progressing to a *minimally conscious state*.

Table 11.3 The appearance of level (wakefulness) and content (awareness) of consciousness as displayed in different normal and abnormal states/conditions

Normal/abnormal states/conditions	Consciousness	
	Level (wakefulness)	Content (awareness)
Healthy (awake) individual	✓	✓
Comatose patient	X	X
Under general anaesthetic	Very low	Very low
From deep sedation/sleep → wakefulness	✓	✓
Vegetative state (VS)	✓ (apparent)	X
REM ('dream') sleep and (other) oneiric (dream-related) experiences	X	✓
Source: Based on Monti, M.M. and Owen, A.M., *The Psychologist*, 23, 478–481, 2010.		

(For a discussion of how we determine that a patient has regained consciousness, see Gross, 2012a.)

So the significant difference is that the VS patient could seem to be aware because of being wakeful whereas an aware patient can dream/experience dreamlike activities (denoting brain function) while not being wakeful. This is confusing and distressing for families of VS patients who perhaps then have false hopes of the patient's recovery.

Genetic aspects of illness

Basic concepts

- *Genetics* is the scientific study of the inheritance of both physical and behavioural traits (Gill and McGrath, 2010).
- *Genes*, the basic units of heredity (or units of genetic information), consist of molecules of *deoxyribonucleic acid* (DNA) and are found inside the nucleus of almost every cell in the human body. They provide the assembly code for the molecules that make up life and enable reproduction of living organisms (Gill and McGrath, 2010).
- Genes are located on *chromosomes*, highly folded and compressed stretches of DNA. Each gene has a specific location on a chromosome.
- Humans normally have 23 pairs of chromosomes (one member of each pair passed from each parent): 22 pairs are called *autosomes* (any non-sex chromosome) and one pair is called *sex chromosomes* (female: XX; male: XY).
- Ridley (1999) asks us to imagine that the genome is a book. The book comprises 23 chapters (corresponding to the 23 *chromosomes*). Each chapter contains several thousand stories (*genes*). (In fact, the number now appears to be about 23, 500 [Le Page, 2010]). Each story is composed of paragraphs (*exons*), which are interrupted by advertisements (*introns*). Each paragraph is made up of words (*codons*). Each word is written in letters (*bases*). (There are an estimated 3 billion bases [Pollard et al., 2009].) There are 1 billion words in the book (as long as 800 Bibles) (see Figure 11.5).

Ridley's (1999) analogy illustrates cleverly the huge potential for differences in human beings – and is a very effective argument for treating each person as an individual!

While, according to Ridley, the idea of the genome as a book is literally true, there are also some important differences. English books are written in words of variable length using 26 letters, genomes are written entirely in three-letter words, using only four letters: A (which stands for *adenine*), C (*cytosine*), G (*guanine*) and T (*thymine*). Also, instead of being written on flat pages, these words are written on long chains of sugar and phosphate called DNA molecules; the bases are attached as side rungs. Each chromosome is one pair of very long DNA molecules. Ridley describes the genome as a 'very clever book': in the right conditions, it can both photocopy itself (*replication*) and read itself (*translation*).

Figure 11.5 Human genome represented as a book. (Based on Ridley, M., *Genome: The Autobiography of a Species in 23 Chapters*, London, Fourth Estate, 1999.)

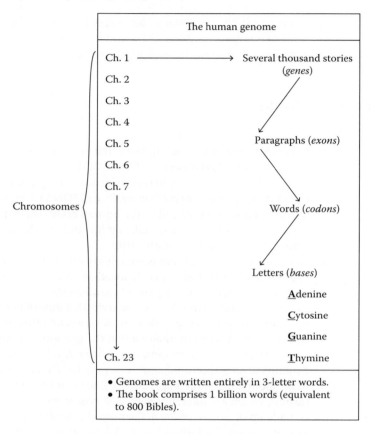

- Mistakes can and do occur when genes are replicated. A letter (base) is occasionally missed out or the wrong letter inserted. Whole sentences or paragraphs are sometimes duplicated, omitted or reversed. These errors are called mutations. As Ridley (1999) points out, many mutations are neither harmful nor beneficial. Human beings accumulate about 100 mutations per generation; in the wrong place even a single one can be fatal.
- For each pair of chromosomes, the form of each gene may be the same on both chromosomes (*homozygous*) or different (*heterozygous*). Alternative forms of a gene at a specific chromosomal location are called alleles.
- With the exception of identical (monozygotic) twins, every individual has a unique set of genes (*genotype*). In any two randomly selected human genotypes, 99.9% of the DNA sequence will be identical: the 0.01% that is different accounts for the genetic contribution to individuality, susceptibility to disease and population diversity (Gill and McGrath, 2010).

Replication and translation

Figure 11.6 Structure of a DNA molecule represented schematically, showing the double-stranded coiled structure.

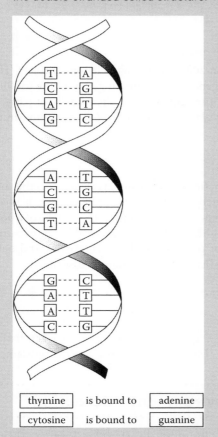

thymine	is bound to	adenine
cytosine	is bound to	guanine

Replication works because of an ingenious property of the four bases: A pairs only with T, and G pairs only with C. So, a single strand of DNA can copy itself by assembling a complementary strand with Ts opposite all the As, As opposite all the Ts, Cs opposite all the Gs and Gs opposite all the Cs. In fact, the usual state of DNA is the famous *double helix* of the original strand and its complementary pair intertwined (see Figure 11.6).

So, making a copy of the complementary strand brings back the original text: the sequence ACGT becomes TGCA in the copy, which transcribes back to ACGT in the copy of the copy. In this way, DNA can replicate indefinitely, while still containing the same information.

The *translation* process is completed when the gene has become converted into a *protein*: every protein is a translated gene. Translation begins with the text of a gene being *transcribed* (translated) into a copy by the same base-pairing process described above. But this time, the copy is made of RNA – a very slightly different chemical. RNA can also carry a linear code and uses the same letters as DNA – except that it uses U (*uracil*) instead of T. This RNA copy (called *messenger RNA*) is then edited by removing all introns and the splicing together of all exons.

Almost everything in the body, from hair to hormones, is either made of proteins or made by them .... (Ridley, 1999)

- An individual's genotype is contrasted with his/her *phenotype*, that is, observable traits or characteristics. Both 'genotype' and 'phenotype' can either refer to a specific trait or characteristic (including a particular disease) or to the complete set of traits or characteristics the individual possesses.
- A common misunderstanding of the influence of genes is that a particular genotype inevitably produces a particular phenotype (i.e., given the inheritance of a particular gene/genes, the individual will develop the associated characteristic). Rose (1997) calls this view *neurogenetic determinism* and is based on the false assumption that causes can be classified

as *either* genetic *or* environmental. What neurogenetic determinism fails to take into account is *gene–environment interaction*. A classic example of gene–environment interaction is *phenylketonuria* (PKU), as described in Box 11.1.

So even in such a biologically influenced matter, some of the few 'mistakes' can be mediated by the environment. This should come much later However, if there is no possibility of correctional environmental intervention (as in AD as yet), there are still psychological and social implications for individuals, families and society. So the BPS model of health care is still more useful than a purely medical one.

Begun in 1990 and completed in 2003, the Human Genome Project (HGP) has successfully identified all the genes in the human genome (the totality of human genes); it has determined the sequences of chemical base pairs that comprise human DNA. (This has also been achieved for many non-human species; see Gross [2012a].)

Molecular genetic research and genetic disorders

As we noted in page 267, neurogenetic determinism largely ignores the role of environmental factors. We also noted that in the case of PKU, there is no one-to-one relationship between genotype and phenotype; if that is true of a potentially fatal bodily disorder, it is highly likely that there will be an even more complex interaction in the case of psychological characteristics and behaviours (such as intelligence, personality and certain mental disorders).

This could presumably include a predisposition to alcohol addiction – like Mr Bates? (*case study 12*) – which is heavily influenced by personality and social context.

The search for genes that 'cause' specific behaviours or characteristics is called *molecular genetic research* (MGR). MGR raises several fundamental

Box 11.1 Phenylketonuria and gene–environment interaction

Genetically speaking, Phenylketonuria (*PKU*) is a simple characteristic: a bodily disorder caused by the inheritance of a single recessive gene from each parent. Normally, the body produces the amino acid phenylalanine hydroxylase, which converts phenylalanine (a substance found in many foods, particularly dairy products) into tyrosine. But in the presence of the two recessive PKU genes, this process fails and phenylalanine builds up in the blood, depressing the levels of other amino acids. Consequently, the developing nervous system is deprived of essential nutrients, leading to severe mental retardation and, without intervention, proves fatal.

The relationship between the *genotype* (the two PKU genes) and the phenotype (high levels of phenylalanine in the blood, and mental retardation) appears to be straightforward, direct and inevitable: given the genotype, the phenotype will occur. However, a routine blood test soon after birth can detect the presence of the PKU genes, and an affected baby will be put on a low-phenylalanine diet. This prevents the disease from developing. In other words, an environmental intervention will prevent the phenotype from occurring.

methodological (see Chapter 1) and ethical issues (e.g., Joseph, 2003). A number of researchers have pointed out that genetic advances in diagnosis and treatment (and sometimes prevention) of physical diseases also present their own ethical quandaries (Hamilton-West, 2011); for example,

1. Is it ethical to offer genetic testing?
2. What information should be given about the limitations and risks of testing?
3. Who should be informed about genetic testing results?
4. Should access to test results be available to outside parties (such as employers and insurers)?

According to Hamilton-West (2011), psychologists, working together with genetic counsellors, may provide a useful service in helping to resolve the (potential) conflict between the autonomy of relatives – who may not wish to participate in genetic testing – and the interests of the patient – for whom relatives' test results could provide important information regarding the nature and location of familial mutation.

Angus is a friend of mine who has Type 1 (the commonest, and mild, form of Von Willebrand disease [VWD]). This is a bleeding disorder which is usually inherited as an autosomal dominant trait which therefore affects both sexes.

Angus only needs treatment if he has surgery or trauma, but when Fiona, his partner, became pregnant recently they decided it would be sensible to find out their baby's VWB status. So, early in the pregnancy they asked their midwife who referred them to a haematology consultant. He was reassuring and explained that if the baby was VWB positive the only risk would be in the event of intervention, e.g. forceps delivery, during the birth. However, it meant the pregnancy must now be obstetric consultant, rather than midwife, led.

Genetic disease: Inherited and acquired mutations

Although the term 'mutation' refers to any change in sequence or structure, it is sometimes taken to mean a change that causes or contributes to a disease or abnormal phenotype.

- If the DNA variant created by a mutation event becomes common within a population over time, then it is known as a *polymorphism* (Gill and McGrath, 2010).
- A mutation that arises during the division of the fertilised embryo (*mitosis* or *mitotic division*) is called a *somatic mutation* and is not heritable.
- Mutations that arise in cells that go on to produce *gametes* (sperm and egg cells), which divide through *meiosis* or *meiotic division*, are called *germ-line mutations* and may be transmitted to the next generation.
- The simplest form of mutations involves a single base pair (a *point mutation*) (Gill and McGrath, 2010).
- Damage to DNA during a person's lifetime (*acquired mutations*) can occur as a result of *endogenous* (i.e., internal) causes (e.g., errors arising in normal

cell replication) or *exogenous* (i.e., external/environmental) causes (e.g., diet, alcohol and environmental toxins, including radiation and hazardous substances) (Gidron et al., 2006).

Disorders that are at least partly caused by genetic factors are classified as follows (Hamilton-West, 2011):

- *Single gene disorders* (such as cystic fibrosis and sickle cell disease) are caused by a mutation in a single gene.
- *Chromosomal disorders* (such as Down's syndrome) result from an abnormal number of chromosomes or structural rearrangement of chromosomes.
- *Complex* (or *multifactorial*) *disorders* (such as schizophrenia and type 1 diabetes) are produced by complex interactions between genes and the environment.

Inheritance of disease

The pattern of inheritance in hereditary diseases is determined by both (i) the type of chromosome the abnormal gene is located on (autosomal or sex chromosome) and (ii) whether the gene itself is *dominant* or *recessive*.

- A *dominant* gene is a mutant gene, only one of which is required to cause the associated disease, that is, even if the corresponding gene inherited from the other parent is normal, the single dominant gene is sufficient to produce the disease. In *autosomal dominant* disease, each individual has a 50% chance of passing the mutant gene to his/her children (since each parent passes just one chromosome of each pair to the offspring). Individuals who inherit a single dominant gene both have the disease and are carriers (i.e., they can pass it on to their own offspring). Examples include Huntington's disease, neurofibromatosis types 1 and 2, Marfan syndrome and hereditary nonpolyposis colorectal cancer.

The Type 1 VWB gene is autosomal dominant and is transmitted through Angus's mother's family. Angus's mother has two sisters, one of whom has the disease and one doesn't; like each of all three siblings Angus's baby has a 1:2 chance of having the disorder.

- In *autosomal recessive* diseases, the child must inherit *two* copies of the mutant gene (one from each parent) to develop the disease. Since each individual has a 50% chance of inheriting the mutant gene from each parent, children of parents who both carry the gene have
  - A 25 per cent chance of inheriting two affected chromosomes (and so inherit the disease)
  - A 25 per cent chance of inheriting two normal chromosomes) (healthy, no disease and not a carrier)
  - A 50 per cent chance of inheriting one affected chromosome and one normal chromosome (healthy, but a carrier)

Examples include cystic fibrosis, sickle cell disease, Tay–Sachs disease, Niemann–Pick disease and spinal muscular atrophy.

Unlike Janet, who, when having an abortion because of genetic testing for Down's syndrome, was concerned with ethical issues (case study 10), Angus and Fiona weren't. However, they had psychological ones. In the event of needing instrumental intervention they would have to make the decision whether to go ahead and it must have added an extra element of anxiety to the birth for them.

Note that inheriting two recessive genes does not make development of the disease inevitable – as we saw in the case of PKU. Diseases may also be linked to the X chromosome. Since men have one X chromosome and one Y chromosome, fathers with an affected X chromosome will *always* pass on the mutant gene, while mothers have a 50% chance of doing so. In the case of a dominant mutant gene (*X-linked dominant inheritance*), a father with the disease will pass on the mutant gene to all his daughters, but none of his sons; if the mother has the disease, she has a 50% chance of passing on the mutant gene to each child.

- In the case of *X-linked recessive inheritance*, females must inherit one mutant gene from each parent to have the disease; if they inherit a single recessive gene (from either parent), they will just be a carrier. Males only need to inherit a single gene on their X chromosome to have the disease; unlike females, there is no corresponding normal gene on their Y chromosome to counteract the effects of the mutant gene. Some of the most common examples of X-linked recessive disorders include haemophilia, Duchenne muscular dystrophy, Becker's muscular dystrophy, X-linked icthyosis (a skin disorder), X-linked agammaglobulinaemia (an immune system deficiency) and colour blindness.

I've found the scientific elements of this chapter difficult, but it has confirmed a 'perspective transformation' for me. Mesirow (1981) identified this as a sudden insight into one's assumptions and a transitional movement to a revision of those assumptions. Mesirow saw the first four of his levels of reflectivity as 'consciousness' and the last three as 'critical consciousness'. The last of these, theoretical reflection (the awareness of reasons for our precipitant judgment or conceptual inadequacy), was the process he considered central to perspective transformation (Bulman and Shutz 2008, pages 231 and 232).

My attempts at reflective writing have increasingly (not suddenly, as Mesirow suggests) made me aware of the complexity of knowledge relating to the biological, psychological, social and ethical aspects of medical and nursing care and how closely integrated they are: the information is never complete and depends on research findings in every area and making links between them. It is why, within the rapidly changing provision of healthcare, caring emotionally for ill people must be based on on-going, critical evaluation of psychology theory in particular, and nursing theory and practice in general. A challenging, but exciting, realisation!

CHAPTER SUMMARY

- Severe *dementia* affects only a minority of elderly people. However, it is the most age-related disabling conditions affecting older people.
- For diagnostic purposes, a broad distinction is made between
  i. cortical *dementias* (such as AD), involving the classic neuropsychological deficit syndromes of *amnesia, aphasia/dysphasia agnosia* and *apraxia* and
  ii. *subcortical dementias* (such as multiple sclerosis and Huntington's disease) involving slowing of cognition, often associated with altered behaviour and personality, and dysexecutive syndrome.
- Common behavioural psychological symptoms of dementia include depression, anxiety and general emotional sensitivity, various psychotic symptoms, aggression, wandering and changes in sleep and eating patterns.
- *Personality* changes (including apathy and neglect of self-care) are a prominent feature of frontal lobe dementias.
- All dementias involve a progressive loss of *motor function* in the end stages.
- *AD* is the most common form of dementia and is one of the most debilitating and dreaded of the common diseases of ageing.
- AD involves brain shrinkage (atrophy), mainly in temporal lobe structures (including the hippocampus) and the neurons develop tangles and plaques (amyloid).
- However, AD, strictly speaking, is a *behavioural syndrome* (not a disease): we cannot yet define its severity in terms of brain pathology.
- In addition to memory loss (initially short-term, then long-term), clinical features include *nominal* and *fluent dysphasia* and impairment of judgement as well as many of the features associated with dementia (including personality change).
- According to OPTIMA, AD is a disease process distinct from normal ageing (and not an accelerated form of normal changes in the ageing brain); however, it is more likely to affect us as we age.
- Coleman and O'Hanlon believe that loss of *automatic intelligence* helps to distinguish AD from other memory disorders resulting from neurological injury.
- A major *stroke* (*CVA*) can mark entry to the 'fourth age'/'old age' proper.
- Major causes of stroke are *ischaemia/infarction* or *intracerebral haemorrhage*; the former can itself be caused by *embolism* or *cerebral thrombosis*, while the latter can be the result of an *aneurysm* or *high BP*.
- Communication problems include *aphasia* (*receptive, expressive* or *mixed*), *dysarthria* and *dyspraxia*. *Paralysis* usually affects only one limb/side of the body.
- *Cognitive problems* include deficits in visual memory or verbal memory, short-term memory and anterograde amnesia, selective and divided attention, executive functioning and social cognition.

- *Emotional/affective changes* include depression and anxiety, emotionalism, anger and personality changes.
- Two main types of vascular dementia related to strokes are MID and SID.
- While strokes are remarkably common, especially in the over-65s, they are becoming increasingly common in the under-30s as a result of taking drugs such as cocaine.
- *Genetics* is the scientific study of the inheritance of both physical and behavioural traits.
- *Neurogenetic determinism* represents a common misunderstanding of the influence of *genes*, namely that a particular *genotype* inevitably produces a particular *phenotype*. It fails to take into account *gene–environment interaction*, as demonstrated by *PKU*.
- The Human Genome Project (HGP) has successfully identified all the genes in the human genome; it has determined the sequence of *chemical base pairs* that comprise human *DNA*.
- Molecular genetic research (*MGR*) raises several fundamental methodological and ethical issues.
- Disorders that are at least partly caused by genetic factors are classified as *single gene, chromosomal* and *complex/multifactorial disorders.*
- The pattern of inheritance in hereditary disease is determined by both the type of chromosome the abnormal gene is located on (*autosome* or *sex chromosome*) and whether the gene itself is *dominant* or *recessive.*
- Abnormal genes can be found on the female (X) chromosomes, as in *X-linked dominant* and *X-linked recessive inheritance.*

12 Substance use and abuse

Introduction and overview

In the context of hospitals and doctors' surgeries, a drug is normally understood to mean a medicine ('pills'/'tablets') and is assumed to be beneficial. According to the World Health Organization (Sykes, 1995), a drug is 'any substance or product that is used or intended to be used to modify or explore physiological systems or pathological states for the benefit of the recipient'.

However, for thousands of years, people have taken substances to alter their perception of reality and societies have restricted the substances their members are allowed to take. These substances, which we usually call drugs, are *psychoactive*, denoting a chemical substance that alters conscious awareness through its effect on the brain. Most drugs fit this definition. Some – for example, aspirin – are *indirectly* psychoactive: their primary purpose is to remove pain, but being headache free lifts our mood. Others, however, are *designed* to change mood and behaviour. These are collectively referred to as *psychotherapeutic* drugs, such as those used in the treatment of anxiety, depression and schizophrenia (see Gross, 2010).

This chapter is concerned with psychoactive drugs used to produce a temporarily altered state of consciousness for the purpose of *pleasure*. These include *recreational drugs*, which have no legal restrictions (such as alcohol, nicotine and caffeine), and *drugs of abuse*, which are illegal. However, just as recreational drugs can be abused (such as alcohol), illegal drugs are taken recreationally (such as ecstasy). 'Substance abuse', therefore, does not imply particular types of drug, but refers to the extent to which the drug is used and the effects – emotional, behavioural and medical – on the abuser. According to Veitia and McGahee (1995):

> Cigarette smoking and alcohol abuse permeate our culture and are widespread enough to be considered ordinary addictions ... The degree to which these drugs permeate our culture and the extent to which they are accepted by our society distinguish them from other addictive but illegal substances such as heroin.

From my diary (12): Year 2/Medical Ward

Mr Bates (Brian) is a 50-year-old man who is alcohol-dependent and has a cirrhotic liver and ascites. Adam, my mentor, knows Brian well as he appears at intervals with haematemesis and/or malaena. When I helped admit him, Brian looked thin, pale, sweaty, dyspnoeic and was in obvious discomfort from his grossly distended abdomen. An ascitic tap was planned for an hour later. He was given oxygen, IV fluids were started and Adam inserted a naso-gastric tube. As his bladder needed to be emptied prior to the tap and Brian couldn't pass urine into a urinal, the F1 ordered an indwelling catheter. Brian began shouting at the doctor that he 'couldn't stand any more tubes', so Adam suggested the doctor should leave the problem with him. He gradually calmed Brian down and we then managed to help him out of bed and on to a commode.

Defining abuse

The concept of addiction

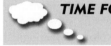 **TIME FOR REFLECTION ...**

- What do you understand by the term 'addiction'?

Until recently, the study and treatment of drug problems were organised around the concept of *addiction*: people with drug problems have problems because they are addicted to the drug (Hammersley, 1999). Addicts are compelled by a physiological need to continue taking the drug, experience horrible physical and psychological symptoms when trying to stop, and will continue taking it despite these symptoms because of their addictive need. Their addiction will also change them psychologically for the worse, they will commit crimes to pay for the drug, neglect their social roles and responsibilities, and even harm the people around them. In addition, some drugs are considered inherently much more addictive than others, and substance users can be divided into addicts and non-addicts.

Criticisms of the concept

- It is an oversimplification. Most professionals who deal with people with any kind of problem – medical, criminal, educational, social – will have seen many clients who are not exactly addicts, but whose drug use seems to have contributed to, or worsened, their other problems (Hammersley, 1999).
- It is based on the *addiction-as-disease model*. Medical models such as this are generally persuasive, because they offer a diagnosis, a definition and a pathology; but they also appear to relieve the 'addict' of responsibility for his/her behaviour (Baker, 2000). This is discussed further below, in relation to alcohol dependence (see pages 288 through 290).

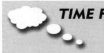 Brian's primary diagnosis is 'alcohol dependency'; he's addicted to the recreational, and legal, drug of alcohol.

According to Hammersley (1999), the more modern view is to see drug problems as two-fold: *substance abuse* and *substance dependence* (hence the title of this chapter). This view is adopted in the American Psychiatric Association's (2000) *Diagnostic and Statistical Manual of Mental Disorders* (DSM-IV-TR – see Boxes 12.1 and 12.2). 'Addiction' is now usually used to refer to a field of study covering substance use, abuse and dependence, rather than to a theory of why people become dependent.

TIME FOR REFLECTION ...

- What do terms such as 'workaholic', 'shopaholic' and 'chocaholic' tell you about the nature of addictive behaviour?
- Can you define addiction in a way that can cover such non-drug behaviours?
- What might they all have in common?

Is there more to addiction than drugs?

Rather than rejecting the concept of addiction, some researchers argue that the concept should be *broadened*, in order to cover certain recent forms of 'addictive' behaviour that do not involve chemical substances at all.

Box 12.1 DSM-IV-TR criteria for substance abuse

- A maladaptive pattern of substance use leading to clinically significant impairment or distress, as manifested by one (or more) of the following, occurring within a 12-month period:
  1. Recurrent substance use resulting in a failure to fulfil major role obligations at work, school or home (e.g. repeated absences or poor work performance related to substance use, substance-related absences, suspensions, or expulsions from school; neglect of children or household)
  2. Recurrent substance use in situations where it is physically hazardous (e.g. driving an automobile or operating a machine when impaired by substance use)
  3. Recurrent substance-related legal problems (e.g. arrests for substance-related disorderly conduct)
  4. Continued substance use despite having persistent or recurrent social or interpersonal problems caused or exacerbated by the effects of the substance (e.g. arguments with spouse about consequences of intoxication, physical fights)
- The symptoms have never met the criteria for substance dependence for this class of substance.

Box 12.2 DSM-IV-TR criteria for substance dependence

- A maladaptive pattern of substance use leading to clinically significant impairment or distress, as manifested by three (or more) of the following, occurring at any time in the same 12-month period:
  1. Tolerance, as defined by either of the following:
     a. A need for markedly increased amounts of the substance to achieve intoxication or desired effect
     b. Markedly diminished effect with continued use of the same amount of the substance.
  2. Withdrawal, as manifested by either of the following:
     a. The characteristic withdrawal syndrome for the substance (varies from substance to substance)
     b. The same (or a closely related) substance is taken to relieve or avoid withdrawal symptoms.
  3. The substance is often taken in larger amounts and over a longer period than was intended.
  4. There is a persistent desire or unsuccessful efforts to cut down or control substance use.
  5. A great deal of time is spent in activities necessary to obtain the substance (e.g. visiting multiple doctors or driving long distances), use the substance (e.g. chain smoking) or recover from its effects.
  6. Important social, occupational or recreational activities are given up or reduced because of substance use.
  7. The substance use is continued despite knowledge of having a persistent physical or psychological problem that is likely to have been caused or exacerbated by the substance (e.g. current cocaine use despite recognition of cocaine-induced depression, or continued drinking despite recognition that an ulcer was made worse by alcohol consumption).

Specify if:
- *With physiological dependence*: evidence of tolerance or withdrawal (i.e. either item 1 or 2 is present).
- *With psychological dependence*: no evidence of tolerance or withdrawal (i.e. neither item 1 nor 2 is present).

For example, Griffiths (2005) maintained that several other behaviours, including gambling, watching television, playing amusement machines, overeating, sex, playing computer games and using the Internet, are potentially addictive.

According to Griffiths (2010), the 'classical' features shared by *all* addictions are as follows:

Salience: the all-consuming importance of the activity to the individual
Mood modification: the experience people report when they carry out their addictive behaviour (the 'rush', 'buzz' or 'high')

Tolerance: the increasing amount of the activity required to achieve the same effect

Withdrawal: the unpleasant feelings and physical effects that occur when the addictive behaviour is suddenly discontinued or reduced

Conflict: either with the people around the addicted person, causing great social misery, or within him/herself

Relapse: the tendency for repeated reversions to earlier patterns of the particular activity to recur and for even the most extreme patterns typical of the height of the addiction to be quickly restored after many years of abstinence or control

Brian fulfils most of Griffiths' criteria and knows alcohol is the cause of his other illnesses, but he persists in his drinking pattern.

Substance use and abuse

According to Hammersley (1999), abuse is the use of a substance in a harmful or risky manner, without medical sanction. The concept is something of a compromise, because it is debatable whether *any* use of a substance can be entirely risk free. It also suggests that some risks are negligible, while others are substantial. Hammersley believes that the health risks of tobacco smoking now seem so substantial that all smoking is probably abuse – there is no negligible-risk use of tobacco. But most other drugs *can* be used in ways that make risks negligible.

Brian obviously abuses alcohol; he's chronically ill, hasn't been employed for years, and has lost his driving licence due to convictions for 'drunk driving'.

Dependence

How does dependence differ from abuse?

Brian's notes record if he doesn't drink he gets the 'shakes', indicating physiological dependency, but also becomes 'stressed' (aggressive) under pressure (e.g. having a catheter inserted), which indicates psychological dependency.

The concept of dependence is based around a constellation of symptoms and problems, not just on the idea of physiological need for a drug. Only items 1 and 2 in Box 12.2 refer to physiological dependence. Anyone who fits three or more of these criteria would be diagnosed as substance dependent. Dependence, therefore, is quite varied, and few people fit all seven criteria (Hammersley, 1999).

Even restricting dependence to physiological dependence, the picture is more complex than it might at first appearance. Different drugs may involve

Figure 12.1 George Best, gifted footballer and famous alcoholic.

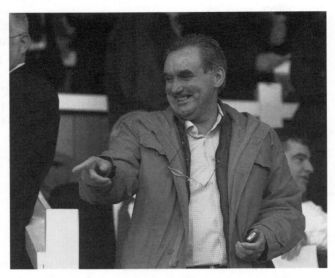

specific effects, such as opiates raising pain thresholds. As Sykes (1995) points out, the search for analgesics that do not have addictive potential continues, but it is possible that the effectiveness of opiates and similar drugs in reducing severe pain is partly due to the pleasurable mood they induce – so the search may fail (see Chapter 3).

Most substance-dependent people have tried to give up several times, always returning to use after weeks, months or even years. They often report strong craving or desire for the substance, and are at particular risk of resuming use when stressed, anxious, depressed, angry or happy. When they relapse, they often return very quickly to their old, often destructive, habits (see Figure 12.1).

 Brian has tried to stop drinking but said he's now given up 'giving up'.

Physiological versus psychological dependence

As Box 12.2 shows, *physiological dependence* is related to *withdrawal* and/or *tolerance* (which relates to the traditional concept of *addiction*), while *psychological dependence* is not. However, being deprived of a substance that is highly pleasurable can induce anxiety. Since the symptoms of anxiety (rapid pulse, profuse sweating, shaking, and so on) overlap with withdrawal symptoms, people may mistakenly believe that they are physiologically dependent. Psychological dependence is, though, part of the overall *dependence syndrome* (see Figure 12.2).

 Whether Brian's 'shakes' are the result of psychological or physiological dependence they must be equally distressing.

Figure 12.2 Summary of major components of dependence syndrome.

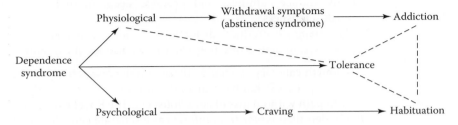

A good example of the difference between the two types of dependence is imipramine, used to treat depression. When it is stopped after prolonged use, there may be nausea, muscle aches, anxiety and difficulty in sleeping, but there was *never* a compulsion to resume taking it (Lowe, 1995). However, Lowe claims that 'psychological' dependence has little scientific meaning beyond the notion that drug taking becomes part of one's habitual behaviour. Giving it up is very difficult, because the person has become *habituated* to it:

> **Habituation is the repeated use of a drug because the user finds that use increases pleasurable feelings or reduces feelings of anxiety, fear or stress. Habituation becomes problematic when the person becomes so consumed by the need for the drug-altered state of consciousness that all his or her energies are directed to compulsive drug-seeking behaviour … (Lowe, 1995).**

Physiologically addictive drugs, such as heroin and alcohol, typically cause habituation *as well*. Most widely used recreational drugs, including cannabis, cocaine, lysergic acid diethylamide (LSD), phencycladine (see Table 12.1) and *methylenedioxymethamphetamine* (*MDMA*, otherwise known as '*ecstasy*'), *do not* cause physiological dependence – but people *do* become habituated.

To help nurses understand habituation, David Cooper (in Alexander et al., 2006) suggests stopping a favourite substance for a week and noting the effects. I tried giving up coffee. The physical symptoms (headache and tiredness) of caffeine withdrawal were mild, but I resented being deprived of the pleasure of drinking it and after two days became very bad tempered!

Classifying drugs

Hamilton and Timmons (1995) identified three broad groups of psychoactive drugs:

1. *Stimulants* temporarily excite neural activity, arouse bodily functions, enhance positive feelings and heighten alertness; in high doses, they cause overt seizures

2. *Depressants* (or *sedatives*) depress neural activity, slow down bodily functions, induce calmness and produce sleep; in high doses, they cause unconsciousness
3. *Hallucinogens* produce distortion of normal perception and thought processes; in high doses, they can cause episodes of psychotic behaviour

A fourth category is *opiates*. These also depress activity in the central nervous system (CNS), but have an *analgesic* property – that is, they reduce sensitivity to pain without loss of consciousness. The Royal College of Psychiatrists (1987) identified *minor tranquillisers* as a separate category, but in Table 12.1, they have been included under the general category of depressants. *Cannabis* does not fall easily into any of these other categories.

 I have to admit that I, and several friends, are habituated to the stimulant drug of caffeine!

Table 12.1 Some examples of the major categories of psychoactive drugs

Major category	Examples/slang names
Depressants (sedatives)	Alcohol
	Barbiturates: 'downers', 'barbs', various other names derived from names or colour of pill/capsule (e.g. 'blueys')
	Tranquillisers: 'tranx'
	Solvents
Stimulants	Caffeine
	Nicotine
	Amphetamines: 'uppers', 'speed', 'sulphate', 'sulph', 'whizz'
	MDMA: 'ecstasy', 'E', plus many names derived from shape and colour of drugs
	Cocaine: 'coke', 'snow', 'crack', 'freebase', 'base', 'wash', 'rock'
Opiates	Morphine: 'junk', 'skag', 'H', 'smack'
	Heroin
	Codeine
	Methadone: 'amps' (injectable), 'linctus' (oral)
Hallucinogens	Lysergic acid diethylamide: 'acid'
	Mescaline
	Psilocybin: 'magic mushrooms', 'mushies'
	Phencycladine: 'angel dust'
Cannabis	Cannabis sativa: 'pot', 'dope', 'blow', 'draw', 'smoke'
	Herbal cannabis: 'grass', 'marijuana', 'ganja'
	Cannabis resin: 'weed', 'the herb', 'skunk'
	Cannabis oil: 'hash', 'hashish'

Source: Cooper, D., *Nursing Times Guides*, 1995.

The effects of drugs

Alcohol

TIME FOR REFLECTION ...

- Either from your own experience, or from observing others, how would you describe the effects of alcohol?

Despite the difficulties in assessing the relationship between level of intake and harmful effects, certain 'safe levels' are widely accepted (Gelder et al., 1999). These are expressed in terms of *units* of alcohol; one unit is equal to 8 g of ethanol (the equivalent of half a pint of beer, a small glass of wine, a glass of sherry or a standard (pub) measure of spirits).

For *men*, up to *28 units* per week, and for *women*, up to *21 units* is considered safe (Ogden, 2004), provided the whole amount is not taken all at once and that there are occasional drink-free days. Anything over 50 and 35 units, respectively, is considered 'dangerous'. The British legal driving blood alcohol limit is 80 mg per 100 ml (equivalent to two or three drinks) (Box 12.3).

Box 12.3 Some physiological effects of alcohol

- Ethanol is a *diuretic*, so you end up *expelling* more water than you drink. It acts on the pituitary gland, blocking production of the hormone *vasopressin*, which directs the kidneys to reabsorb water that would otherwise end up in the bladder. So, the body borrows water from other places, including the brain, which shrinks temporarily. Although the brain itself cannot experience pain, it is thought that dehydration shrivels the *dura* (a membrane covering the brain). As this happens, it tugs at pain-sensitive filaments connecting it to the skull. Water loss might also account for pains elsewhere in the body (see Chapter 3).
- Frequent trips to the toilet also result in loss of essential sodium and potassium ions, which are central to how nerves and muscles work. Subtle chemical imbalances caused by ion depletion could account for a cluster of symptoms, including headaches, nausea and fatigue.
- Alcohol also depletes our reserves of sugar, leading to hypoglycaemia. The body's store of energy-rich glycogen in the liver is broken down into glucose; this quickly becomes another constituent of urine. This can account for feelings of weakness and unsteadiness the morning after.

Source: New Scientist, *New Scientist, 164*(2214), 34–36, 1999.

📋 The increased abuse of alcohol by young people indicates changing psychosocial/environmental causes; Brian's medical history showed he started drinking heavily as a teenager, with a gang of friends. This reminds me of 16-year-old Josh (case study 8, page 86) and is an example of the 'normative' social and environmental elements of the Theory of Planned Behaviour Model (see Chapter 10). Brian's present drinking cronies and past unsuccessful attempts to give up his drinking would affect his 'perceived behavioural control'.

Heavy drinkers suffer malnutrition: since alcohol is high in calories, appetite is suppressed. It also causes vitamin deficiency, by interfering with absorption of vitamin B from the intestines; long term, this causes brain damage. Other physical effects include liver damage, heart disease, increased risk of a stroke and susceptibility to infections due to a suppressed immune system (see Chapter 5). Women who drink while pregnant can produce babies with *foetal alcohol syndrome*.

📋 Brian is undernourished and on admission was dehydrated. His immune system is being weakened by internal stress and his frequent hospital admissions are evidence his health is deteriorating.

Alcohol and memory

Alcohol interferes with normal sleep patterns. Although it causes sedation, alcohol also suppresses rapid eye movement sleep (where most dreaming takes place) by as much as 20 per cent (see Gross, 2010). There also appears to be a link between alcohol-induced sleepiness and memory loss. People who get drunk and then forget what happened have memory impairments similar to those suffered by people with sleep disorders, such as daytime sleepiness (Motluk, 1999). In both cases, the person cannot recall how they got home, or what happened while at work or at the pub.

It is the transfer of information into long-term memory that seems to be disrupted. The GABA signals that induce the sleepiness can interfere with both the early and late stages of memory formation (*stimulus registration* and *consolidation*, respectively). Chemicals that mimic GABA can do this, and there are many GABA receptors in the hippocampus. Another memory disorder associated with chronic alcohol consumption is *Korsakoff's syndrome*.

📋 We recently had a patient with Korsakoff's syndrome waiting for a care home bed. This is a memory disorder associated with prolonged and heavy use of alcohol causing inability to process new information into long-term memory (anterograde amnesia) and remember past events (retrograde amnesia) (See Gross, 2010, page 265). Eddie was 61 and had to be taken to the toilet as he was confused and forgot where it was; one night he was found passing urine in the visitor's room. The night nurse admitted she was furious and had to make a big effort to remind herself Eddie can't help his behaviour.

Cocaine

Cocaine hydrochloride is a powerful CNS stimulant extracted from the leaves of the coca shrub, native to the Andes mountains in South America. When smoked, the drug reaches the brain in 5–10 seconds, much faster than the other methods. It can also be swallowed, rubbed on the gums or blown into the throat.

Typically, the user experiences a state of euphoria, deadening of pain, and increased self-confidence, energy and attention. There is also a 'crash' when the drug wears off.

The growing pandemic of cocaine use in Western society is overshadowing the traditional risk factors for stroke, such as high blood pressure. This is much more common in older people, as are strokes, but it is becoming increasingly common for people under 30 to suffer strokes after taking drugs (Laurance, 2000) (see Chapter 11).

Cocaine (and amphetamines) produces a surge in blood pressure. People with abnormal blood vessels in their brain, such as a cerebral aneurysm, are at greatest risk. But, it is also possible that the drug taking caused the deformed blood vessels (Laurance, 2000). Repeated inhalation constricts the blood vessels in the nose. The nasal septum may become perforated, necessitating cosmetic surgery.

Formication refers to the sensation that 'insects' ('coke bugs') are crawling beneath the skin. Although this is merely random neural activity, users sometimes try to remove the imaginary insects by cutting deep into their skin. Cocaine definitely produces *psychological dependence*, but there is much more doubt regarding *physiological dependence, tolerance* and *withdrawal.* The effects of *crack* are more rapid and intense than that of cocaine, but the 'crash' is also more intense.

Unlike heroin-dependent people, most cocaine users will get over their drug problem *without* professional help (Hammersley, 1999).

Morphine and heroin

As shown in Table 12.1, morphine and heroin belong to the *opiate* group of psychoactive drugs. Opiates are derived from the unripe seed pods of the opium poppy ('plant of joy'); one constituent of opium is morphine, from which codeine and heroin can be extracted.

In general, the opiates depress neural functioning and suppress physical sensations and responses to stimulation.

Heroin can be smoked, inhaled or injected intravenously. Puffing the heated white powder ('chasing the dragon') is now the preferred method, because syringes are seen as dirty and dangerous (Khan, 2003). The immediate effects (the 'rush') are described as an overwhelming sensation of pleasure, similar to sexual orgasm but affecting the whole body. Such effects are so pleasurable that they override any thoughts of food or sex. Heroin rapidly decomposes into morphine, producing feelings of euphoria, well-being, relaxation and drowsiness (Box 12.4).

Long-term users become more aggressive and socially isolated, as well as less physically active. Opiates in general may damage the body's immune system, leading to increased susceptibility to infection. The impurity of the heroin used, users' lack of adequate diet, and the risks from contaminated needles all increase health risks. Overdoses are common.

Box 12.4 Heroin and endorphins

- The brain produces its own opiates (*opioid peptides* or *endorphins* – see Chapter 3).
- When we engage in important survival behaviours, endorphins are released into the fluid that bathes the neurons. Endorphin molecules stimulate *opiate receptors* on some neurons, producing an intensely pleasurable effect just like that reported by heroin users.
- Regular use of opiates overloads endorphin sites in the brain and the brain stops producing its own endorphins (Snyder, 1977). When the user abstains, neither the naturally occurring endorphins nor the opiates are available. Consequently, the internal mechanism for regulating pain is severely disrupted, producing some of the withdrawal symptoms described earlier.

Heroin produces both *physiological* and *psychological dependence. Tolerance* develops quickly. *Withdrawal symptoms* initially involve flu-like symptoms, progressing to tremors, stomach cramps, and alternating chills and sweats. Rapid pulse, high blood pressure, insomnia and diarrhoea also occur. The skin often breaks out into goose bumps resembling a plucked turkey (hence '*cold turkey*' to describe attempts to abstain). The legs jerk uncontrollably (hence '*kicking the habit*'). These symptoms last about 1 week, reaching a peak after about 48 hours.

Addiction to prescription drugs is not uncommon, but McCaffery and Beebe (1994, in Alexander et al., 2006) argue that this dependence rarely appears in a clinical setting, since analgesic opioids are usually titrated and gradually reduced as pain diminishes. However, I remembered Clare (case study 9, page 367), who had been in hospital very frequently prior to her ileostomy with acute abdominal pain. She usually had a cannula in situ as IV drugs were more comfortable, but on one occasion Caroline (ward manager) raised the issue of possible dependency and the F2 changed the morphine prescription to IM.

Methadone

This is a synthetic opiate (or opioid) created to treat the physiological dependence on heroin and other opiates. Methadone acts more slowly than heroin and does not produce the heroin 'rush'. While heroin users may be less likely to take heroin if they are on methadone, they are likely to become at least *psychologically dependent* on it. By the early 1980s, long-term prescribing of methadone (methadone maintenance) began to be questioned, both in terms of effectiveness and the message it conveyed to users.

However, the HIV/AIDS epidemic has made harm minimisation a priority. The dispensing of injecting equipment and condoms in 'needle exchange' schemes has been combined with attempts to persuade users to substitute oral methadone for intravenous heroin. This reduces the risk of transmitting both HIV and other blood-borne viruses, such as hepatitis B (Lipsedge, 1997).

Cannabis

This is second only to alcohol in popularity. The *cannabis sativa* plant's psychoactive ingredient is *delta-9-tetrahydrocannabinil* (THC). THC is found in the branches and leaves of the male and female plants (*marijuana*), but is highly concentrated in the resin of the female plant. *Hashish* is derived from the sticky resin and is more potent than marijuana (see Table 12.1). '*Skunk*' is herbal cannabis grown from selected seeds by intensive indoor methods and is twice as potent as hash or weed.

When smoked, THC reaches the brain within 7 seconds. Small amounts produce a mild, pleasurable 'high', involving relaxation, a loss of social inhibition, intoxication and a humorous mood. Speech becomes slurred and coordination is impaired. Increased heart rate, reduced concentration, enhanced appetite and impaired short-term memory are also quite common effects. Some users report fear, anxiety and confusion.

Large amounts produce hallucinogenic reactions, but these are not full blown as with LSD. THC remains in the body for up to a month, and both male sex hormones and the female menstrual cycle can be disrupted. If used during pregnancy, the foetus may fail to grow properly, and cannabis is more dangerous to the throat and lungs than cigarettes.

While tolerance is usually a sign of physiological dependence, with cannabis *reverse tolerance* has been reported: regular use leads to a *lowering* of the amount needed to produce the initial effects. This could be due to a build-up of THC, which takes a long time to be metabolised. Alternatively, users may become more efficient inhalers and so perceive the drug's effects more quickly. *Withdrawal* effects (restlessness, irritability and insomnia) have been reported, but they seem to be associated only with continuous use of very large amounts. *Psychological dependence* almost certainly occurs in at least some people.

TIME FOR REFLECTION ...

- Do you agree with the government's decision to reclassify cannabis back to a Class B drug in 2009? (It was 'reduced' to a Class C drug, alongside tranquillisers and steroids, in 2004.)
- Do you think it should be legalised (decriminalised)?
- Why/why not?

When Josh was admitted after getting drunk last year, his mother was worried he was also smoking cannabis. She appeared to think this much worse than alcohol which (perhaps as it's legal) she didn't seem to think of as a drug.

Theories of dependence

According to Lowe (1995), 'It is now generally agreed that addictive behaviours are multiply determined phenomena, and should be considered as biopsychosocial entities'. Similarly, Hammersley (1999) maintained that

Figure 12.3 Five main theories of addiction. (From Hammersley, R., Substance use, abuse and dependence, In D. Messer and F. Jones (eds.), *Psychology and Social Care*, London, Jessica Kingsley Publishers, 1999.)

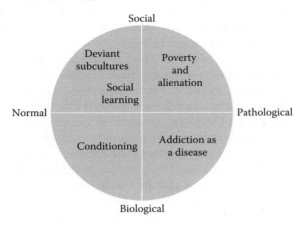

dependence is a complex behaviour that takes several years to develop. So, it is unlikely that one theory or factor could account for all of it. Most researchers believe that social, personal, family and lifestyle factors are important, as well as the action of the drug itself. However, it is not yet understood fully how these work and interact. According to Hammersley, theories of dependence have two dimensions. These are concerned with the extent to which dependence is

1. Supposedly caused by *biological*, as opposed to *social*, factors
2. The result of *abnormal/pathological* processes, as opposed to the *extreme end* of *normal* processes (Figure 12.3)

Stages of substance use

The traditional approach to 'breaking the habit' (whether this involved alcohol or tobacco) was total abstinence, and this is still the philosophy of Alcoholics Anonymous (AA). However, this relatively unsuccessful approach has now largely been replaced by a research emphasis on cessation *as a process*, as demonstrated in Prochaska and DiClemente's (1984) *Stages of Change (SoC) model* (Box 12.5).

 Brian indicated he's unlikely to return to the 'action' stage.

Theories of alcohol dependence

The disease model

Rush, widely regarded as the father of American psychiatry, is commonly credited with being the first major figure to conceptualise alcoholism as a 'disease', in the early 1800s. At about the same time, the British doctor, Trotter,

Box 12.5 SoC model and the nurse's role

1. *Precontemplation*: the person is basically unaware of having a problem/fails to acknowledge it (denial). Most nurses (especially those in A&E) see people in this stage. Misusers are not health seeking (as are most patients) and the nurse's main role is *harm reduction*, as in providing information leaflets regarding needle exchanges.
2. *Cotemplation*: the person begins to recognise that they have a problem and becomes prepared to do something about it.
3. *Preparation*: the person is now seriously considering taking some action to change their behaviour.
4. *Action*: some initial behaviour change takes place.
5. *Maintenance*: the behaviour change is sustained for a period of time.
6. *Relapse*: eventually, most of those who relapse will return to the action stage.

The SoC model helps explain how a person can remain ambivalent about change over many years (Crouch, 2003). Individuals do not progress through the stages in a straightforward, linear fashion, but may switch back and forth (the 'revolving door'); this illustrates the *dynamic* nature of cessation (Ogden, 2004).

Source: Prochaska, J.A. and DiClemente, D.D., *The Transtheoretical Approach: Crossing Traditional Boundaries of Therapy*, Homewood, IL, Dow Jones Irwin, 1984; Crouch, D., *Nursing Times*, 99(33), 20–23, 2003.

likened alcoholism to a mental disorder. Both men saw it as a product of a distinct biological defect or dysfunction, much like cancer, diabetes or TB (Lilienfeld, 1995).

In 1935, a doctor and former alcoholic, Smith and Wilson (a stockbroker) founded Alcholics Anonymons (AA) in the United States. AA assumes that certain individuals possess a physiological susceptibility to alcohol analogous to an allergy: a single drink is sufficient to trigger an unquenchable desire for more, resulting in an inevitable loss of control.

Perhaps the most influential champion of the disease model was Jellinek, a physiologist. Based on questionnaire data with AA members, Jellinek (1946, 1952) proposed that alcoholism was a biological illness with a highly characteristic and predictable course.

Evaluating the disease model

According to Lilienfeld (1995), the course of alcoholism appears to be far more variable than Jellinek proposed (there are no clear-cut stages that alcoholics go through), and many drinkers do not fit into any of Jellinek's 'species'. For example, Cloninger (1987) proposed that:

Group 1 alcoholics are at risk for 'Type 1' alcoholism: they drink primarily to reduce tension, are predominantly female and prone to anxiety and depression and tend to have relatively late onset of problem drinking.

By contrast, *Group 2* alcoholics are at risk for 'Type 2' alcoholism: they drink primarily to relieve boredom, give free rein to their tendency towards risk taking and sensation-seeking, are predominantly male and prone to anti-social and criminal behaviour, and tend to have relatively early onset of drinking behaviour.

Although the evidence for Cloninger's model is tentative and indirect, it challenges the disease model in a quite fundamental way. If he is correct, alcoholism may represent the culmination of two very different (and, in fact, essentially opposite) pathways (Lilienfeld, 1995).

Nevertheless, the disease model was the single most influential theory for much of the 20th century. It is still the dominant view underlying psychiatric and other medically-orientated treatment programmes, but has been much less influential among psychologically-based programmes since the 1980s.

Alcohol dependence syndrome (ADS) (Edwards, 1986) is a later version of the disease model. It grew out of dissatisfaction with 'alcoholism' and with the traditional conception of alcoholism as disease. 'Syndrome' adds flexibility, suggesting a group of concurrent behaviours that accompany alcohol dependence. They need not always be observed in the same individual, nor are they observable to the same degree in everyone. For example, instead of loss of control or inability to abstain, ADS describes 'impaired control'. This implies that people drink heavily because, at certain times and for a variety of psychological and physiological reasons, they choose not to exercise control (Lowe, 1995). Simple disease models have now been largely replaced by a more complex set of working hypotheses based not on irreversible physiological processes but on learning and conditioning, motivation and self-regulation, expectations and attributions (Lowe, 1995).

Lowe's approach is more compatible with the biopsychosocial model of health and illness and is concerned with time and process elements (like the Health Action Process Approach model – see Chapter 3). This is too late to help Eddie, and probably (although not inevitably) for Brian, but it could be very effective in the early stages, e.g. for Josh and his friends.

Preventing alcohol dependence

Prevention and early detection

The importance of tackling alcohol misuse early cannot be overestimated and nurses play a key role in providing health education and prevention (Davies, 2012). Evidence shows that heavy drinking in adolescence increases the likelihood of binge drinking in adulthood (Jefferis et al., 2005). According to Foxcroft et al. (2008), the Traditional Public Health Model (Blane, 1976) proposes three useful *levels of prevention*: *primary* (incidence and prevalence), *secondary* (early identification) and *tertiary* (treatment).

Primary prevention (PP) is appropriate when dealing with adolescents who misuse alcohol. Adolescents often binge drink (rather than being alcohol dependent); they have not been drinking long enough to have become dependent, so PP targets current alcohol misuse and aims at preventing future dependence (Davies, 2012).

PP begins with an initial assessment, during which nurses should evaluate the individual's level of motivation or desire to change his/her alcohol-related behaviour. This can be achieved via *motivational interviewing* (MI) (Miller and Rollnick, 2002), a person-centred style of communication designed to guide the person towards choosing to change his/her behaviour, rather than imposing expectations of change on the individual (see Chapter 2). MI helps adolescents (and older alcohol misusers) realise that they have a problem that needs to be addressed (Marlatt et al., 1998).

Treating alcohol dependence

Theory of planned behaviour and adolescent drinkers

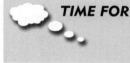

TIME FOR REFLECTION ...

- Look back at Chapter 10 (pages 232 and 233) and the discussion of the TPB.
- How might nurses apply it to change adolescents' misuse of alcohol?

Nurses can apply the TPB by

a. Targeting perceived behavioural control (PBC) through boosting adolescents' self-confidence to tackle alcohol misuse
b. Targeting social norms (such as peer pressure and drinking to fit in)

The importance of individual beliefs regarding alcohol consumption has led to the recommendation that the TPB should be used to understand alcohol misuse and help develop interventions (French and Cooke, 2012). The model can help nurses identify the multi-factorial issues surrounding adolescents' misuse of alcohol: targeting adolescents' attitudes and beliefs might be a more effective approach than solely targeting the problem behaviour. This approach has been successful with smoking campaigns (Davies, 2012).

Holistic care

According to Davies (2012), for nurses to provide holistic care, it is important to explore beyond the issue of alcohol misuse; they need to take account of the adolescent's life circumstances and level of social support. This can be achieved by working with staff in schools, careers services, housing associations, and other community agencies. In addition, it is important to investigate whether the young person is misusing any other substances. Those who misuse alcohol are more likely to also take illegal drugs, especially amphetamines and cocaine (IAS, 2007).

A person-centred approach is required when working collaboratively with adolescents to develop an agreed plan of action. While abstinence might be the nurse's goal, it may not be the young person's. In such cases, it is vital that nurses provide harm-reduction information. For example, if adolescents insist on using alcohol, they should be advised to choose the lowest percentage drinks (Davies, 2012).

 *So Josh's mother was right to be worried? As he was still at school he was referred to the school nurse; if he wasn't, would help have been more difficult to obtain?*

The AA approach

According to Powell (2000), the more general concept of addiction as a 'disease of the will' has become popular. It has been broadly applied to other forms of addiction and is adopted by the AA's 'sister' organisations, Narcotics Anonymous, Gamblers Anonymous, Workaholics Anonymous, Sex Addicts Anonymous and even Survivors of Incest Anonymous.

Strictly, what AA offers is not 'treatment' at all. Instead, it adopts a spiritual framework, requiring alcoholics to surrender their will to a 'higher power' (or God), confess their wrongs and try to rectify them. This requires an acceptance of abstinence as a goal, and usually works better for those who are heavily dependent (Hammersley, 1999).

TIME FOR REFLECTION ...

- Look back at Chapter 4 (pages 91 and 92) and the account of the treatment of anticipatory nausea and vomiting in cancer patients undergoing chemotherapy.
- Apply these same principles of classical conditioning to describe how nausea and vomiting would be made a conditioned response (CR) to alcohol.

 This may be effective but isn't it just substituting one dependency for another?

Aversion therapy

In *aversion therapy* (a form of behaviour therapy based on classical conditioning – see Chapter 2), some undesirable response to a particular stimulus is removed by associating the stimulus with another, aversive (literally, 'painful') stimulus. For example, alcohol is paired with an emetic drug (which induces severe nausea and vomiting), so that nausea and vomiting become a CR to alcohol (See Figures 12.3 and 12.4).

Meyer and Chesser (1970) found that about half their alcoholic patients abstained for at least 1 year following treatment, and that aversion therapy is better than no treatment at all. Lang and Marlatt (1982) concluded that use of antabuse was more effective than electric shock, but it requires the patient to take the drug and also ignores the multiplicity of reasons behind their drinking problem. According to Tucker et al. (1992), aversion therapy, if used at all, seems best applied in the context of broadly based programmes that address the patient's particular life circumstances, such as marital conflict, social fears and other factors often associated with problem drinking.

Choosing Johns and Freshwater's 2005 Model of Structured Reflection (Bulman and Schutz 2008, page 229) for this reflective record provided an interesting insight into my personal learning. As

Figure 12.3 Diagrammatic illustration of aversion therapy for treating alcoholism.

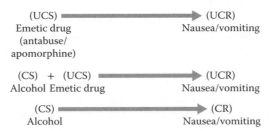

Figure 12.4 Malcolm McDowell in a scene from *Clockwork Orange*. His eyes are clamped open, forcing him to watch a film portraying acts of violence and sadism, as part of aversion therapy. He had earlier been given an emetic drug, so that extreme nausea and violence will become associated.

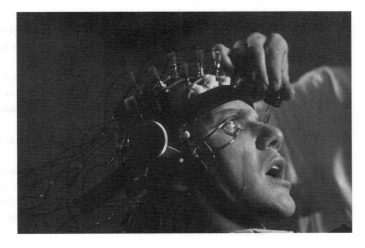

the model suggests, I used Carper's 1978 'ways of knowing' (see page 304) to analyse knowledge. I realised that in caring for Josh, Brian and Eddie I had, at different times, learned how to meet the nursing needs of three different stages of alcohol addiction (Aesthetic, or experiential knowledge). In each case, I had learned biological, psychological and social facts associated with their conditions (empirical knowledge). Learning about the physiological elements of the condition has made me more sympathetic to patients who are dependent and helped me communicate better with them and their relatives (personal knowledge). Lowe's (1995) biopsychosocial approach to alcohol dependency makes me realise that many individual experiences (peer pressure, stress) may start a reactive process that becomes for some (the reason is still unknown) out of control. By the time they get to Eddie's stage, it is too late so it is important that health education should be a significant aspect of their care (ethical knowledge).

However, in his model, Johns added 'reflexivity' to the ways of knowing – a new term to me. It was his reflective cue 'How does this experience connect with previous experiences?' that prompted me to record Brian's admission and discover that the separate bits of this particular experiential jigsaw fit together to make a more meaningful and comprehensive understanding of alcohol dependency. Does this mean I am, at last, progressing towards becoming an 'experienced practitioner'?

13 Death and dying

Introduction and overview

The loss, through death, of loved ones (*bereavement*) can occur at any stage of the life cycle. However, it becomes more likely as we get older. Some losses are more 'non-normative' than others, such as the loss of a child. This can occur at any stage from conception through to childhood and adolescence, and beyond. Miscarriage, stillbirth and neonatal death are all forms of bereavement, as are terminations.

The psychological and bodily reactions that occur in people who suffer bereavement (whatever form it takes) are called *grief*. The 'observable expression of grief' (Parkes and Weiss, 1983) is called *mourning*, although this term is often used to refer to the social conventions surrounding death (such as funerals and wearing black clothes). (See Figure 13.1.)

But grief can 'begin' before the actual death (*anticipatory grief*), and those who are dying can also grieve for their own death. Nurses have a crucial role to play in helping patients with a terminal illness to accept their condition. They are in the privileged position of being able to listen to patients talking about their hopes and fears, and their experience, knowledge and skills may enable patients to explore their feelings and come to terms with their condition (Dean, 2002). The patients may be children, adolescents (see Chapter 17) or adults (including elderly adults – see Chapter 19).

 From my diary (3): Year 1/Community/District Nurse

Today, with Sally, my community nurse mentor, was my first visit to Gail' a 35-year-old terminally ill patient with ovarian cancer.

Lydia, her mother and a retired nurse, is caring for her at home and when we arrived, said that Gail was bathed and ready to get up when Sally had changed her syringe driver. Gail muttered that she wasn't going to get up and Lydia said brightly that of course she must, it wouldn't be good for her to stay in bed all day. Suddenly, Gail sat up, flung her hairbrush across the room towards her mother and shouted angrily that there was no point and why didn't we all just leave her to die in peace. I hurriedly picked up the brush, feeling very nervous at the mention of death and uncertain of how to respond. I felt sorry for Lydia; in spite of her apparent control as she gathered up the laundry, she looked distraught.

Sally calmly went on getting the drug ready and asked Gail if she'd had a bad night. Gail fell back against the pillows and closed her eyes, saying every night was a bad night. On her way out, Lydia suggested I go and ask Ron (her husband) to make us all a cup of tea and I was so glad to escape. After introducing myself, I asked how he was coping 'with all this' and he said quite cheerfully, "Oh, I'm fine – I'm just the tea-maker," but as he turned away, I thought he looked close to tears so I said I'd like to have my tea in the kitchen with him, if he didn't mind. I did think too that Sally might want to talk privately to Gail.

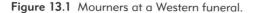

As Holland and Hogg (2001) observe, death, dying and grief are personal experiences that become very public when they occur in a hospital setting:

> … The beliefs, rituals and customs associated with death in different cultures are extremely varied. This includes the nurse's own professional culture where, for a student nurse, meeting death for the first time is part of their initiation into the profession … (Holland and Hogg, 2001).

As our society becomes more multicultural, both nurses and other health care professionals are exposed to a wider range of spiritual and religious beliefs; this, in turn, increases the need for care practices to become culturally orientated.

Figure 13.1 Mourners at a Western funeral.

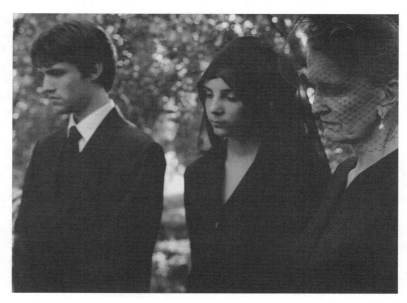

While psychologists are increasingly working alongside health care professionals with patients at various stages of their illness trajectories, relatively few work with people reaching the end of their life and their families (end-of-life care) (Nydegger, 2008). However, many of the issues for people reaching the end of their life are of a psychosocial nature and psychologists have much to offer them (Professional Practice Board of the BPS, 2008).

This was a very private setting and perhaps easier in some ways for the family but obviously there were tensions. Talking to Ron, I asked if they were getting any outside support and discovered that her parents were committed Christians but Gail 'had given up on religion' which was a source of distress to them. So this was an example of different beliefs within the same small unit of a culture.

Approaches to the understanding of grief

According to Archer (1999), grief has been variously depicted as

1. *A natural human reaction*: Grief is a *universal* feature of human existence, found in all cultures. But its form and the intensity of its expression vary considerably (see pages 312 through 314).
2. *A psychiatric disorder*: Although grief itself has never been classified as a mental disorder, 'The psychiatric framework emphasises the human suffering grief involves, and therefore provides a useful balance to viewing it simply as a natural reaction' (Archer, 1999). (We should note that DSM-5 – due for publication in May 2013,—includes a new disorder, 'Anxiety Disorder Related to Bereavement.)
3. *A disease process*: Although there may be increased rates of morbidity (health deterioration) or mortality (death) among bereaved people, these are not necessarily directly caused by the grief process. For example, the effects of change in lifestyle (such as altered nutrition or drug intake), or increased attention to physical illness, which predated the bereavement, might be mistaken for the effects of grief itself. However, there is substantial evidence that bereaved spouses are more at risk of dying themselves compared with matched non-bereaved controls. This is true mainly for widowers (Stroebe and Stroebe, 1993), and especially for younger widowers experiencing an unexpected bereavement (Smith and Zick, 1996).

All three approaches contain an element of truth.

The fact that an emotion can contribute to physical illness supports the psychoneuroimmuniological (PNI) model of health (Chapter 3, page 44). As Gail was divorced and had no children, her parents would be the ones most affected by her death – and possibly at increased risk of illness?

Stage or phase accounts of grief

According to Archer (1999), a widely held assumption is that grief proceeds through an orderly series of stages or phases, with distinct features. While different accounts vary in the details of particular stages, the two most commonly cited are those of Bowlby (1980) and Kübler-Ross (1969) (Box 13.1).

> ### Box 13.1 Bowlby's phase theory of grief
>
> According to Bowlby (1980), adult grief is an extension of a general distress response to separation commonly observed in young children (see Chapter 14). Adult grief is a form of *separation anxiety* in response to the disruption of an attachment bond.
>
> - *Phase of numbing:* Numbness and disbelief, which can last from a few hours up to a week, may be punctuated by outbursts of extremely intense distress and/or anger.
> - *Yearning and searching:* These are accompanied by anxiety and intermittent periods of anger, and can last for months or even years.
> - *Disorganisation and despair:* Feelings of depression and apathy occur when old patterns have been discarded.
> - *Reorganisation:* There is a greater/lesser degree of recovery from bereavement and acceptance of what has occurred.

Thinking about grief as the breaking of the attachment bond is enlightening as Gail was becoming increasingly dependent on her mother – a return to behaviour more characteristic of early attachment; when Gail dies this may make Lydia's loss even more acute.

Kübler-Ross's stage theory: Anticipatory grief

Kübler-Ross's (1969) stage account was based on her pioneering work with more than 200 terminally ill patients. She was interested in how they prepared for their imminent deaths (*anticipatory grief*), and so her stages describe the *process of dying*. But she was inspired by an earlier version of Bowlby's theory (Parkes, 1995) and her stages were later applied (by other researchers) to *grief for others*. Her theory remains very influential in nursing and counselling, with both dying patients and the bereaved (Archer, 1999).

Kübler-Ross helps to explain the family's behaviour that morning. Gail's reaction seemed a mixture of anger and perhaps preparatory depression; she wanted to be left alone, which could indicate withdrawal. Lydia may have been using denial as a coping mechanism and Ron seemed sadly accepting; he confessed he felt inadequate to help either of them.

Almost all the patients she interviewed initially denied they had life-threatening illnesses, the drifting in and out of denial. Denial was more common when someone had been given the diagnosis in an abrupt or insensitive way, or if they were surrounded by family and/or staff who were also in denial.

Depression is a common reaction in the dying. For example, Hinton (1975) reported that 18% of those who committed suicide suffered from serious physical illnesses, with 4% having illnesses that probably would have killed them within 6 months.

Elderly people who have lived full lives have relatively little to grieve for – they have gained much and lost few opportunities. But people who perceive lives full of mistakes and missed opportunities may, paradoxically, have *more* to grieve for as they begin to realise that these opportunities are now lost forever. This resembles Erikson's despair (Chapter 19, page 434), as does *resignation*, which Kübler-Ross distinguished from acceptance. The detachment and stillness of those who have achieved acceptance comes from calmness, while in those who have become resigned, it comes from despair. The latter cannot accept death, nor can they deny its existence any longer (March and Doherty, 1999). Kübler-Ross found that there are a few patients who fight to the end, struggle and keep hoping, which makes it almost impossible for them to achieve true acceptance.

Hope (for a cure, a new drug or a miracle) is the constant thread running through all these stages and is necessary to maintain the patient's morale through the illness. Hope is rationalisation of suffering for some and a means of much-needed denial for others. Kübler-Ross found that if a patient stopped expressing hope, it was usually a sign of imminent death (Parkinson, 1992).

As a nurse, Lydia must have known Gail hadn't long to live but as a mother, and perhaps because of her Christian faith, may not have been able to give up her own hope. Gail's mood seemed more like despair than acceptance. It could be she felt regretful and depressed about her broken marriage and lack of children which she'd wanted, but had had several miscarriages.

It is within these awareness contexts that interactions between patients, relatives and staff take place and can affect the management of the dying patient. Kübler-Ross favours the open awareness context, arguing that the question is not 'Do I tell my patient?' but 'How do I share this knowledge with my patient?' She suggests that whether the patient is told explicitly or not about the terminal illness, s/he will come to this awareness independently. If the news can be transmitted in an empathic and hopeful manner before this stage is reached, the patient will have time to work through the different reactions; this will enable him/her to cope with this new situation and develop confidence in carers. It is also within open awareness that she has identified the stages described in Box 13.2. Patients can only ask 'Why me?' if they know their diagnosis/prognosis. In reality, the question is a statement of their deepest *spiritual pain* – 'I am hurting terribly' (Morrison, 1992; see Chapter 3 and pages 317 and 318).

From discussions with her consultant and oncology nurse Gail and her parents were all aware of her prognosis but perhaps, until now, there was 'mutual pretence awareness' between them. Gail's angry outburst could have been the first step towards the 'open awareness' stage.

An evaluation of stage theories of grief

- Generally, stage models have not been well supported by subsequent research. Both Bowlby's and Kübler-Ross's accounts were proposed before any prolonged, detailed follow-up studies of bereaved people had been undertaken (Archer, 1999).
- According to March and Doherty (1999), they represent generalisations from the experience of some individuals, and lack the flexibility necessary to describe the range of individual reactions. Grief *is not* a simple, universal process we all go through (Stroebe et al., 1993).

Box 13.2 Kübler-Ross's stages of dying

- *Denial (No, not me):* This prevents the patient from being overwhelmed by the initial shock and is used by most patients not only at this early stage of their illness but also later on. Denial acts as a buffer system, allowing the patient time to develop other coping mechanisms. It can also bring isolation. The patient may fear rejection and abandonment in suffering and feel that nobody understands what the suffering is like. Avoidance by staff, for whatever reasons, can exacerbate this feeling of isolation in terminal illness (Parkinson, 1992). Searching for a second opinion was a very common initial reaction, representing a desperate attempt to change the unpredictable world they had just been catapulted into, back into the world they knew and understood (March and Doherty, 1999).

- *Anger (It is not fair – why me?):* This may be directed at doctors, nurses, relatives, other healthy people who will go on living or God. This can be the most difficult stage for family and staff to deal with. They may react personally to the patient's anger and respond with anger of their own; this only increases the patient's hostile behaviour (Parkinson, 1992).

- *Bargaining (Please God let me …):* This is an attempt to postpone death by 'doing a deal' with God (or fate, or the hospital), much as a child might bargain with its parents to get its own way. So, it has to include a prize for 'good behaviour' and sets a self-imposed 'deadline' such as a son or daughter's wedding; the patient promises not to ask for more time if this postponement is granted.

- *Depression (How can I leave all this behind?):* This is likely to arise when the patient realises that no bargain can be struck and that death is inevitable. S/he grieves for all the losses that death represents. This is *preparatory depression*, a form of preparatory grief that helps the patient to prepare him/herself for the final separation from the world. *Reactive depression* involves expressions of fear and anxiety and a sense of great loss – of body image (as in disfigurement – see Chapter 16), job, financial security or ability to continue caring for children.

- *Acceptance (Leave me be, I am ready to die):* Almost devoid of feelings, the patient seems to have given up the struggle for life, sleeps more and withdraws from other people, as if preparing for 'the long journey'.

- Some researchers prefer to talk about the *components of grief.* Ramsay and de Groot (1977), for example, have identified nine such components, some of which occur early and others late in the grieving process. These are *shock, disorganisation, denial, depression, guilt, anxiety, aggression, resolution* and *reintegration.*

- However, many stage theorists have explicitly *denied* that the stages are meant to apply equally and rigidly to everyone. For example, Bowlby (1980) himself said that 'These phases are not clear-cut, and any one individual may oscillate for a time back and forth between any two of them.' Similarly, Kübler-Ross's stages can last for different periods of time and can replace each other or coexist (Parkinson, 1992).

- Stages provide us with a framework for understanding the experiences of bereaved and dying individuals, while at the same recognising that there is a huge variability in the ways individuals react. Stages do not prescribe where an individual 'ought' to be in the grieving process (March and Doherty, 1999).

 Kübler-Ross's concept of 'anticipatory grief' helps me understand the complexity of Gail's feelings; Gail appeared to be experiencing both anger and depression, which Bowlby (1980) said might happen. Ramsay and de Groot (1977) identified agression as a component of grief which explains Gail's episode with the hairbrush. And was Lydia perhaps fluctuating between denial and acceptance of what she knew was inevitable?

Nurses, death and dying

According to Hare and Pratt (1989), until recently a death on the ward was a violent reminder of the failings of nursing/medicine. But major developments, such as growth of the hospice movement, suggest that the emphasis is changing from curing to caring. March maintains that 'Nursing appears to be redefining itself to include the wholehearted care of dying and bereaved people …' (see pages 318 through 320).

Western culture generally has been moving since the 1960s towards open communication about death and dying, with paternalistic notions that patients would be too upset to discuss death slowly changing (Field and Copp, 1999).

TIME FOR REFLECTION …

- Do you think much about your own death and that of your loved ones?
- Are your attitudes towards death influenced by religious beliefs?
- Do you think your attitudes and feelings about death affect how you (might) communicate with terminally ill patients?

According to March (1995), 'Most nurses are confronted with the reality of death with a regularity that lay people would find shocking …'.

Dying is a major crisis, which can be painfully distressing, unfamiliar and frightening (Baker Miller, 1976). To help patients and their families through this process, nurses need to develop awareness of their own attitudes and ability to face terminal illness and death, and their particular prejudices and convictions (Parkinson, 1992).

 This was my first experience of caring for a terminally ill patient and I felt apprehensive, and inadequate; I was distressed by Gail's anger towards her mother, but I didn't know what to say. It was, I confess, scary to think of someone not much older than I am dying and the thought of my own daughter dying was devastating. It's a 'non-normative' loss and for Gail's parents just as painful as that of any child.

Talking to dying patients

Research suggests that a proportion of patients do not wish to talk about the terminal nature of their condition (Hunt and Meerabeau, 1993). They may cope by avoiding having to focus on their prognosis (Rifkin, 2001), or seeking escape in light-hearted conversation.

In spite of Kubler-Ross's conviction the patient should be told the prognosis it would be wrong surely to impose it; shouldn't we take our lead from the patient? I already know Sally is good at that and over the next few weeks I learned a great deal from observing how she behaved with Gail and her parents. I often felt inexperienced and inadequate so was encouraged when I discovered Carper's (1978, 1992) 'patterns of knowing' in Bulman and Schulz (2008, pages 39 and 40). She identified four types:

1. Empirical (theoretical and research based)
2. Aesthetic (gained through situations)
3. Personal (ability to build therapeutic relationships)
4. Ethical (what ought to be done in particular situations)

It made me realise I was learning in more ways than I thought.

Webster (1981) observed nurses communicating with dying patients in four English hospitals. They often displayed 'blocking' behaviour, avoiding intimate conversations by changing the subject, ignoring cues, making jokes or tailoring their responses to the least distressing aspect of the issues raised. Such light-hearted interactions allowed the nurses to sidestep potentially difficult conversations, keeping them on emotional 'safe ground'. Wilkinson (1991) observed similar behaviour in 54 cancer nurses. For example, the psychosexual impact that gynaecological, bladder or bowel malignancy may have had on patients' lives was never discussed during the observed interactions. This was confirmed by Costello (2000; see also Chapter 16).

Dean (2002) proposes that nurses develop communication skills that not only allow them to talk sensitively about death and dying with patients but also give them the capacity to assess whether or not this is what the patient wants. Similarly, Parkinson (1992) maintains that providing opportunities to talk with patients so that they can express their fears, anger or depression should comprise a major focus of the nurse's work.

I realise now that even when discussing Gail with Sally I 'sheltered' behind questions focusing on 'treatment': pain control, etc. Without exploring this 'theoretical' knowledge I wouldn't have recognised I was avoiding dealing with Gail's, and everyone else's, emotions.

Communicating with dying children

… Adults' protective concern for children over issues around death clearly reflects their own fears and use of denial, in a society where the taboo may be lifting in a widespread social and intellectual sense, but not necessarily in a personal or private sense (Judd, 1989).

Having theoretical understanding of Piaget's cognitive developmental stages (case study 5a, page 352 and 5b, page 353) I understand that, for the very young child, separation is as disturbing as death. Recently a teacher at my daughter's school was killed in a road accident but I didn't connect it to Maia's insistence on having a light on when she goes to sleep. I will explore this with her now.

Children's understanding of death

- Evidence suggests that children develop a concept of death from an early age, and by the age of eight or nine this will be complete (Chesterfield, 1992).
- In Piaget's sensorimotor stage (birth to two – see Chapter 15), 'out of sight' is seen as the equivalent of death. Early games of peek-a-boo are often considered the first stage of learning about death (the word 'peek-a-boo' stems from the old English word meaning 'alive and dead') (Chesterfield, 1992).
- The egocentrism of the preoperational child (aged 2–7) means that s/he does not understand the finality of death, often seeing it as a kind of sleep. The toddler will attribute inanimate objects in general with life and will (*animism*). They often feel guilty because they believe that death is related to something they have done or wished for. They may show great interest in the practical aspects of death, such as what the dead person will eat. The clearest and most feared implication for younger children is separation from their attachment figures (see Chapter 14) and the belief that dead people/animals cannot move (Judd, 1993).
- During the concrete operational stage (ages 7–11), children recognise death as an immediate possibility that may happen to themselves as a consequence of 'badness'. Personification of death and a fear of the dark are common, and the ability to articulate feelings develops.
- In the formal operational stage (age 11–15), the adolescent may have an adult's cognitive abilities, but it is unlikely that s/he will have acquired the life skills or experience to cope with death as an adult would. The young person may regress at times of stress to egocentrism, magical thought, rages and dependency (see Chapter 17).
- According to Bowlby (1980), adults in Western societies hold beliefs about life and death that are ambiguous and inconsistent, so it is no wonder that children's beliefs also vary widely. Anthony (1971) also maintains that children are influenced by beliefs about death that are generally accepted by their culture, especially adults' own animistic beliefs.
- According to Rochlin (1967), children clearly know at a very early age about death as the extinction of all life. But they then use a range of defence mechanisms to avoid the full implications of this awareness.

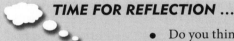

TIME FOR REFLECTION ...

- Do you think children should be told that they are terminally ill?
- Should it be the parents' decision whether or not medical staff are honest with the child?

Children with a life-threatening illness sense that it is serious and that they might die or are dying, even if they are not explicitly told (Judd, 1993). Their anxiety levels are markedly higher than those of chronically ill children, even if undergoing the same number and duration of treatments (Spinetta et al.,

1973). This anxiety and sense of isolation persists when the child is not in hospital and even during periods of remission in children with leukaemia (Spinetta, 1975).

Judd (1993) believes that there is a more open and honest attitude on children's wards in most hospitals, where death and dying are often discussed openly in response to parents' questions and sometimes with the children, depending on the ethos of the unit.

Effective communication with dying children will be influenced by nurses' values, attitudes and beliefs, which in turn are influenced by past experience and religious, cultural and societal beliefs (Chesterfield, 1992). Chesterfield cites studies showing that doctors and nurses become skilled at withdrawal and distancing techniques; these strategies may help protect the practitioner from distress but inhibit effective communication with the dying child. The family may not want the child's impending death discussed openly, shielding the child from distress or because of their own fears (Lansown and Benjamin, 1985; Lombardo and Lombardo, 1986). This mutual pretence – Kübler-Ross's mutual pretence awareness (see Box 13.3) – can prove functional in maintaining hope and the roles of individual family members (Bluebond-Langner, 1978).

Clearly, the dying child needs an age- and developmentally appropriate opportunity to share its fears and concerns. This does not mean imposing a discussion, but involves attempting to be open to the child's willingness (or otherwise) to talk (Judd, 1993). If the child seems to be 'somewhere else' emotionally – but not depressed – this may be a very understandable way of achieving separation from the world around them. This choosing to withdraw may be the one area of control the child has left (see Figure 13.2).

Box 13.3 Awareness of death contexts

An important consideration within the process of dying is *awareness* of death. Awareness is what each interacting person knows of the patient's defined status, combined with the patient's recognition of others' awareness of his/her defined status. Glaser and Strauss identify four awareness contexts:

1. *Closed awareness:* The patient does not recognise s/he is dying, although everyone around does
2. *Suspected awareness:* The patient suspects s/he may be dying and attempts to find out what the prognosis is
3. *Mutual pretence awareness:* Everyone knows the patient is dying but they all pretend they do not
4. *Open awareness:* The patient, relatives and staff all admit that death is inevitable, and speak and act accordingly.

Source: Glaser, B.G. and Strauss, A.L., *Time for Dying*, Chicago, IL, Aldine, 1968.

Figure 13.2 This child is too young to have any concept of death or dying.

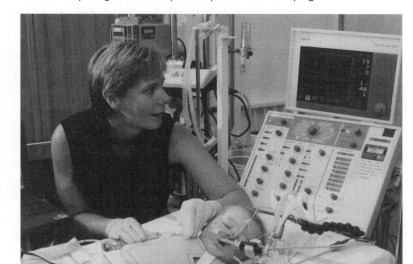

In this case we would also have to defer to parents' values, cultural background and beliefs. However, shouldn't a professional carer act as an advocate for the patient, however young? I can see there might be difficult ethical problems where there is this sort of conflict; it makes good communication between nurses, parents and the child patient even more essential.

Different kinds of bereavement

The stage accounts of grief discussed earlier (Bowlby, 1980; Kübler-Ross, 1969) are both 'attachment models' (March, 1995). According to Parkes (1986), Bowlby's account applies to both dying and bereaved people:

> Most people who are dying have people around them who are mourning their death. The feelings and behaviour of dying and bereaved people are a function of the relationship between them and should not therefore be considered in isolation from each other. Indeed, one of the guiding principles of the new hospice movement is 'the unit of care is the family'.

While anticipatory grief may be helpful for the long-term adjustment of the bereaved, it may cause problems for the dying patient:

> As loved ones come to accept the inevitability of death, they may begin to withdraw from the patient and begin

to consider life after the patient's death. This ... may leave the dying patient feeling rejected and isolated ... (March, 1995).

But the reverse can also happen: the patient may begin to accept his/her own death and withdraw from loved ones, who remain overwhelmed by grief. The patient's withdrawal may only increase their grief (March, 1995). According to Bowlby (1980):

The loss of a loved person is one of the most intensely painful experiences any human being can suffer, and not only is it painful to experience but also painful to witness, if only because we are impotent to help.

Similarly, Parkes (1972) states that

Pain is inevitable in such a case and cannot be avoided. It stems from the awareness of both parties that neither can give the other what he wants. The helper cannot bring back the person who's dead, and the bereaved person cannot gratify the helper by seeming helped.

The nurse's pain, like the relatives', may be more difficult to handle when there has been little or no time to prepare for the patient's death.

After our visit, Sally said the dynamics had changed in the family and from now on, they'd all need more emotional support; she was going to contact the Macmillan nurse and consult her about this and also managing Gail's increased pain. Then she told me I'd done well to notice Gail's father was upset and to talk to him, which pleased me as it means I am, if hesitantly, improving my communication skills.

Death in accident and emergency departments

The news of death can provoke an alarm reaction: the world suddenly becomes a threatening, unpredictable place. Anything that makes the loss unreal (such as a sudden, unexpected death and/or one that occurs in unusual or violent circumstances) is likely to make it more difficult to accept; this can produce a more prolonged and complicated grief reaction (Parkes and Weiss, 1983). Nurses in accident and emergency (A&E) are likely to have to deal with a higher proportion of such deaths than those working in other areas. Indeed, one-third of all deaths in hospital occur within the first few hours of a patient's arrival (Ewins and Bryant, 1992).

According to Smith (1997), the hospice and palliative care movements have done much to prepare nurses as well as patients for death and for the terminal phase of conditions such as cancer and AIDS (see pages 314 and 315). However, many nurses in acute care still feel unprepared and unsupported.

Staff caring for the newly bereaved should be able to provide support early on and help build a foundation for the relatives' recovery process (Cooke et al., 1992). But nursing and medical staff often feel inadequately prepared to meet relatives' needs. In A&E, the situation is complicated by the fact that staff and relatives meet at a time of crisis, and the meeting is usually brief, unexpected and may not have any follow-up. In contrast, a ward environment often allows time for a relationship and rapport to develop. The ethos of A&E is to save life, so when the patient dies this often leads to feelings of failure.

 *I'm grateful my first experience of a patient dying is in a supportive situation where I have a mentor, and time, to explore psychological reactions; unlikely in A&E. I imagine sudden, unexpected death would mean dealing more with the early shock, disorganisation and denial stages; all the more reason to learn what to anticipate and how to respond in such situations.*

TIME FOR REFLECTION ...

- Another issue confronting nurses working in A&E in particular is organ donation.
- What might be some of the major emotional issues surrounding this?

Death of a child

According to Raphael (1984):

> The loss of a child will always be painful, for it is in some way a loss of part of the self ... In any society, the death of a young child seems to represent some failure of family or society and some loss of hope.

Inevitably, the parents will feel cheated of the child's life and future. Often the death is sudden and unexpected (from accident, injury or medical emergency). Much less often it is caused by progressive, debilitating or malignant conditions, which do allow anticipatory grief to take place. But whatever their nature, all childhood deaths are abhorrent and so are especially stressful.

Parents' relationship with their child begins long before birth. For each parent there is the fantasy child s/he will have, which builds on the pre-conception images of what a baby – this baby – will be. Of course, many pregnancies are unplanned or unwanted (initially or even throughout), which makes the relationship with the unborn baby highly ambivalent (Raphael, 1984). But, in all cases, the loss of a baby will need to be grieved for, at whatever stage of pregnancy this might occur.

Miscarriage (spontaneous abortion)

According to Raphael (1984), the level of the mother's grief will be affected by whether or not the baby was wanted. This can be true even with an early miscarriage (i.e. before the baby is viable). But after the baby's movements have been felt, it is more likely to be seen as the loss of a 'person'. The loss is not 'nothing' or 'just a scrape' (dilatation and curetage) or 'not a life', but the beginning of a baby. The use of technical terms to describe the baby – products of conception, conceptus, embryo, foetus – might be perceived as an attempt to deny the existence of a baby the woman already loved, and thus to deny the reality of the grief she experiences for that baby (Buggins, 1995).

The sadness of the loss is often compounded by fear and panic, as in any emergency situation. There is rarely time to deal with these emotions, and many women report feelings of total helplessness (Sherr, 1989). Even if the mother does not have a very clear concept of her lost baby, as with other losses it can never be replaced (by another pregnancy).

Gail's life has been full of loss; the babies I assume she so much wanted – and eventually her husband who, I learned, refused to consider IVF. Although it happened several years ago, exploring unresolved feelings about it now might help her. Lydia too may be feeling cheated of her child's future and grandchildren.

Termination (therapeutic or induced abortion)

The 1967 Abortion Act defined therapeutic termination as one undertaken before the gestational age of 28 weeks. But advances in technology have greatly improved the chances of survival for premature babies, and a reduction to 24 weeks was approved by Parliament in 1990. The Abortion Act made it possible for a woman to have an abortion legally, provided two doctors independently agreed that the termination was necessary to prevent

- The likelihood of the woman's death
- Permanent illness (physical or psychological)
- Damage to a woman's existing children
- Abnormality in the baby

The Act stopped far short of endorsing the idea that a woman has an absolute right to control her body. Practically, the law relies on individual doctors exercising discretion as to who qualifies for an abortion.

Despite its legality, abortion is still a very 'live' moral issue. But the debate has also involved empirical concerns about the links between unwanted pregnancy, abortion and long-term mental health. Specifically, several authors have proposed that abortion may have adverse mental health effects owing to guilt, unresolved loss and lowered self-esteem (Fergusson et al., 2006). According to Raphael (1984), the pattern of grief is similar to that for miscarriage, but suppression or inhibition of grief is much more likely.

However rational the decision to have an abortion, it might still generate instinctive emotional reactions. It's also likely to be complicated by religious, cultural or ethical conflicts.

Stillbirth

According to Sherr (1989), a stillbirth occurs when a baby born after 27 weeks fails to breathe. Knowledge of the fact that there is no live baby at the end of the labour can magnify the experience of pain (see Chapter 3). The increased use of drugs may reflect the feeling that the labour is futile, but it is unclear whether parents want greater intervention or staff simply tend to take greater control and perceive the birth as a medical event to protect them from the reality. According to Sherr,

> Parents cannot 'wipe out' this baby – and may gain strength from the ritual of hello and farewell which will be the only interaction they will have with this child ... this is still their baby, even if it has died.

The baby should not be whisked away or shielded from the parents, even if there is physical abnormality. Sherr believes it is much worse for parents to fear an imaginary baby than to view the real one: they seem to see the baby as beautiful no matter what.

If the stillbirth was not expected, the situation will be more traumatic for everyone, including the staff (Sherr, 1989). But if there is a congenital abnormality or intrauterine event that makes it obvious that the baby was not viable or that it has already died, there may be an opportunity for some anticipatory grieving (Raphael, 1984).

Neonatal death

This refers to babies in special care baby units (SCBUs) and neonatal intensive care units (NICUs), where the threat of death may hang over the parents, as well as babies who are full term and/or born healthy but then become ill later (see Figure 13.3).

In the former, parents may have experienced some anticipatory grieving, but they grieve both for the expected healthy baby that they never had and the sick baby that they will soon have no more. Many babies will have spent their lives on SCBUs, and so will never have truly 'belonged' to their parents (Sherr, 1989). As Sherr observes, 'The environment of SCBU is in itself difficult. This ... is a strange environment of incubators, ventilators, uniforms, tubes and high background noise.'

Many of the characteristics of grief following neonatal death are similar to those for stillbirth, except that in the former the parents have had some

Figure 13.3 A baby being cared for in NICU.

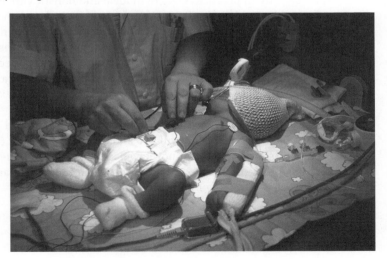

opportunity, however limited, to know and bond with their real child. The two have often been studied together as 'perinatal' death (Raphael, 1984). Raphael describes adoption (the relinquishing of one's baby) and the birth of a baby with some abnormality or disability as losses that, like death, must be grieved for.

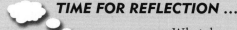 Although subtly different, these deaths are non-normative, which heightens the grief. However, I wonder if the longer and deeper the attachment to the child, the greater the sense of loss?

Cultural aspects of death, dying and grief

Because of the huge individual variability, trying to distinguish 'normal' from 'abnormal' grief seems quite arbitrary (Schuchter and Zisook, 1993). According to Middleton et al. (1993), the validity of the concept of *pathological grief* must be considered in terms of *cultural norms*. Although grief is a universal response to major loss, its meaning, duration and how it is expressed are all culturally prescribed.

'Culture' itself can refer to different things. The focus of the discussion regarding cultural influences on death and grief is usually what DeSantis (1994) calls *patient culture* (the patient's own individual belief systems reflecting his/her religious background and spirituality).

TIME FOR REFLECTION ...

- What do you understand by 'spirituality'?
- Explain how religion and spirituality may differ?

Individuals with no religious affiliations may have spiritual beliefs that contribute to their health. According to Naryanasamy (1991), the provision of spiritual care in practice is less than ideal and holistic care is therefore not an achieveable goal (see the discussion of psychological care and spiritual pain in Chapter 3). For example, a patient may tell the nurse, when asked for details about religion, that s/he is not religious but may later say that s/he goes to the park every day and sits there thinking about the day and feeling in tune with the world. This could imply a 'spiritual well-being' which can give the patient an inner strength to cope with life events such as death without the need to believe in and pray to God (Holland and Hogg, 2001)

DeSantis claims that the nurse–patient encounter can be viewed as an interaction between patient culture and (1) *nursing culture* (the culture based on the nurse's professional knowledge) and (2) *organisational culture* (the culture of the organisation or situation in which the patient and nurse actually meet, such as hospital or home).

And what about the nurse's beliefs? Having abandoned most of my parents' Hindu beliefs I found myself empathising more with Gail; however, seeing her parents' distress makes me more sensitive to the importance of respecting theirs.

Patient culture: The meaning of death, dying and grieving between and within cultures

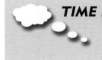

TIME FOR REFLECTION ...

- What is your definition of 'death'?
- Do you think it is possible for death to be defined in more than one way?

In Western societies, the common sense understanding of 'death' reflects the influence of the biomedical model (see Box 13.4 and Chapter 3): 'death' is equated with physical or bodily death (although how doctors define physical death has changed over the decades). However, even in Western culture, 'death' can have different meanings. For example, Sudnow (1967) distinguished between 'clinical death' (equivalent to physical/bodily death) and 'social death'; the latter refers to 'when the individual is treated essentially as a corpse although still clinically and biologically alive' (Bond and Bond, 1986). An example of social death can be seen in hospitals where patients are moved from the main ward area into a side room if there is any possibility of them dying (Holland and Hogg, 2001).

Religious beliefs have a major influence on caring for dying patients and their families, especially their attitudes to and beliefs regarding death itself (see, e.g. Holland and Hogg, 2001).

Box 13.4 Western and non-Western conceptions of death

- Determining the precise moment in time at which death occurs is an important issue in today's 'technologically advanced' society, especially when someone else can benefit (as in organ donation) (Holland and Hogg, 2001).
- The Muslim Law Council (1996) accepts 'brainstem death as constituting the end of life for the purpose of organ transplant', which it supports as a 'means of alleviating pain or saving life on the basis of the rules of Shariah'. This process can also be regarded as a form of 'social death', such as when relatives are asked if the dying person is a donor and if not would they, as next of kin, consent to organ donation taking place.
- However, not all cultures and religions accept this biomedical model interpretation of death. For example, many cultures (e.g. the Chinese) regard death as a transition: as such it is a time for rituals ('rites of passage'), which mark the move from one social status to another. These rituals ensure that those who are dying or bereaved know what is expected of them.
- This means that how individuals experience death will have a major impact on how nurses and other health care professionals support the patient's family; it may also affect how they cope with their own feelings when someone they may have been caring for dies.

Figure 13.4 The degree to which weeping is acceptable or encouraged at funerals varies between religious and cultural groups.

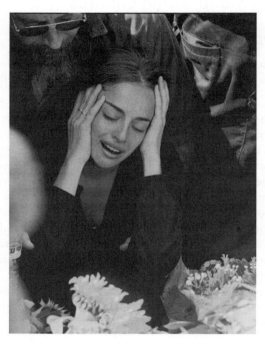

Cultures also differ in what they consider to be appropriate expressions of grief. According to Rosenblatt (1993), culture is such a crucial part of the context of bereavement that it is often impossible to separate an individual's grief from culturally required mourning (see Figure 13.4).

Nursing culture

As we noted earlier, the first encounter with death is part of the student nurse's 'initiation' into the world of nursing; for the majority, this encounter will take place in a hospital. According to Kiger (1994), the main causes of concern are the expected additional difficulties of caring for dying patients, such as the pain of seeing them suffer (see Chapter 3), the shock of seeing a dead body, and having to deal with bereaved relatives.

According to Smith (1992), death and dying in hospital can be regarded as the nurse's ultimate 'emotional labour' (see Chapters 3 and 4). Smith also found that there were clearly defined technical skills involved in dealing with death-related situations (e.g. resuscitation during cardiac arrest and laying out the body). These essential skills are very much part of the student's training experience, taught by tutors/mentors who usually have more experience of death. While death and dying may represent the ultimate emotional labour, all nurses find their own ways to cope with it (such as the development of certain 'rituals' around laying out the body) (Chapman, 1983).

Such rituals may become necessary in a Western cultural setting because death is seen as a very private experience, almost a taboo subject. Nurses are expected not only to cope with the dying person and his/her family but also to undertake the 'last offices'. However, how they manage this is highly dependent on how nurses themselves see death and what they believe takes place at death (Lawler, 1991).

But this also depends on culture? I found the main beliefs listed briefly in Clinical Skills in Adult Nursing, ed. Randle, Coffey and Bradbury, 2009. For instance, a traditional Hindu family might want to take care of the person who's died themselves. They would wish the eldest son to be present at death and may wish to lay the dying patient on the floor to be nearer to Mother Earth.

It also reminds me that Gibbs' Reflective cycle is based on experiential learning – i.e. 'learning by doing' (Bulman and Schutz, 2008, page 225) and that particular skills leading to practical competence (as well as aesthetic knowledge) can be learned only in placements.

Organisational culture: Hospital and community

All the care given to the patient and his/her family will be highly dependent on the effectiveness of the hospital or community responding to the needs of a multicultural-multiracial community (Holland and Hogg, 2001). Hospitals that acknowledge the cultural needs of patients – as part of their individualised care – are likely to have not only a chapel but also a mosque and a temple (or their equivalent) for prayer or alternatively, a 'multi-faith' room. It is also recommended that symbols of Christianity should be removed from chapels of rest where these are being used by non-Christians (Black, 1991).

Providing individualised settings is ideal but I imagine there is an economic issue involved in this! However, in the interests of equality, providing a neutral one seems essential.

Care plans and other documentation, both in hospital and the community, should reflect an awareness of cultural differences. Many National Health Services (NHS) trusts have produced guidelines on the spiritual and bereavement needs of different cultures; these have been developed through collaborative multi-professional and multicultural groups (Holland and Hogg, 2001).

End-of-life care

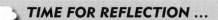

> **TIME FOR REFLECTION …**
>
> What do you understand by
> - 'End-of life care'?
> - 'Palliative care'?
> - 'Hospice'?
> - 'Terminal' illness? (Box 13.5)

> **Box 13.5 Palliative and end-of-life care**
>
> - *Palliative care* is concerned with reducing the suffering, maintaining the dignity and quality of life, and addressing the care needs of people at the end of their lives. It is about the management of physical symptoms and psychological, social and spiritual problems, and coordination and continuity of care in different settings and across the disease trajectory.
> - This involves input from different health care professionals, as well as volunteer services. It includes carers, both in their role as partners in the team and as family members, who themselves require care and support (Radbruch, 2008).
> - Palliative care is life-affirming and regards death as a normal process; its aim is to achieve a 'good death' and neither to quicken nor prolong it.
> - Traditionally in the United Kingdom, palliative care has been associated with the *hospice movement* focusing on the needs of those with advanced cancer and their families. This reflects the pioneering work of Dame Cicely Saunders, who founded St. Christopher's Hospice in London in the 1960s for patients with terminal cancer.
> - However, *hospice care* is no longer confined to hospices; nor is it given only to those with incurable cancer. In the United States, for instance, hospice care is largely home-based. In the United Kingdom, patients receiving hospice care may be suffering from ischaemic heart disease, cerebrovascular disease (including stroke), chronic obstructive pulmonary disease, lower respiratory infections (four of the top five predicted causes of death in the United Kingdom for 2020 – the other being lung, trachea and bronchial cancer, muscular sclerosis and motor nerone disease).
> - 'Palliative care', 'hospice care', 'terminal care' and 'end-of-life care' are often used interchangeably. Since 1975, 'palliative care' has increasingly been used to describe hospice-type services.
> - 'Terminal care' is often used when it is clear that the patient is in a progressive state of decline, and this is part of' palliative care'. 'End-of-life care' is increasingly used in the United Kingdom as an alternative to 'palliative care to encompass the last few years of life and extends to all dying people regardless of their diagnosis (Department of Health, 2008).
>
> *Source:* Hall, S. and Payne, S., Palliative and End-of-Life Care, In D. Fench, K. Vedhara, A.A Kaptein and J. Weinmen (eds.), *Health Psychology* (2nd edn.), Oxford, BPS Blackwell, 2010.

Our hospital now has a palliative care consultant and a team of specialist nurses which I presume does reflect how hospice care is influencing general nursing. However, Sue Duke, a nurse consultant in palliative care, states she wanted to articulate palliative care **nursing** knowledge when palliative medicine was becoming a speciality. It seemed to her that symptom management was being given more importance than psychological and spiritual care as the emphasis was placed on empirical knowledge and the medical voice (Bulman and Schutz, 2008, pages 191 and 192).

Distress at the end of life

According to Hall and Payne (2010),

> From a psychological perspective, dying creates a dual crisis: coping with current ill-health (living the life left) and simultaneously making meaning of the life lived...

There are many sources of distress faced by people reaching the end of life; these include

- Grief about current and anticipated losses
- Concerns about being a burden
- Fear and uncertainty about the future
- Unresolved issues from the past
- Concerns about loved ones

Worries about family members are a major feature of life-threatening illness for most patients (Greisinger et al., 1997). Others include problems with work, finances, housing, transportation and legal matters (see Chapter 4).

While psychological distress is common in people reaching the end of life, assessing it can be challenging. For example, it may be mistaken for appropriate sadness (Thekkumpurath et al., 2008); alternatively, some of the common symptoms, such as fatigue, difficulties with sleeping and eating, and loss of concentration and energy, may be seen as indicating depression.

Spiritual and existential distress

Some definitions of spirituality illustrate the overlap between it and religion; for example, 'relationship to God, a spiritual being, a Higher Power, or a reality greater than the self'. However, others show the difference between them, such as 'transcendence or connectedness unrelated to a belief in a higher being' (Unruh et al., 2002). Clearly, spirituality is broader than religion. For example, 'the spirit' is a dimension of personhood, while religion is a human construct (Kearney and Mount, 2000) (Key Study 13.1).

KEY STUDY 13.1

Spiritual needs amongst dying patients

- Murray et al. interviewed 20 people dying of lung cancer or heart failure, and their carers, in Scotland.
- Spiritual concerns were important to many patients in both groups, both early and later in their illness.
- They felt a need for love, meaning and purpose, and sometimes transcendence, regardless of whether they held religious beliefs.
- Signs of spiritual well-being included inner peace and harmony and finding meaning; signs of spiritual neediness included feeling that life was not worthwhile and asking 'what have I done to deserve this?'
- Both patients and carers were often reluctant to raise spiritual issues with 'busy' health professionals; some sought to disguise their spiritual distress.

Source: Murary, S.A. et al., *Palliative Medicine*, 18, 39–45, 2004.

The increasing diversity of populations in many countries makes it essential to develop interventions that acknowledge the distinctive spiritual beliefs, images and meanings valued in different cultures (Hall and Payne, 2010).

 Gail's agnosticism taught me to make no assumptions about a person's belief. The fact that spiritual needs are universal while religious ones vary is highly significant for nurses when considering the needs of dying patients.

TIME FOR REFLECTION …

- In what ways can spirituality be regarded as relevant to care of the dying?
- What do you understand by the term 'dignity' in the context of nursing?

It was Cicely Saunders who first claimed that suffering is the result of psychological, social and spiritual factors as well as physical symptoms. (This, of course, is consistent with the biopsychological model of health and illness as opposed to the biomedical model; see Chapter 3.) She used the multidimensional concept of 'total pain' to describe how life-threatening illness can impact on the patient and advocated *holistic care* to treat pain effectively (again, see Chapter 3).

According to Brady et al. (1999), spiritual and existential issues can have an important influence on the well-being of people reaching the end of their life, such as finding a sense of purpose and meaning in life. In relation to illness, this involves the ability to tolerate psychosocial symptoms and acquiring a sense of satisfaction with the quality of their life.

TIME FOR REFLECTION …

How does the attainment of a sense of purpose and meaning in life relate to
- Erikson's concept of 'ego integrity'?
- Butler's process of 'life review'?
(See Chapter 19.)

Poor spiritual well-being is associated with a desire for hastened death, hoplessness and suicidal thoughts/ideation (McClain et al., 2003). Loss of meaning in life is often cited by doctors caring for the dying as a reason for patients to request assisted suicide (Meier et al., 1998; see discussion in pages 321 and 322). Consequently, there has been an increasing emphasis on the importance of spiritual care as an essential part of holistic care, especially in palliative care and nursing (Hall and Payne, 2010).

Spirituality from the nurse's perspective

According to Wright and Neuberger (2012),

>…Spirituality cultivates a deepening of our understanding of what it is to be human, of resources we can draw on to connect with and serve others. It

encourages us to feel comfortable in the world and to be more likely to respond to the things life throws at us from a position of love and respect, rather than fear.

Wright and Neuberger claim that spirituality 'is every bit as relevant to patient-centred care as having the right skills and resources to do the job'. Also, it is integral to the well-being of all human beings, whether or not we are conscious of that need for reflection and wholeness. Spirituality is 'the lifelong process through which we find our centre in the world, how we establish our relationships, find love, meaning, connection'.

Wright and Neuberger argue that an affirmation of spirituality in nursing at every level is long overdue: it is the key to minimising the profession's long history of patient abuse and neglect. Transforming nurses' 'inner process' is just as important as transforming the way they deliver care. To this end, they propose a 'manifesto for change', a seven-point plan for integrating spirituality into health care. This is summarised in Box 13.6.

I think this is referring to what Duke, in Bulman and Schutz (2008, page 192), calls 'changes in conceptual perspective' – as when she began to view her experience (her aesthetic knowledge) as central to her learning more about her practice.

Box 13.6 Seven-point plan for integrating spirituality into health care

1. Spiritual care is not a luxury or added extra, but goes to the heart of care. It means never viewing patients as 'other' and has nothing to do with religious beliefs.
2. Educational programmes undertaken by nurses must provide in-depth understanding of what spirituality means and how to deliver spiritual care.
3. Imaginative educational programmes for nurses relating to spiritual care and their own spirituality should be provided as part of a lifelong process of learning; they should be both sponsored by employers and form part of nurses' own independent commitment to the highest standards in nursing care.
4. Nurses' workplaces should, ideally, provide all patients with access to spiritual support: the creation of settings that welcome the heart and body, mind and soul of the nurse – and those of the patient – is essential to holistic care.
5. Spirituality has a direct effect on health and well-being, making it a proper area of research and action for all involved in health care settings: from the patient's perspective, *everyone* is 'front line'
6. Too many nurses don't understand what it is to provide spiritual care. Care for people with long-term conditions, palliative care and mental health care is essential for the ongoing training of all nurses.
7. Spiritual care is also part of enhancing the healing environment. All nurses can add their voice to calls for improving the physical environment for patients and staff.

Source: Wright, S. and Neuberger, J., *Nursing Standard*, 26(40), 19–21, 2012.

📋 I can see this has huge implications for nurse education, the extent of the supporting role of counsellors and psychologists, and the nursing environment. It offers ethical guidelines but has little to say
about how to 'deliver spiritual care'.

Dignity

While the concept of dignity from a nursing perspective has been defined in a
variety of ways, a common theme is respecting a patient as a person (Franklin
et al., 2006). Maintaining dignity is given a high priority in health care strategy documents in most European countries and this represents an 'overarch-
ing value or goal of palliative care' (Hall and Payne, 2010). For some, 'dying
with dignity' is synonymous with the right to assisted suicide and euthanasia
(hence 'Dignitas'; see pages 321 and 322).

One approach to dignity-oriented care provision, which focuses specifically
on the terminally ill, is the *dignity conserving model* (Chochinov et al., 2002)
(see Figure 13.5).

The model was developed in Canada from interviews with 50 patients with
advanced cancer, focusing on what supports and what undermines their dignity. The three major categories (*illness-related concerns, dignity conserving
repertoire, social dignity inventory*) refer to broad issues that determine how
individuals experience a sense of dignity as they approach death. Each involves
several themes and sub-themes.

There is some empirical support for the model (Hall et al., 2009), which provides direction for how to develop interventions that enhance a sense of dignity

Figure 13.5 The dignity model. (From Chochinov, H.M., Hack, T., Hassard, T., Kristjanson, L.J., McClement, S.
and Harlos, M. *J Clin Oncol*, 23, 5520–5525.)

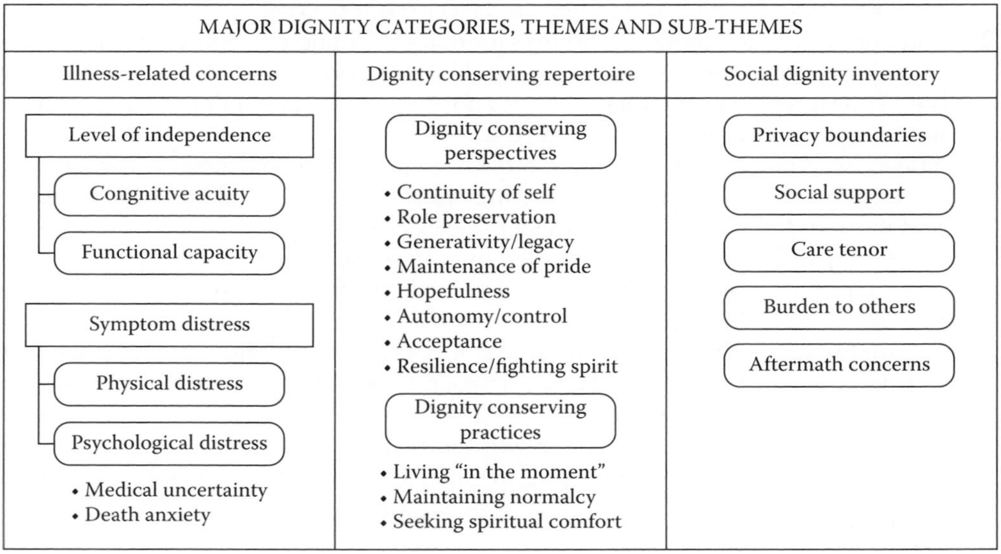

MAJOR DIGNITY CATEGORIES, THEMES AND SUB-THEMES		
Illness-related concerns	Dignity conserving repertoire	Social dignity inventory
Level of independence	Dignity conserving perspectives	Privacy boundaries
Congnitive acuity	• Continuity of self • Role preservation	Social support
Functional capacity	• Generativity/legacy • Maintenance of pride	Care tenor
Symptom distress	• Hopefulness • Autonomy/control	Burden to others
Physical distress	• Acceptance • Resilience/fighting spirit	Aftermath concerns
Psychological distress	Dignity conserving practices	
• Medical uncertainty • Death anxiety	• Living "in the moment" • Maintaining normalcy • Seeking spiritual comfort	

(Chochinov, 2006). For example, the model offers a framework for developing forms of psychotherapy aimed at promoting a sense of dignity and reducing psychological and spiritual distress for people who are dying (Chochinov et al., 2005). One example is dignity therapy (DT).

Dignity therapy

DT is brief and can be delivered at the bedside by a trained health care professional to people who are very close to death. The individualised therapy aims to address physical, psychosocial, existential and spiritual concerns or distress. The person is interviewed regarding important aspects of his/her life, including

- The times they felt most alive
- Characteristics they would like their family to know and remember about them
- Important roles they performed
- Concerns that have been left unspoken
- Any advice or messages for their loved ones

The interview is recorded, promptly transcribed (i.e. written down, word-for-word), edited, then presented to the patient (who can revise it if they wish). Much of the benefit of DT is thought to derive from creating this lasting paper legacy document, which individuals can share with or bequests to people of their choosing. In this way, DT aims to help both those who are dying and those they leave behind.

This is helpful: a positive and practical way to deliver spiritual care and a universally acceptable therapy tool. It would help Gail to focus on the achievements of her life (which I understand ego-integrity to mean) rather than the disappointments. And it would surely also be a comfort to her parents after her death? It's something I shall 'file away' for future use.

Assisted dying

The past decade has seen vigorous campaigning for the legalisation of 'assisted dying' (a term used by the pro-euthanasia lobby group, Dignity in Dying [Dyer, 2009]). Parliament has so far resisted changing the law to licence doctors to prescribe drugs to terminally ill people with the intention of causing death.

While there are proponents and opponents of assisted dying within the nursing profession, the Royal College of Nursing (RCN) has chosen to adopt a neutral position (RCN, 2009). Articles by Haigh (2012) and Robinson and Scott (2012) appeared in the *Nursing Standard* (January, 2012), in which the cases for and against, respectively, were argued.

TIME FOR REFLECTION ...

- What do you understand by the term 'assisted dying'?
- Try to formulate some arguments for and against assisted dying.
- Where do you stand with respect to this debate?

The issue of mental capacity/competence is fundamental to the assisted suicide debate (Robinson and Scott). According to Dignity in Dying (2010), 'Assisted dying (legalised and regulated in the U.S. States of Oregon and Washington) only applies to terminally ill, mentally competent adults and requires the dying patient, after meeting strict legal safeguards, to self-administer life-ending medication'.

Haigh considers the 'slippery slope' anti-assisted dying argument: if there is legislation legalising assisted dying for terminally ill people, there is a risk that vulnerable groups, such as older people or people with learning difficulties and mental illness, will be encouraged by their families to take this course of action against their will so that the family can be relieved from the burden of caring for them.

Robinson and Scott discuss (1) the protection of vulnerable groups; (2) assessment of mental capacity (i.e. the ability to make decisions); and (3) responding to patients' desire to die. As far as (2) is concerned, they argue that

> …it can be challenging to assess mental capacity in advanced disease when temporary, fluctuating or permanent cognitive impairment can hinder people's ability to make informed choices as a result of, for example, overwhelming fatigue, depression, infection, hypoxia and side effects of medication (Addington-Hall, 2002; Basovich, 2010).

Other factors that can influence requests for hastened death in terminally ill patients include hopelessness (negative expectations about the future), intractable pain and other symptoms, lack of dignity, fears about the dying process and death, loss of control and autonomy, lack of social support, spiritual distress, and feeling a burden on carers (Robinson and Scott, 2012).

While all these arguments are valid it is important to respect those to whom they don't apply; don't we, in every other sense, involve patients in their treatment?

Postscript.

Gail died three weeks after I recorded this incident; reconciled to a loving relationship with her parents, if not their religion. I feel privileged to have experienced the sensitive and dedicated care she was given, which could be considered a positive alternative to 'assisted dying'.

Reflecting positively on a sad experience, I'm pleased that I was able to use and develop the personal knowledge and (communication) skills I already had; one day I managed to get Gail to talk about her job as a school secretary (which she obviously loved) and although I found it difficult, tried to be more open to talking to her parents about their feelings. I've researched a great deal of theoretical information and, working with Sally – and Lydia – gained valuable aesthetic and ethical palliative care knowledge to help me in future.

CHAPTER SUMMARY

- *Bereavement* is a non-normative influence, but it becomes more likely as we get older.
- *Grief* has been portrayed as a natural, universal human reaction to bereavement, a psychiatric disorder and a disease process.
- The two most commonly cited *stage theories* of grief are those of Bowlby and Kübler-Ross. While both can be applied to the dying and the bereaved, Kübler-Ross's theory is an explicit account of *anticipatory grief* and describes the *process of dying*.
- Kübler-Ross distinguishes *acceptance* from *resignation*; the latter is similar to Erikson's concept of *despair*. Hope is a theme running through all the stages.
- Kübler-Ross favours the *open awareness context*, in which the patient, relatives and staff all admit that death is inevitable, and interact accordingly.
- Stage theories have been criticised on the grounds that grief is not a simple, universal process, which is the same for everyone. However, stages provide a framework for understanding bereaved people's experiences, which display a huge variability.
- Also, many stage theorists have explicitly denied that the stages are meant to apply equally and rigidly to everyone.
- Nurses' ability to help dying patients deal with their feelings will be influenced by awareness of their own attitudes towards death and dying. They sometimes sidestep potentially difficult conversations, keeping interactions emotionally 'safe'.
- These withdrawal and distancing techniques are also used by staff dealing with dying children. But children with a life-threatening illness usually sense that they might be dying and they need an age- and developmentally appropriate opportunity to share their fears.
- Nurses in A&E are likely to have to deal with a higher proportion of sudden/unexpected deaths, which may occur in unusual or violent circumstances. Many nurses in acute care feel unprepared and unsupported.
- The death of a child can take the form of *miscarriage* (*spontaneous abortion*), *termination* (*therapeutic/induced abortion*), *stillbirth* or *neonatal death* (babies in SCBUs/NICUs). Each is a bereavement that needs to be grieved for, but termination is more likely to cause mental health problems in the mother.
- Although grief is a universal response to major loss, its meaning, duration and expression are all *culturally prescribed*. Cultures differ in how they define death, and it is often impossible to separate an individual's grief from culturally required mourning.
- All the world's major religions teach that there is some kind of *afterlife*. They also comfort the bereaved by helping to make sense of death and by providing 'milestones' that allow a gradual time to adjust to life without the deceased.

- Part of *nursing culture* is the expectation that nurses will undertake the 'last offices'.
- The hospital or community setting represents the *organizational culture*.
- *'Palliative care'*, *'hospice care'*, *'terminal care'* and *'end-of-life care'* are often used interchangeably.
- Spiritual and existential issues (such as finding a sense of purpose or meaning) can affect the well-being of people at the end of their lives.
- Maintaining the patients *dignity* is a fundamental goal of palliative care.

14 Early experience and social development

Introduction and overview

The study of attachments and their loss or disruption represents an important way of trying to understand how early experience can affect later development. Although Freud had emphasised the importance of early experience in the late 1800s (see Chapter 2), it is really only since the 1950s that developmental psychologists have systematically studied the nature and importance of the child's tie to its mother.

This began with the English psychiatrist John Bowlby. He was commissioned by the World Health Organization to investigate the effects on children's development of being raised in institutions (in the aftermath of the Second World War). The central concept discussed in his report (*Maternal Care and Mental Health*, 1951) was *maternal deprivation*, which has become almost synonymous with the harmful effects of not growing up within a family.

However, Bowlby has been criticised for exaggerating the importance of the mother–child relationship. Fathers are attachment figures in their own right, as are siblings. Children's social development involves the expansion of the network of relationships to include teachers, neighbours and classmates, some of whom will become their friends.

There is now a considerable body of research into attachments beyond infancy and childhood, especially between adult sexual partners, and many psychologists have questioned the deterministic nature of the early years (see Gross, 2010, 2012b).

According to Schaffer (2004), 'relationships provide the context in which all of a child's psychological functions develop … Understanding relationship formation is thus an essential part of understanding child development.'

From my diary (4): Year 1/Community (Health Visitor)

As part of my Primary Care experience with a Health Visitor (Chris) I made a home visit to a family on the Child Protection Register. Nicky is 21 and has two children – Ben (22 months), from a previous relationship, and Julie (10 weeks), from her present one. When Nicky answered the door I could hear the baby crying. Ben hid behind her and clung to her legs but once inside, she sat him in front of the TV, which was already on. Ben huddled there, thumb in mouth and clutching a rather grubby little toy rabbit as he stared blankly at an episode of Tracy Beaker; I felt so sorry for him. The baby's nappy was soaked when we undressed her; her weight was under the lowest percentile for her age. Nicky didn't seem concerned but said the baby 'didn't seem to want' all her feeds; she also hadn't noticed Julie had a 'sticky eye'. Chris suggested Nicky dress the baby while she 'had a chat' with Ben, but I saw she was also observing Nicky. The baby was smiling but Nicky hardly responded at all and didn't talk to her. Afterwards Chris checked how Nicky made up the feeds (she wasn't measuring the food properly) and showed her how to bathe the baby's eyes with cool, boiled water. She also encouraged her to talk to the baby more. When we left, I felt very anxious about both the children.

The development and variety of attachments

What is attachment?

According to Kagan et al. (1978), an attachment is

> … an intense emotional relationship that is specific to two people, that endures over time, and in which prolonged separation from the partner is accompanied by stress and sorrow.

While this definition applies to attachment formation at any point in the life cycle, our first attachment acts as a *prototype* (or model) for all later relationships. Similarly, although the definition applies to any attachment, the crucial first attachment is usually taken to be with the mother.

Phases in the development of attachments

The attachment process can be divided into several phases (Schaffer, 1996a), as follows:

1. The *pre-attachment phase* lasts until about 3 months of age. From about 6 weeks, babies develop an attraction to other human beings in preference to physical aspects of the environment. This is shown through behaviours such as nestling, gurgling and smiling (the *social smile*), which are directed to just about anyone.
2. At about 3 months, infants begin to discriminate between familiar and unfamiliar people, smiling much more at the former (the social smile has now disappeared). However, they will allow strangers to handle them without becoming noticeably distressed, provided they are cared for adequately. This *indiscriminate attachment phase* lasts until around 7 months.

3. From about 7 or 8 months, infants begin to develop specific attachments. This is shown through actively trying to stay close to certain people (particularly the mother) and becoming distressed when separated from them (*separation anxiety*). This *discriminate attachment phase* occurs when an infant can consistently tell the difference between its mother and other people, and has developed *object permanence* (the awareness that things – in this case, the mother – continue to exist even when they cannot be seen; see Chapter 15). Also at this time, infants avoid closeness with unfamiliar people and some display the *fear-of-strangers response*. This includes crying and/or trying to move away, which are usually triggered only when a stranger tries to make direct contact with the baby (rather than when the stranger is just 'there').

4. In the *multiple attachment phase* (from about 9 months onwards), strong additional ties are formed with other major caregivers (such as the father, grandparents and siblings) and with non-caregivers (such as other children). Although the fear-of-strangers response typically weakens, the strongest attachment continues to be with the mother.

Baby Julie is in the pre-attachment phase; when I took her from Nicky and began to talk to her, she responded with smiles and little excited movements. By hiding from us, Ben showed he didn't trust strangers.

Theories of the attachment process

'Cupboard love' theories

According to *psychoanalytic* accounts, the infant becomes attached to its caregiver (usually the mother) because of his/her ability to satisfy its instinctual needs. For Freud (1926),

> The reason why the infant in arms wants to perceive
> the presence of its mother is only because it already
> knows that she satisfies all its needs without delay.

Freud believed that healthy attachments are formed when feeding practices satisfy the infant's needs for food, security and oral sexual gratification (see Chapter 2). Unhealthy attachments occur when infants are *deprived* of food and oral pleasure, or are *overindulged*. Thus, psychoanalytic accounts stress the importance of feeding, especially breastfeeding, and of the maternal figure (see Figure 14.1).

Chris said that Nicky had breastfed Ben for a few weeks, but didn't succeed with Julie; it was clear she wasn't responding well to the baby's physical or psychological needs.

TIME FOR REFLECTION ...

- What do you think the *behaviourist* account of attachment might be (see Chapter 2)?

Figure 14.1 Is this really all there is to attachment formation?

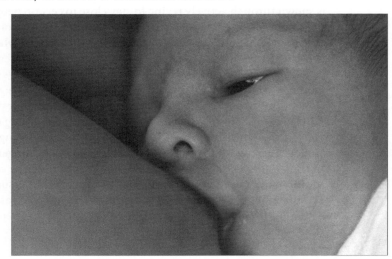

The *behaviourist* view of attachment also sees infants as becoming attached to those who satisfy their physiological needs. Infants associate their caregivers (who act as *conditioned* or *secondary reinforcers*) with gratification/satisfaction (food being an *unconditioned* or *primary reinforcer*), and they learn to approach them to have their needs met. This eventually generalises into a feeling of security whenever the caregiver is present.

In that case, the baby should attach to Nicky as she is the only one feeding her. The father appears periodically but doesn't stay for more than a day or two at a time.

An evaluation of 'cupboard love' theories

- Both behaviourist and psychoanalytic accounts of attachment as 'cupboard love' were challenged by Harlow's studies involving rhesus monkeys (e.g., Harlow, 1959; Harlow and Zimmerman, 1959). In the course of studying learning, Harlow separated newborn monkeys from their mothers and raised them in individual cages. Each cage contained a 'baby blanket', to which the monkey became intensely attached, showing great distress when it was removed. This apparent attachment to its blanket, and the display of behaviour comparable to that of an infant monkey actually separated from its mother, seemed to contradict the view that attachment comes from an association with nourishment.
- Harlow also found that baby monkeys showed a distinct preference for a cloth (terry towelling) surrogate mother to a wire mother – regardless of which one provided milk. While this also challenges the cupboard love explanation, these babies became extremely aggressive adults, rarely interacted with other monkeys, made inappropriate sexual responses and were difficult (if not impossible) to breed. So, in monkeys at least, normal

development seems to depend on factors other than having something soft and cuddly to provide comfort, one of these being *interaction with other members of the species* during the first 6 months of life.

Ben had his 'attachment' article – it presumably gave him that feeling of warmth and security. As well as food, breastfeeding provides warmth and softness naturally for the baby; bottle feeding can be, though of course not necessarily, less intimate. During our visit there was very little interaction of any kind between Nicky and the baby, or Ben.

- Research on attachment in humans also casts doubt on 'cupboard love' theories (Key Study 14.1).

  Schaffer and Emerson (1964) concluded that the two features of a person's behaviour that best predicted whether s/he would become an attachment figure for the infant are

  1. *Responsiveness* to the infant's behaviour
  2. The *total amount of stimulation* s/he provided (such as talking, touching and playing)

  For Schaffer (1971), 'cupboard love' theories of attachment put things the wrong way round. Instead of infants being passive recipients of nutrition (they 'live to eat'), he prefers to see them as *active seekers of stimulation* (they 'eat to live').

Chris intends to bring a video on massage to encourage Nicky to have more tactile contact with the baby. Both the baby and Ben need to be talked to and cuddled, not just fed.

KEY STUDY 14.1

Feeding is not everything for Scottish infants

- Sixty infants were followed up at four weekly intervals throughout their first year, and then again at 18 months.
- Mothers reported on their infants' behaviour in seven everyday situations involving separations, such as being left alone in a room, with a babysitter, and being put to bed at night. For each situation, information was obtained regarding whether the infant protested or not, how much and how regularly it protested, and whose departure elicited this reaction.
- Infants were clearly attached to people who did not perform caretaking activities (notably the father). Also, in 39% of cases, the person who usually fed, bathed and changed the infant (typically the mother) was *not* the infant's primary attachment figure.

Source: Schaffer, H.R. and Emerson, P.E., The development of social attachments in infancy, *Monographs of the Society for Research in Child Development*, 29 (whole No. 3), 1964.

Ethological theories

The term 'attachment' was actually introduced to psychology by *ethologists* (zoologists who study the evolutionary functions of the 'natural' behaviour of non-human animals). Lorenz (1935) showed that some non-humans (including geese) form strong bonds with the first moving objects they encounter (usually, but not always, the mother). Since this *imprinting* occurs simply through perceiving the caregiver without any feeding taking place, it too makes a 'cupboard love' account of attachment seem less valid, at least in goslings.

RESEARCH QUESTION ...
- How relevant are Harlow's and Lorenz's findings with rhesus monkeys and goslings, respectively, to understanding human attachments?

Most psychologists would agree that the only way to be sure about a particular species is to study that species. To generalise the findings from rhesus monkeys and goslings to human infants is dangerous (although less so in the case of rhesus monkeys). However, Harlow's and Lorenz's findings can suggest how attachments might be formed in humans. Indeed, Bowlby, whose theory represents the most comprehensive account of human attachment formation, was greatly influenced by Lorenz's concept of imprinting.

Well, normally, the baby is given to the mother immediately after birth for skin-to-skin contact to encourage attachment, as Maia, my little girl, was. I discovered subsequently Julie went to intensive care for 24 hours on delivery, which might be significant.

Bowlby's theory

Bowlby (1969, 1973) argued that because newborn human infants are entirely helpless, they are *genetically programmed* to behave towards their mothers in ways that ensure their survival (Box 14.1).

Baby Julie demonstrated all these behaviours. Ben wrapped himself around Nicky's legs so his whole body was in contact with her and, when he was removed, comforted himself by non-nutritive sucking. Freud would say it was satisfying an oral sexual need; a behaviourist would say it was a conditioned response eliciting the security experienced during feeding!

The mother also inherits a genetic blueprint that programmes her to respond to the baby. There is a critical period during which the *synchrony of action* between mother and infant produces an attachment. In Bowlby's (1951) view, mothering is useless for all children if delayed until after 2½ to 3 years, and for most children if delayed until after 12 months.

Bowlby believed that infants display a strong innate tendency to become attached to one particular adult female (not necessarily the natural mother), a tendency he called *monotropy*. This attachment to the mother figure is *qualitatively* different (different in kind) from any later attachments. For Bowlby

---

Box 14.1 Species-specific behaviours used by infants to shape and control their caregivers' behaviour

Sucking: While sucking is important for nourishment, *non-nutritive sucking* seems to be an innate tendency, which inhibits a newborn's distress. In Western societies, babies are often given 'dummies' (or 'pacifiers') to calm them when they are upset.

Cuddling: Human infants adjust their postures to mould themselves to the contours of the parent's body. The reflexive response that encourages front-to-front contact with the mother plays an important part in reinforcing the caregiver's behaviour.

Looking: An infant's looking behaviour acts as an invitation to its mother to respond. If she fails to do so, the infant becomes upset and avoids further visual contact. By contrast, mutual gazing is rewarding for an infant.

Smiling: This seems to be an innate behaviour, since babies can produce smiles shortly after birth. Although the first 'social smile' does not usually occur before 6 weeks (see page 326), adults view the smiling infant as a 'real person', which they find very rewarding.

Crying: Young infants usually cry only when hungry, cold or in pain, and crying is most effectively ended by picking up and cuddling them. Caregivers who respond quickly during the first 3 months tend to have babies that cry *less* during the last 4 months of their first year than infants with unresponsive caregivers (Bell and Ainsworth, 1972).

(1951), 'Mother love in infancy is as important for mental health as are vitamins and proteins for physical health.'

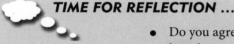 Chris is concerned that this doesn't seem to be happening with Julie, who clearly isn't a 'thriving' baby. Also, Ben isn't getting enough attention and stimulation.

An evaluation of Bowlby's theory

TIME FOR REFLECTION ...

- Do you agree with Bowlby that the infant's relationship with its mother is unique, or are men just as capable as women of providing adequate parenting and becoming attachment figures for their young children?

- Infants and young children display a whole range of attachment behaviours towards a variety of attachment figures other than their mothers. In other words, the mother is not special in the way the infant shows its attachment to her (Rutter, 1981).

- Although Bowlby did not deny that children form multiple attachments, he saw attachment to the mother as being unique: it is the first to develop and is the strongest of all. However, Schaffer and Emerson's (1964) study (see Key Study 14.1) showed that multiple attachments seem to be the rule rather than the exception. For example, at about 7 months, 29% of infants had already formed several attachments simultaneously, and by 10 months, 59% had developed more than one attachment.

- While there was usually one particularly strong attachment, only half of the 18-month olds were most strongly attached to their mothers and almost one-third were most strongly attached to their fathers.

When Ben was six months old his father left and there are no grandparents locally. Nicky said when Julie's dad is around he's 'good with Ben' but that's infrequently. So, other than Nicky, Ben is lacking attachment figures.

For Bowlby, the father is of no direct emotional significance to the young infant, but only of indirect value as an emotional and economic support for the mother. *Evolutionary psychologists* (see Gross, 2010) see mothers as having a greater *parental investment* in their offspring and hence they are better prepared for child rearing and attachment (Kenrick, 1994). However, Bowlby's views on fathers as attachment figures are disputed by findings such as those of Schaffer and Emerson (1964) (Critical Discussion 14.1).

This is a reminder of the need to evaluate research findings in their social/historical context. Bowlby was writing when mothers (like mine) were the main carers – whatever their inclination. Now, according to government figures, 66.5% of mothers are working (Jane Matinson, Guardian, posted 31.3.2011). When Nicky said her partner was 'good with Ben', did she mean he just plays with him, or helps care for him too? In this situation, shouldn't we assess Julie's father's relationship with both children?

Individual variations in attachment

Ainsworth et al.'s (1971, 1978) *Strange Situation (SS)* is widely accepted as the 'gold standard' measure of security in early life. The SS is a standardised observational technique comprising eight brief episodes as described in Table 14.1 (and see Figure 14.2).

Figure 14.2 One of the eight episodes in the 'Strange Situation'.

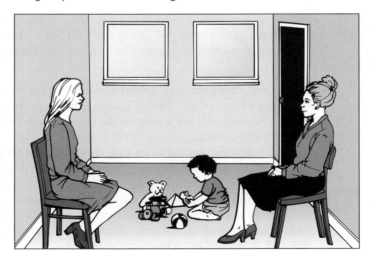

CRITICAL DISCUSSION 14.1

•••

How good are fathers at being mothers?

•••

- Framing the question this way, of course, rests on the implicit assumption that women are 'natural' parents. This view of women is reflected in Bowlby's theory of monotropy and the complementary responsiveness of mothers to their babies (the 'maternal instinct').

- Based on this view of women-as-mothers, any departure from the traditional division of labour in child care has been greeted with suspicion – men inevitably will provide inferior parenting (Schaffer, 2004).

- Although men as principal parents is still a minority phenomenon, fathers' participation in child rearing has certainly become much more common and an increasing number of children now live in father-headed families.

- There is considerable cultural variation in the extent of fathers' involvement in child care. This suggests that whatever sex differences exist in this respect are a matter of *social convention* and not an 'immutably fixed part of being male or female' (Schaffer, 2004) or *biology*.

- Although the evidence is sparse, there is no indication that the development of children brought up by a man differs in any way from others. Direct observation of men in their fathering role has shown them to be as capable of as much warmth and sensitivity as women (Schaffer, 2004).

- Rather than being poor substitutes for mothers, fathers make their own unique contribution to the care and development of infants and young children (at least in two-parent families). Children's developmental outcome is affected not by the parents' gender but by the kind of relationship that exists within each individual parent–child couple (Parke, 2002) (see Figure 14.3).

Figure 14.3 Does the baby really mind that the person who feeds it is not female?

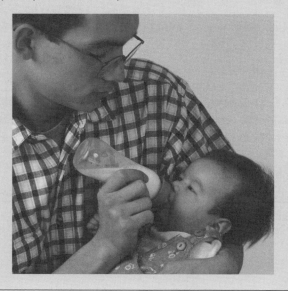

Table 14.1 The eight episodes of the 'Strange Situation'

Episode	Persons present	Duration	Brief description
1	Mother, baby, observer	30 seconds	Observer introduces mother and baby to experimental room, then leaves.
2	Mother, baby	3 minutes	Mother is non-participant while baby explores; if necessary, play is stimulated after 2 minutes.
3	Stranger, mother, baby	3 minutes	Stranger enters. First minute: stranger silent. Second minute: stranger converses with mother. Third minute: stranger approaches baby. After 3 minutes, mother leaves unobtrusively.
4	Stranger, baby	3 minutes or less[a]	First separation episode. Stranger's behaviour is geared to the baby's.
5	Mother, baby	3 minutes or more[b]	First reunion episode. Stranger leaves. Mother greets and/or comforts baby, then tries to settle baby again in play. Mother then leaves, saying 'bye-bye'.
6	Baby	3 minutes or less[a]	Second separation episode.
7	Stranger, baby	3 minutes or less[a]	Continuation of second separation. Stranger enters and gears her behaviour to babys.
8	Mother, baby	3 minutes	Second reunion episode. Mother enters, greets baby, then picks up baby. Meanwhile, stranger leaves unobtrusively.

Source: Ainsworth, M.D.S. et al., *Patters of Attachment: A Psychological Study of the Strange Situation*, Hillsdale, NJ, Lawrence Erlbaum Associates Inc., 1978; Krebs, D. and Blackman, R., *Psychology: A First Encounter*, New York, Harcourt Brace Jovanovich, 1988)

[a] Apply style Episode is ended early if baby is unduly distressed.
[b] Episode is prolonged if more time is required for baby to become reinvolved in play.

In the SS technique, although every aspect of the participants' reactions is observed and videotaped, it is the child's response to the mother's return that is given the most attention (i.e., *reunion behaviours*). This provides a clearer picture of the state of attachment than even the response to separation itself (Marrone, 1998) (see Table 14.2).

The dynamics of the attachment relationship can be seen in terms of a balance between (1) exploratory behaviour directed towards the environment and (2) attachment behaviour directed towards the caregiver. Looked at in this light, securely attached babies have got the balance right (Meins, 2003). But in both patterns of insecure attachment, the balance is tipped to one or other extreme: the anxious-avoidant baby shows high levels of environment-directed behaviour to the detriment of attachment behaviour, while the anxious-resistant baby is preoccupied with the caregiver to the detriment of exploration and play.

Table 14.2 Behaviour associated with three types of attachment in one-year-olds using the 'Strange Situation'

Category	Name	Sample (%)
Type A	Anxious-avoidant	15
Typical behaviour: Baby largely ignores mother, because of *indifference* towards her. Play is little affected by whether she is present or absent. No or few signs of distress when mother leaves, and actively ignores or avoids her on her return. *Distress is caused by being alone*, rather than being left by the mother. Can be comforted as easily by the stranger as by the mother. In fact, *both adults are treated in a very similar way.*		
Type B	Securely attached	70
Typical behaviour: Baby plays happily while the mother is present, whether the stranger is present or not. Mother is largely 'ignored', because she can be trusted to be there if needed. Clearly distressed when the mother leaves, and play is considerably reduced. Seeks immediate contact with mother on her return, quickly calms down in her arms and resumes play. The *distress is caused by the mother's absence*, not by being alone. Although the stranger can provide some comfort, *she and the mother are treated very differently.*		
Type C	Anxious-resistant	15
Typical behaviour: Baby is fussy and wary while the mother is present. Cries a lot more than types A and B, and *has difficulty using mother as a safe base*. Very distressed when she leaves, seeks contact with her on her return, but simultaneously shows anger and resists contact (may approach her and reach out to be picked up, then struggles to get down again). This shows the baby's *ambivalence* towards her. Does not return to play readily. *Actively resists stranger's efforts to make contact.*		

Although not in a 'Strange Situation', Ben's behaviour was more like the anxious-resistant group; he kept checking his mother was in sight and didn't respond to my attempt to talk to him about the TV programme.

The role of maternal sensitivity

The crucial feature determining the quality of attachment is the mother's *sensitivity*. The sensitive mother sees things from her baby's perspective, correctly interprets its signals, responds to its needs, and is accepting, cooperative and accessible. By contrast, the insensitive mother interacts almost exclusively in terms of her own wishes, moods and activities. According to Ainsworth et al., sensitive mothers tend to have babies who are *securely attached*, whereas insensitive mothers have *insecurely attached* babies (either *anxious-avoidant/detached* or *anxious-resistant/ambivalent*).

During the past 20 years or so, several studies with larger samples have tested, and supported, the original claim that parental sensitivity actually *causes* attachment security (van Ijzendoorn and Schuengel, 1999). However, sensitivity is not an *exclusive* condition for attachment security – other parenting qualities play a part (e.g., DeWolff and van Ijzendoorn, 1997). Conversely, even abusive parents do not necessarily produce deviant forms of attachment. According to Schaffer (2004), although maltreated children are clearly at risk:

- They usually show some signs of attachment to their abusing parents, although this may be confused and disorganised; the attachment system seems to be so powerful that even in the absence of consistent love and emotional warmth, children persist in trying to form attachments.
- There are always some children (although a small minority – about 15%) who form secure attachments; they enjoy good relationships with peers and others, and by no means do all abused children become abusing adults.

Schaffer's (2004) conclusions and reference to the attachment system as 'powerful' suggest an infant's instinctive need to attach. But the **development** of attachment seems to depend on the sensitivity and responsiveness of the carer, whoever it is.

Deprivation and privation

Bowlby's maternal deprivation hypothesis

As noted earlier, Bowlby argued for the existence of a critical period in attachment formation. This, along with his theory of monotropy (see page 330), led him to claim that the mother–infant attachment could not be broken in the first few years of life without serious and permanent damage to social, emotional and intellectual development. For Bowlby (1951), 'An infant and young child should experience a warm, intimate and continuous relationship with his mother (or permanent mother figure) in which both find satisfaction and enjoyment.'

Bowlby's *maternal deprivation hypothesis* (MDH) was based largely on studies conducted in the 1930s and 1940s of children brought up in residential nurseries and other large institutions (such as orphanages), notably those of Goldfarb (1943), Spitz (1945, 1946), and Spitz and Wolf (1946).

Bowlby, Goldfarb, Spitz and Wolf explained the harmful effects of growing up in an institution in terms of what Bowlby called maternal deprivation. In doing so, they failed

- To recognise that poor, unstimulating environments are generally associated with learning difficulties and retarded language development (vital for overall intellectual development); hence, a crucial variable in intellectual development is the amount of *intellectual stimulation* a child receives, *not* the amount of mothering (Rutter, 1981)
- To distinguish between the effects of deprivation and privation. Strictly, *deprivation* ('de-privation') refers to the *loss*, through separation, of the maternal attachment figure (which assumes that an attachment has already developed); *privation* refers to the *absence* of an attachment figure – there has been no opportunity to form an attachment in the first place (Rutter, 1981)
- These studies are most accurately thought of as showing the effects of *privation*. However, Bowlby's own theory and research were mainly concerned with *deprivation*. By using only the one term (deprivation), he confused two very different types of early experience, which have very different types of effect (both short-and long-term). See Figure 14.4.

Figure 14.4 Examples of the difference between deprivation and privation, including their effects.

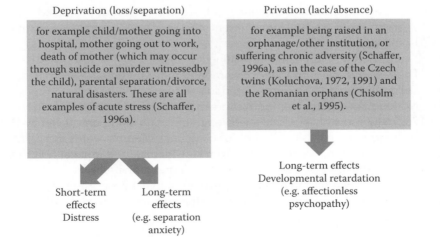

Nicky's children both have an attachment figure **physically** present so are not suffering from privation or maternal deprivation – but they do seem to be suffering from poor quality of care.

Deprivation (separation or loss)

Short-term deprivation and its effects

One example of short-term deprivation (days or weeks, rather than months or years) is that of a child going into a nursery while its mother goes into hospital. Another is that of the child itself going into hospital (see Critical Discussion 14.2). Bowlby and Robertson showed that when young children go into hospital, they display *distress*, which typically involves three components or stages Box 14.2.

CRITICAL DISCUSSION 14.2

Children in hospital

- In many children's wards in the mid-1950s, visiting was restricted to a couple of hours at the weekend.
- James Robertson, a psychoanalyst who worked with Anna Freud and Dorothy Burlingham in the 1940s, made films of children before, during and after hospital admission – including *A Two-Year-Old Goes to Hospital* (1952) and *Going to Hospital with Mother* (1958). These are still used to train paediatric staff.
- The films captured the stages of distress and helped sow the seeds of a revolution that ensured children have a better hospital of experience. Robertson argued that parents should be allowed to be with their children throughout their stay.
- The two films were used in evidence to the committee that produced the Platt Report (1959), the first of several government circulars and reports during the 1960s and 1970s, all recommending that
  - There should be unrestricted visiting.
  - There should be overnight accommodation for parents.
  - Children shouldn't be nursed on adult wards.
- The National Association for the Welfare of Children in Hospital (NAWCH) first reported (in 1962) that most hospitals still allowed afternoon visiting only. Even by 1982, parents were still regarded as visitors in half of all acute children's wards in England, overnight accommodation for parents was far from satisfactory, and at least half the wards nursing children were not part of comprehensive paediatric units.
- In 1986, NAWCH reported a huge improvement in the proportion of wards with entirely unrestricted access for parents. But conditions are still far from ideal.

Source: Devlin, R., *Nursing Times*, 85(5), 18, 1989.

Box 14.2 Components or stages of distress

- *Protest:* The initial, immediate reaction takes the form of crying, screaming, kicking and generally struggling to escape, or clinging to the mother to prevent her from leaving. This is an outward and direct expression of the child's anger, fear, bitterness and bewilderment.
- *Despair:* The struggling and protest eventually give way to calmer behaviour. The child may appear apathetic, but internally still feels all the anger and fear previously displayed. It keeps such feelings 'locked up' and wants nothing to do with other people. The child may no longer anticipate the mother's return, and barely reacts to others' offers of comfort, preferring to comfort itself by rocking, thumb-sucking and so on.
- *Detachment:* If the separation continues, the child begins to respond to people again, but tends to treat everyone alike and rather superficially. However, if reunited with the mother at this stage, the child may well have to 'relearn' its relationship with her and may even 'reject' her (as she 'rejected' her child).

Factors influencing distress

Many institutions used to be run in a way that made the development of substitute attachments very difficult (see page 342). One *long-term* effect of short-term separation is *separation anxiety.* This is also associated with long-term deprivation (see Figure 14.5 and page 340).

TIME FOR REFLECTION ...

- Distress (especially protest and despair) can be thought of as an extreme display of attachment behaviours. Looked at this way, what factors do you think are likely to make separation most distressing for the child?

Evidence suggests that not all children go through the stages of distress, and that they differ in how much distress they experience. Separation is likely to be most distressing

- When there is no mother substitute to take the mother's place
- Between the ages of 7 and 8 months (when attachments are just beginning to develop) and 3 years, with a peak at 12–18 months (Maccoby, 1980). This is related to the child's inability to retain a mental image of the absent mother, and its limited understanding of language
- For boys (although there are also wide differences within each gender)
- If there have been any behaviour problems, such as aggression, that existed before the separation; such problems are likely to be accentuated by separation
- If the mother and child have an extremely close and protective relationship, in which they are rarely apart; children appear to cofe best if their relationship with the mother is close but not too close, and if they have other attachment figures (such as their fathers) who can provide love and care

Figure 14.5 John (17 months) experienced extreme distress while spending 9 days in a residential nursery when his mother was in hospital having a second baby. According to Bowlby, he was grieving for the absent mother. Robertson and Robertson (1969) (who made a series of films called *Young Children in Brief Separation*) found that the extreme distress was caused by a combination of factors – multiple caretakers, lack of a mother substitute, loss of the mother and strange environment and routines.

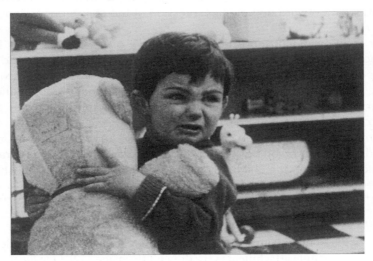

This was an example of the medical model of nursing not being challenged until (Bowlby's) research-based evidence stimulated change – which took 30 years! It's also an example of the difficulty of changing entrenched attitudes (see Chapter 6) and how social and political forces can bring it about. Thankfully, when Maia was four and in hospital, I could stay with her, including overnight.

Long-term deprivation and its effects

Long-term deprivation includes the permanent separation resulting from *parental death* and the increasingly common separation caused by *divorce*. Perhaps the most common effect of long-term deprivation is what Bowlby called *separation anxiety* – the fear that separation will occur again in the future.

Day care is also regarded by some as another form of long-term deprivation (see Gross, 2010).

As so many nurses (including me) are now both divorced and working parents, I found this worrying. However, Schaffer (2004) argues it depends on mediating factors, e.g quality of parenting and contact with the father and concludes 'the fear that children are scarred for life by parental divorce is thus not justified as a generalisation' (Box 32.3, page 503, Gross 2010)', which is reassuring!

Privation

As we noted above, privation is the failure to develop an attachment to any individual. Given the importance of the child's first relationship as a model or prototype of relationships in general, failure to develop an attachment of any kind is likely to adversely affect all subsequent relationships.

Affectionless psychopathy

According to Bowlby, maternal deprivation in early childhood causes *affectionless psychopathy*. This is the inability to care and have deep feelings for other people and the consequent lack of meaningful interpersonal relationships, together with the inability to experience guilt (Key Study 14.2).

Bowlby et al. admitted that 'part of the emotional disturbance can be attributed to factors other than separation', such as the common occurrence of illness and death in the sanatorium children's families. So, there was very little evidence for the link between affectionless psychopathy and *separation* (or *bond disruption*). However, Bowlby may have provided evidence for an association with privation instead (a failure to form bonds in early life). According to Rutter (1981), privation is likely to lead to

- An initial phase of clinging, dependent behaviour
- Attention-seeking, and uninhibited, indiscriminate friendliness
- A personality characterised by lack of guilt, an inability to keep rules, and an inability to form lasting relationships

📄 *Although Julie is with Nicky all the time, unless she responds more to the baby they are unlikely to bond satisfactorily.*

KEY STUDY 14.2

Growing up with tuberculosis

- Bowlby et al. studied 60 children aged 7–13, who had spent between 5 months and 2 years in a tuberculosis sanatorium (which provided no substitute mothering) at various ages up to 4.
- About half had been separated from their parents before they were 2 years old.
- When compared with a group of non-separated 'control' children from the same school classes, the overall picture was that the two groups were more similar than different.
- The separated children were more prone to 'daydreaming', showed less initiative, were more overexcited, rougher in play, concentrated less well and were less competitive. But they were not more likely to show affectionless psychopathy, regardless of when their separation had occurred (before or after the age of 2).

Source: Bowlby, J., et al., *British Journal of Medical Psychology*, 24(3/4), 211–247, 1956.

Are the effects of privation reversible?

There are (at least) three kinds of study which show that it is possible to undo the effects of early privation.

1. *Case studies* of children who have endured extreme early privation, often in near complete isolation. Examples include the Czech twins studied by Koluchova (1972, 1991) and concentration camp survivors (Freud and Dann, 1951; see Gross, 2010) (see Figure 14.6).
2. Studies of *late adoption*: children raised in institutions are adopted after Bowlby's critical period for attachment development (12 months for most children, up to 2½–3 years for the rest). Studies include those of Tizard and her colleagues (e.g., Hodges and Tizard, 1989; see Key Study 14.3) and Chisolm et al. (1995; again see Figure 14.6 and Gross, 2010).
3. Studies of developmental pathways (see pages 342–346).

Studies of late adoption

Tizard (1977) and Hodges and Tizard (1989) studied children who, on leaving care between the ages of 2 and 7, were either adopted or returned to their own families. The institutions they grew up in provided good physical care and appeared to provide adequate intellectual stimulation, but by age 2, they had been looked after for at least a week by an average of 24 different caregivers. The children's attachment behaviour was very unusual and, in general, the first opportunity to form long-term attachments came when they left the institutions and were placed in families.

By age 8, most of the adopted children had formed close attachments to their adoptive parents (who very much wanted a child), despite the lack of early attachments in the institutions (Tizard and Hodges, 1978). But only some of those children returned to their own families had formed close attachments. As reported by their teachers, the ex-institutional children as a whole displayed attention-seeking behaviour, restlessness, disobedience and poor peer relationships (see Key Study 14.3).

Based on a follow-up of these ex-institution children into adulthood (average age 31 years), Hodges (personal communication, 2000) states that, 'the evidence seems to support both the view that the effects of earlier adversity fade given the right later circumstances, and the view that there are some enduring effects producing continuities in personal characteristics (Key Study 14.4).'

Again, the overall evidence seems to indicate that it's the **quality** of care the child receives that matters, both with, or without, maternal attachment.

Developmental pathways

Quinton and Rutter (1988) wanted to find out whether children deprived of parental care become depriving parents themselves. They observed one group of women, brought up in care, interacting with their own children, and compared them with a second group of non-institutionalised mothers. The women brought up in care were, as a whole, less sensitive, supportive and warm towards their children.

Figure 14.6 A simplified adaptive chain of circumstances in institution-raised women. (Based on Quinton, D. and Rutter, M., *Parental Breakdown: The Making and Breaking of Intergenerational Links.* London: Gower, 1988; Rutter, M., *Journal of Child & Psychology & Psychiatry, 30,* 23–25, 1989.)

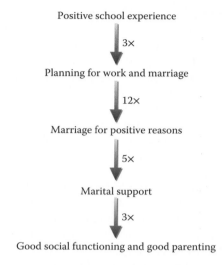

Positive school experience

3×

Planning for work and marriage

12×

Marriage for positive reasons

5×

Marital support

3×

Good social functioning and good parenting

KEY STUDY 14.3

Ex-institution children at age 16

- At age 16, the family relationships of most of the adopted children seemed satisfactory, for both them and their parents. They differed little from a non-adopted comparison group who had never been in care. Hence, early institutional care had not necessarily led to a later inability to form a close attachment to parents (contrary to Bowlby's predictions).
- By contrast, those children returned to their families still suffered difficulties and poor family relationships, including mutual difficulty in showing affection; the parents reported feeling closer to the children's siblings than to the returned children.
- *Outside* the family, *both* the adopted and returned children showed similar relationships with peers and adults. Compared with a control group, they were
  - Still more likely to seek adult affection and approval
  - Still more likely to have difficulties in their relationships with peers
  - Less likely to have a special friend or to see peers as sources of emotional support
  - More likely to be friendly to any peer rather than choosing their friends
  These findings *are* consistent with Bowlby's MDH.

Source: Hodges, J. and Tizard, B., *Journal of Child Psychology & Psychiatry, 30,* 77–97, 1989.

However, there was also considerable variability *within* the group brought up in care, with some women displaying good parenting skills. This could be explained in terms of *developmental pathways* (what Schaffer, 2004, calls *developmental trajectories*). For example, some of the women had more positive

KEY STUDY 14.4

Late adoption of Romanian orphans

- Rutter and the English and Romanian Adoptees (ERA) study team (1998) reported their findings from a study of 111 Romanian children raised in poor to appalling 'hospitals' or 'orphanages' and adopted before the age of 2 by English families (educationally and occupationally above general population norms).

- The Romanian children were compared with 52 control group children (within-U.K. adoptees, who had not suffered early privation). The Romanian children, as a whole, were more severely deprived – physically and psychologically - than almost any other sizeable group of children previously studied; they showed major developmental retardation.

- By age 4, the Romanian adoptees showed 'spectacular' *developmental catch-up* (especially cognitive), particularly marked in those adopted before 6 months. However, two follow-ups suggest that there is a continuing strong effect of their early privation.

- In the first follow-up, they were studied up to the age of 6 (Rutter and the ERA study team, 2004). Many children displayed *disinhibited attachment* (DA), which in many ways resembles the attachment behaviour of Hodges and Tizard's ex-institution sample: a lack of close confiding relationships; rather indiscriminate friendliness; a relative lack of differentiation in response to different adults; a tendency to go off with strangers; and a lack of checking back with a parent in anxiety-provoking situations. DA is one form of *reactive attachment disorder*.

- This pattern persisted from ages 4 to 6, and Rutter (2006) argued that it might represent some form of biological programming, that is, an effect on brain structure and functioning, which occurs as a form of adaptation to an abnormal environment during a sensitive period of development. On this basis, we would expect this pattern of behaviour to continue into middle childhood/early adolescence.

- Indeed, parents' reports of a persistence of DA from age 6–11 were confirmed by Rutter et al. (2007) – but it did become less frequent.

Source: Rutter, M., *The Development of Social Engagement: Neurobiological Perspectives.* New York: Oxford University Press, 2006; Rutter, M. and The English and Romanian Adoptees (ERA) study team, *Journal of Child Psychology & Psychiatry,* 39(4), 465–476, 1998; Rutter, M. et al., *Journal of Child & Psychology & Psychiatry,* 48(1), 17–30, 2007.

school experiences than others. This made them three times more likely as adolescents or young adults to make proper career and marriage partner choices (Rutter, 1989). Such positive experience represents an escape route from the early hardships associated with being brought up in care (see Figure 14.6).

Similar adverse childhood experiences can have multiple outcomes (Schaffer, 1996b, 2004). *Starting off* at a disadvantage doesn't necessarily mean having to *finish up* at a disadvantage. In other words, early disadvantage does not inevitably set off a chain reaction of more and more disadvantage. Periodically, individuals reach *turning points* where choices must be made, and the path that is taken can either reinforce or help to minimise the consequences of previous experience (Schaffer, 2004).

The developmental pathways concept makes me feel more optimistic about Nicky, who, at 13, after being in three different foster homes, ended up in care. And Chris emphasised that if Nicky had proper support now and responds well she could 'turn her life around'.

TIME FOR REFLECTION ...

- What do you think the effects on children brought into the world by such 'unnatural' means as described in Critical Discussion 14.3 might be?

CRITICAL DISCUSSION 14.3

Effects of 'reduced' or 'minimal parenting'

- Due to advances in reproductive technologies, it has become possible for children to be conceived and born 'artificially' to parents who would otherwise remain childless.
  - *In vitro fertilisation* (IVF): sperm and egg are provided by the father and mother, but they are combined in the laboratory.
  - *Egg donation: the father's sperm fertilises another woman's egg – so the child will be genetically related only to him.*
  - *Donor insemination (DI)/artificial insemination by donor (AID): the mother is impregnated by the sperm of a male other than the husband – so the child will be genetically related only to her.*
  - *Embryo donation: both egg and sperm are donated, so that neither parent is genetically related to the child. This is like adoption, except that the parents experience the pregnancy and the child's birth.*
  - *Surrogacy: one woman hosts a pregnancy for another woman. Non-genetic surrogacy uses the egg of the mother who will raise the child; in genetic surrogacy, the surrogate mother both hosts the pregnancy and provides the egg.*
  - *It is now possible for a child to have five parents: an egg donor, a sperm donor, a surrogate mother who hosts the pregnancy, and the two social parents whom the child knows as mum and dad (Golombok, 2010).*
  - *Almost 18,000 babies have been born in the United Kingdom through donated gametes (sperm and eggs) and embryos since the Human Fertilisation and Embryology Authority (HFEA) was created in 1991. Currently, birth certificates reveal nothing about the genetic father, and the law, as it stands, prevents revelation of the donor's identity. However, like adopted people, people have the right to ask the HFEA if they were conceived via donor eggs or sperm and, if conceived after 2005, the donor's identity. Since 2009, donors have new rights to access information about themselves and their donation.*
  - *There are various potential problems that may arise, including the absence of a genetic link with one or both parents involved in some of the techniques used (Schaffer, 2004).*

- In the first psychological study of assisted reproduction families, almost 500 children in the Netherlands, Italy, Spain and the United Kingdom were assessed at ages 6 (Golombok et al., 1995, 1996), 12 (Golombok et al., 2001, 2002a, b) and 18 years (Golombok et al., 2009). Children born following IVF or donor insemination were compared with adopted and naturally conceived children.
- Contrary to the concerns that had been raised about assisted reproduction families, there was no evidence that these new reproductive technologies have negative consequences – for either child or parent. Neither lack of genetic relationship nor manner of conception had any implications for their well-being.

> …Whether created by IVF, donor insemination, egg donation or surrogacy, and whether headed by same-sex or opposite-sex parents, what seems to matter most for children's psychological well-being is not the structure of the family but the quality of family life. (Golombok, 2010).

The research continually emphasises the importance of quality of care. Hodges and Tizard's research seems to indicate that children who suffered from early adversity did have relationship difficulties but **can** recover if their later attachments are carefully nurtured. I hope this applies to Nicky.

Conclusions

Schaffer (1998) believes that psychological development is far more flexible than was previously thought. Our personalities are not fixed once and for all by events in the early years and, given the right circumstances, the effects of even quite severe and prolonged deprivation can be reversed. As Clarke and Clarke (2000) conclude, 'For most children … the effects of such experiences represent no more than a first step in an ongoing lifepath ….'

Discussing the visit afterwards, Chris said she was arranging for Nicky to attend a local Sure Start group; it will provide important social interaction for Nicky, help her develop her parenting skills and provide play opportunities for Ben.

This experience has reinforced the fact that nursing isn't only about solving medical problems. In some cases it is psychological and social factors that lead to health problems and, referring to level three of Goodman's reflective framework (case study 10, page 244), it is psychological, social and political care that can solve, or avoid, them. In Julie's case, early intervention may prevent Nicky's situation becoming a worse problem; it was a good example of the 'proactive' approach within the biopsychosocial model of health that is a basic principle of health visiting.

CHAPTER SUMMARY

- *Attachments* are intense, enduring emotional ties to specific people. The *mother–child relationship* is usually taken as a model for all later relationships.
- The attachment process can be divided into *pre-attachment, indiscriminate, discriminate* and *multiple attachment phases*.
- The development of specific attachments is shown through *separation anxiety*. Some babies also display the *fear-of-strangers response*.
- According to *'cupboard love'* theories, attachments are learned through satisfaction of the baby's need for food. However, Schaffer and Emerson found that not only were infants attached to people who did not perform caretaking activities, but those who did weren't always their primary attachment figures.
- According to Bowlby, newborn humans are *genetically programmed* to behave towards their mothers in ways that ensure their survival. There is a *critical period* for attachment development, and attachment to the mother figure is based on *monotropy*.
- The Strange Situation (SS) is used to classify the baby's basic attachment to the mother into three main types: *anxious-avoidant, securely attached* and *anxious-resistant*. The crucial feature determining the quality of attachment is the mothers' *sensitivity*.
- Bowlbys' material deprivation hypothesis (MDH) was used to explain the harmful effects of growing up in institutions. But this fails to recognise the understimulating nature of the institutional environment, and to disentangle the different kinds of retardation produced by different types of *privation*.
- According to Bowlby's theory, short-term deprivation produces *distress*. Privation produces *long-term developmental retardation* (such as *affectionless psychopathy*).
- Parental death and divorce are examples of *long-term deprivation* and are associated with long-term effects, particularly separation anxiety. Another example is day care.
- Case studies of children who have endured extreme privation represent one kind of study showing that the effects of early privation are *reversible*.
- Another source of evidence is *late adoption* studies (such as the longitudinal studies of Hodges and Tizard, and Rutter and the ERA study team's study of Romanian orphans). However, many of these children displayed *disinhibited attachment* (DA), a form of *reactive attachment disorder* (RAD).
- Quinton and Rutter's study of *developmental pathways* also indicates that the effects of early privation are reversible.
- Varieties of *'reduced'* or *'minimal parenting'* include *in vitro fertilisation* (IVF), *egg donation, donor insemination* (DI), *artificial insemination by donor* (AID), *embryo donation* and *surrogacy* (genetic or non-genetic).
- Research by Golombok and others has concluded that these new reproductive technologies do not have negative consequences – for child or parent.

Cognitive development

Introduction and overview

According to Meadows (1993, 1995), cognitive development is concerned with the study of 'the child as thinker'. However, different theoretical accounts of how the child's thinking develops rest on very different images of what the child is like

- Piaget sees the child as an organism adapting to its environment, as well as a scientist constructing its own understanding of the world.
- Vygotsky, in contrast with Piaget, sees the child as a *participant in an interactive process*, by which socially and culturally determined knowledge and understanding gradually become *individualised*.
- Bruner, like Vygotsky, emphasises the *social* aspects of the child's cognitive development (see Gross, 2010).

Some years ago, Piaget's theory was regarded as the major framework or paradigm within child development. Despite remaining a vital source of influence both in psychology and education, many fundamental aspects of Piaget's theory have been challenged, and fewer and fewer developmental psychologists now subscribe to his or other 'hard' stage theories (Durkin, 1995). Nonetheless, Piaget's is still the most comprehensive account of how children come to understand the world (Schaffer, 2004). Arguably, however, it was a little too 'cold' – that is, concerned with purely *intellectual* functions that supposedly can be studied separately from socio-emotional functions. Vygotsky tried to redress the balance (Schaffer, 2004).

 From my diary (5a): Year 1/Community/Health Visitor

As I'd been a nursery/reception class assistant prior to starting nursing Chris (the HV) suggested that on our next visit to Nicky (see my diary entry on page 326), I should concentrate on Ben (nearly 2 years old) while she saw Nicky and baby Julie. When we arrived, Ben was (again) watching TV – until I produced a toy tractor I'd brought for him! When

he agreed to switch off the TV, we could see his reflection in the blank screen and I asked him who it was. He paused, then pointed to himself and said, 'That Ben!' I asked him who had a tractor like his and he replied, 'Bob Builder!' He became more animated as we talked about Bob and when I asked, 'Can we fix it?' he laughed and completed the catch-phrase by adding, 'Yes, we can!'

He then seemed happy to play 'find the treats' with me. I 'hid' a tiny packet of raisins under a cup; he found and ate them. I did it again, using another cup, and he did the same. The third time I put the raisins under one cup and the empty box under a nearer one. He found the empty box, looked puzzled for a few seconds, then turned up the other cup and – to his delight – found them. He seemed to enjoy the attention so much I felt sad to leave him.

Piaget's theory: The child-as-scientist

Rather than trying to explain individual differences (why some children are more intelligent than others), Piaget was interested in how intelligence itself changes as children grow. He called this *genetic epistemology*.

According to Piaget (see Figure 15.1), cognitive development occurs through the interaction of innate capacities with environmental events, and progresses through a series of *hierarchical, qualitatively different stages*:

- All children pass through the stages in the *same sequence* without skipping any or (except in the case of brain damage) regressing to earlier ones (they're *invariant*).
- The stages are also the *same for everyone* irrespective of culture (they're *universal*).
- Underlying the changes are certain *functional invariants*, fundamental aspects of the developmental process, which remain the same and work in

Figure 15.1 Jean Piaget (1896–1980)

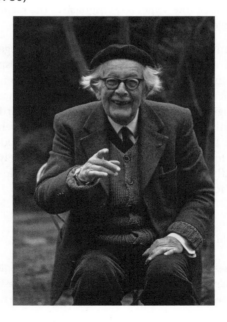

the same way through the various stages. The most important of these are *assimilation, accommodation* and *equilibration*.

- The principal *cognitive structure* that changes is the *schema* (plural *schemas* or *schemata*).

Schemas (or schemata)

A *schema* (or *scheme*) is the basic building block or unit of intelligent behaviour. Piaget saw schemas as mental structures, which organise past experiences and provide a way of understanding future experiences. Life begins with simple schemas that are largely confined to inbuilt reflexes (such as sucking and grasping). These operate independently of other reflexes, and are activated only when certain objects are present. As we grow, so our schemas become increasingly complex.

Assimilation, accommodation and equilibration

Assimilation is the process by which we incorporate new information into existing schemas. For example, babies will reflexively suck a nipple and other objects, such as a finger. To learn to suck from a bottle or drink from a cup, the initial sucking reflex must be modified through *accommodation*.

When a child can deal with most, if not all, new experiences by assimilating them, it is in a state of *equilibrium*. This is brought about by *equilibration*, the process of seeking 'mental balance'. But if existing schemas are inadequate to cope with new situations, cognitive *disequilibrium* occurs. To restore equilibrium, the existing schema must be 'stretched' to take in (or 'accommodate') new information. The necessary and complementary processes of assimilation and accommodation constitute the fundamental process of *adaptation* (see Figure 15.2).

So the **process** by which we learn doesn't change, but the way we organise our experience does. Baby Julie's 'drinking schema' consists only of sucking, whereas Ben's has accommodated drinking from a bottle and a cup and through a straw.

Figure 15.2 Relationship between assimilation, equilibrium, disequilibrium and accommodation in the development of schemas.

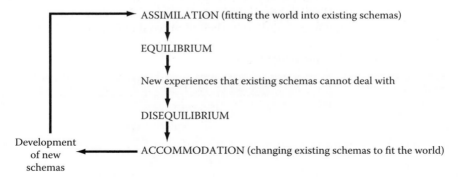

Stages of cognitive development

Each of Piaget's four stages represents a stage in the development of intelligence (hence *sensorimotor intelligence, preoperational intelligence,* and so on) and is a way of summarising the various schemas a child has at a particular time. The ages shown in Table 15.1 are approximate, because children move through the stages at different rates due to differences in both the environment and their biological maturation. Children also pass through transitional periods, in which their thinking is a mixture of two stages.

The sensorimotor stage

This lasts for approximately the first two years of life. Infants learn about the world primarily through their senses ('sensori-'), and by doing ('motor'). Based on observations of his own children, Piaget (1952) divided the sensorimotor stage into six sub-stages.

Object permanence

Frequent interaction with objects ultimately leads to the development of *object permanence.* In the second sub-stage (*primary circular reactions*: 1–4 months), an infant will look where an object disappears for a few moments, but would not search for it and apparently loses interest ('out of sight is out of mind').

In the third sub-stage (*secondary circular reactions*: 4–10 months), an infant will reach for a partially hidden object, suggesting that s/he realises that the rest of it is attached to the visible part. But if the object is completely hidden, infants make no attempt to retrieve it. In the fourth sub-stage (*the coordination of secondary circular reactions*: 10–12 months), a hidden object will be searched for ('out of sight' is no longer 'out of mind'), but the infant will persist in looking for it where it was last hidden, even when it is hidden somewhere else.

So this explains why attachment peaks at this age: the older child can retain an image of the attachment figure and will make efforts to 'find' him or her.

While after 12 months infants will look for an object where they last saw it hidden, object permanence is not yet fully developed. Suppose an infant sees an object placed in a matchbox, which is then put under a pillow. When it is not looking, the object is removed from the matchbox and left under the pillow. If the matchbox is given to the infant, it will open it expecting to find the object. On not finding it, the infant would not look under the pillow. This is

Table 15.1 Piaget's four stages of cognitive development

Stage	Approximate age
Sensorimotor	0–2 years
Pre-operational	2–7 years
Concrete operational	7–11 years
Formal operational	11 years onwards

because it cannot take into account the possibility that something it has not actually seen might have happened (*failure to infer invisible displacements*). Once the infant can infer invisible displacements (after 18 months), the development of object permanence is complete.

Julie and Ben are at different sub-stages within the sensorimotor stage. Julie 'passively explores', for instance, her fingers 'caressing' her bottle as Nicky fed her. By continuing his search for the raisins in my 'game', Ben showed he can infer invisible displacement.

The general symbolic function

- Other cognitive structures that have developed by the end of the sensorimotor stage include *self-recognition* (see Chapter 16) and *symbolic thought* (such as *language*).
- *Deferred imitation* is the ability to imitate or reproduce something that has been perceived but is no longer present (Meltzoff and Moore, 1983).
- *Representational* (or *make-believe*) *play* involves using one object as though it were another. Like deferred imitation, this ability depends on the infant's growing ability to form mental images of things and people in their absence (to *remember*).

Ben recognised his reflection as himself. Names and words are symbols representing objects, so he can use symbolic thought; his quoting 'Yes we can!' showed deferred imitation of Bob the Builder and going to the Sure Start nursery will help develop his rather limited language skills.

The preoperational stage

Probably, the main difference between this and the sensorimotor stage is the continued development and use of internal images (or '*interiorised*' *schemas*), symbols and language, especially important for the child's developing sense of self-awareness (see Chapter 16). However, the child tends to be influenced by how things *look*, rather than by logical principles or operations (hence the term 'preoperational').

Piaget subdivided the stage into the *preconceptual* (ages 2 to 4) and the *intuitive sub-stages* (ages 4 to 7). The *absolute* nature of the preconceptual child's thinking makes relative terms such as 'bigger' or 'stronger' difficult to understand (things tend to be 'biggest' or just 'big'). The intuitive child can use relative terms, but its ability to think logically is still limited.

 From my diary (5b): Year 1/Children's Ward

I'd enjoyed looking after two children with 'special needs' at school and thought I might like to care for sick children, so Chris arranged for me to spend three days on a children's ward. The first day I helped a Staff Nurse (Laura) look after three patients: Peter (2½ years old) had severe eczema, Lucy (6) was in for surgery to pin back her ears, and Jacob (12½) was in traction for a fractured femur. Peter kept following me around, wanting to be picked up; Lucy wanted to chat a lot but Jacob didn't seem to want to speak to anybody. During my lunch break I realised it was an opportunity to observe children in different stages of cognitive development. Peter is in the preconceptual sub-stage and Lucy in the intuitive sub-stage of Piaget's preoperational stage.

Seriation and artificialism

In *seriation*, the preconceptual child has difficulty arranging objects on the basis of a particular dimension, such as increasing height (Piaget and Szeminska, 1952). *Artificialism* is the belief that natural features have been designed and constructed by people. For example, the question 'Why is the sky blue?' might produce the answer 'Somebody painted it'.

Transductive reasoning and animism

Transductive reasoning involves drawing an inference about the relationship between two things based on a single shared attribute – for example, if both cats and dogs have four legs, then cats must be dogs. This sort of reasoning can lead to *animism* – the belief that inanimate objects are alive. (This is relevant to the child's understanding of death; see Chapter 13.)

TIME FOR REFLECTION …

- Can you think of any examples of adults displaying animistic thinking?
- Do you ever think this way yourself?

Centration

Centration involves focusing on only a single perceptual quality at a time. A pre-conceptual child asked to divide apples into 'big and red' ones and 'small and green' ones will either put all the red (or green) apples together irrespective of their size, or all the big (or small) apples together irrespective of their colour. Until the child can *decentre*, it will be unable to classify things logically or systematically. Centration is also associated with the *inability* to conserve (see discussion in page 355).

 Laura said that to avoid confusing Lucy, we needed to do her 'magic ointment' (to stop the needle hurting) preparation and the post-operative (bandaging of her ears) preparation at different times.

Egocentrism

According to Piaget, preoperational children are *egocentric*, that is, they see the world from their own standpoints and cannot appreciate that other people might see things differently. They cannot put themselves 'in other people's shoes' to realise that other people do not know or perceive everything they themselves do. Consider the following example (Phillips, 1969) of a conversation between an experimenter and a 4-year-old boy:

Experimenter:	'Do you have a brother?'
Child:	'Yes.'
Experimenter:	'What's his name?'
Child:	'Jim.'
Experimenter:	'Does Jim have a brother?'
Child:	'No.'

📄 Just after the 'pretend' local anaesthetic was applied to her hand, Lucy's father rang and she said proudly, 'See, I have a plaster!' and then, 'No – it's Tigger!' in a surprised tone as if he should have known.

Conservation

Conservation is the understanding that any quantity (such as number, liquid quantity, length, or substance) remains the same despite physical changes in the arrangement of objects. Preoperational children cannot conserve because their thinking is dominated by the *perceptual* nature of objects (their 'appearance').

The inability to conserve is another example of centration. With liquid quantity, for example, the child centres on just one dimension of the beaker, usually its height, and fails to take width into account (see Figure 15.3).

Only in the concrete operational stage do children understand that 'getting taller' and 'getting narrower' tend to cancel each other out (*compensation*). If the contents of the taller beaker are poured back into the shorter one, the child will again say that the two shorter beakers contain the same amount. But it cannot perform this operation mentally and so lacks *reversibility* (understanding that what can be done can be undone without any gain or loss). These same limitations apply to other forms of conservation, such as number (using two rows of counters) and substance/quantity (using plasticine).

📄 This happened sometimes in the reception class at school – I soon learned to give them identical beakers at snack time!

Figure 15.3 The conservation of liquid quantity. Although the child agrees that there is the same amount of liquid in A and B, when the contents of B are poured into C, the appearance of C sways the child's judgement so that C is now judged to contain more liquid than A ('it looks more' or 'it's taller'). Although the child has seen the liquid poured from B into C and agrees that none has been spilled or added in the process (what Piaget calls 'identity'), the appearance of the higher level of liquid in the taller, thinner beaker C is compelling.

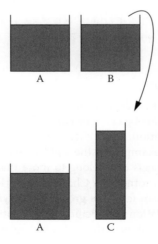

Imaginary friends

- Swendsen (1934) defined an imaginary friend as 'an invisible character named and referred to in conversation with other persons, or played with directly for a period of time … having an air of reality for the child but no apparent objective basis'. It may be a toy or doll, especially a favourite one, or a creature or animal.
- Most researchers agree that imaginary friends first appear at around 2½ years and disappear around 5 or 6. This corresponds to Piaget's preoperational stage. Swendsen claims that girls are three times more likely than boys to have an imaginary friend.
- The child tends to attribute adult qualities to the friend, such as knowledge, authority and power. It may be given an ordinary boy's or girl's name or a pet (invented) name.
- Young children will often use their imaginary friend to help them bridge the gap between external controls (usually the parents) and the internal ones represented by the superego (see Chapter 2). The child may ask the friend what to do in a particular situation. The imaginary friend can also become a very convenient scapegoat for the child's naughtiness. This is not simply a case of the young child lying to avoid punishment, but an important stage in the developing process of self-criticism and self-control (Nagera, 1969).
- Several researchers have claimed that only children, or those who have been neglected or rejected, are more likely to have an imaginary friend. For example, Nagera gives several accounts of children who have created their imaginary friend shortly after parental divorce or after the birth of a new baby.

Source: Darbyshire, P., *Nursing Times*, 40–42, 1986a.

Going into hospital is another stressful situation in which imaginary friends may appear. It is tempting for a nurse to use the friend as a means of reassuring the child. But the child may become confused if the nurse later tries to deny the nature of the friend; for instance, when the child says she is not taking that medicine because X says it is horrible.

Yes, it was when her father left that my daughter, Maia's, two imaginary clowns appeared (at bedtime) to play with her; they stayed until she started school.

The concrete operational stage

The child is now capable of performing logical operations, but only in the presence of actual objects. S/he can conserve, and show reversibility and more logical classification.

Further examples of the child's ability to decentre include his/her appreciation that objects can belong to more than one class (as in the case of Andrew being Bob's brother *and* Charlie's best friend). There is also a significant *decline* in egocentrism (and the growing *relativism* of the child's viewpoint), plus the onset of seriation and reciprocity of relationships (such as knowing that adding one to three produces the same amount as taking one from five) (Key Study 15.1).

KEY STUDY 15.1

What are nurses like?

- Price (1988) reports the findings from a survey of 203 7- to 12-years old (corresponding to the whole of the concrete operational stage and the early part of the formal operational stage).
- Their mother might put on a uniform and become a nurse, but this does not prevent her from returning that night as mummy once more. Even though she wears a uniform and is a nurse, she is still mummy 'underneath'. This shows conservation (specifically, the idea of reversibility – see discussion in page 355).
- Children were asked to complete a written questionnaire, which included six open-ended questions on nurses and one on doctors.
- 'What nurses do' produced responses that Price classified as (1) *the expressive/feminine role* (such as giving cuddles or making a fuss of children when they feel lonely or sore; they read bedtime stories and play); (2) *nurses as clinicians* (nurses use skills such as 'give you stitches and operations', 'operate on you' and 'dus tings lck sowe your stumoc together' [*sic*] they also give injections, medicines and pills); (3) *nurses as doctors' assistants* (nurses often help the doctor, in the operating theatre, clinic and treatment room). A total of 27 children said that nurses explain what the doctor does, and 9 felt that the doctors help the nurses!
- The 'nice' things that nurses do centred on the expressive communication role, such as explaining, 'chat', tactile comfort, storytelling and being honest.
- Surprisingly, there were few 'nasty' things that nurses do. These centred on giving injections and lying about operations/procedures that 'would not hurt'.
- The most important qualities for nurses to have are patience (76), kindness (63) and bravery (57). They were also thought to be 'brainy', 'clever' and talkative.
- These qualities were to be displayed in a wide range of settings: hospital, surgery, old people's homes, 'around the district', hospices, in aeroplanes and at accidents. They expected to see nurses in their own homes, at school and in the army.
- Drawings of nurses always included a uniform, usually with red crosses on it, a fob watch, and often a belt and hat. Typical accoutrements included syringes, stethoscopes, first-aid boxes and a saw!
- Because children at this stage are reasoning from what they have actually experienced, the role of the nurse as communicator has never been more important. The findings suggest that nurses can expect a degree of trust from children, but that they should act as an 'interpreter' of nursing events. Failure to do so will traumatise the child (Price, 1988).

Source: Price, B., *Nursing Times*, 84(1), 42–43, 1988.

📄 The Price (1988) survey seems to sum up what should be our role behaviour: patience, kindness and tactile comfort, communication and honesty. (Might a survey of adult patients produce a similar result?)

📄 Price also says children reason from experience (Piaget's concrete operational stage) which is why Laura asked me to help prepare Lucy for post-operative bandaging through role-play. We played being nurse; Lucy let me bandage her head and then she bandaged mine; when I pretended I couldn't hear anything at all it made her laugh.

The formal operational stage

While the concrete operational child is still concerned with manipulating things (even if this is done mentally), the formal operational thinker can manipulate *ideas* or *propositions*, and can reason solely on the basis of verbal statements ('first order' and 'second order' operations, respectively). 'Formal' refers to the ability to follow the form of an argument without reference to its particular content. In *transitivity problems*, for example, 'If A is taller than B, and B is taller than C, then A is taller than C' is a form of argument whose conclusion is logically true, regardless of what A, B and C might refer to.

Formal operational thinkers can also think *hypothetically* – that is, they can think about what *could be* as well as what *actually is*. This ability to imagine and discuss things that have never been encountered is evidence of the continued decentration that occurs beyond concrete operations.

📄 As Jacob (in the formal operational stage) didn't speak much, I watched him play a game on his laptop for a bit, then asked how it worked; he explained it so enthusiastically! Afterwards, when I asked him about school, he admitted (casually) he was 'just wondering' if anything might go wrong with his leg because he was in the school football team; he's clearly thinking 'what could be'.

An evaluation of Piaget's theory

As we noted in the *Introduction and Overview*, Piaget's theory has had an enormous impact on our understanding of cognitive development. However, as Flavell (1982) and others (e.g. Siegal, 2003) have remarked, 'some of us now think that the theory may in varying degrees be unclear, incorrect and incomplete'.

Egocentrism

Gelman (1979) has shown that 4-year-olds adjust their explanations of things to make them clearer to a blindfold listener. This is not what we would expect if children of this age are egocentric. Nor would we expect 4-year-olds to use simpler forms of speech when talking to 2-year-olds (Gelman, 1979).

Critics of the 'Swiss mountain scene' test (Key Study 15.2) see it as an unusually difficult way of presenting a problem to a young child. Borke (1975) and Hughes (cited in Donaldson, 1978) have shown that when the task is presented in a meaningful context (making what Donaldson calls 'human sense'), even 3½-year-olds can appreciate the world as another person sees it. These are all

KEY STUDY 15.2

'Swiss mountain scene' test of egocentrism

- The three papier-mâché model mountains shown in Figure 15.4 are of different colours. One has snow on the top, one a house and one a red cross.
- The child walks round and explores the model, and then sits on one side while a doll is placed at some different location. The child is shown 10 pictures of different views of the model and asked to choose the one that represents how the doll sees it.
- Four-year-olds were completely unaware of perspectives other than their own, and always chose a picture which matched *their* views of the model. Six-year-olds showed some awareness, but often chose the wrong picture. Only 7- and 8-year-olds consistently chose the picture that represented the *doll's* view.
- According to Piaget, children below the age of 7 are bound by the *egocentric illusion*. They fail to understand that what they see is *relative to their own* positions, and instead take it to represent 'the world as it really is'.

Figure 15.4 Piaget and Inhelder's three-mountain scene, seen from four different sides. (From Smith, P.K. and Cowie, H., *Understanding Children's Development*, Oxford, Basil Blackwell, 1988.)

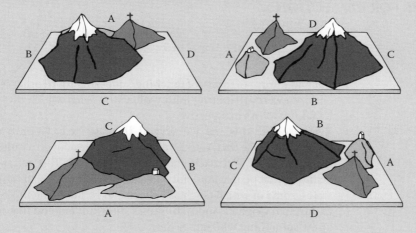

Source: Piaget, J. and Inhelder, B., *The Psychology of the Child*, London, Routledge & Kegan Paul, 1956.

examples of *perspective-taking* (PT). While young children are not egocentric all of the time, their PT skills clearly improve during childhood (Siegal, 2003) (see Box 15.1).

- Typically, 3-year-olds said that John would think it was a sponge (which it is), while 4- to 5-year-olds said he would think it was a rock (because he had

TIME FOR REFLECTION ...

- How do you think the 3-year-olds answered?
- How do you think the 4- to 5-year-olds answered?

not had the opportunity of touching/squeezing it). In other words, the older children were attributing John with a *false belief*, which they could only do by taking John's perspective.

- Evidence like this has led several theorists (e.g. Gopnik and Wellman, 1994) to propose that 4- to 5-year-olds have developed a quite sophisticated *theory of mind* (Premack and Woodruff, 1978). This refers to the understanding that people (and not objects) have desires, beliefs and other mental states, some of which (such as beliefs) can be false (*cognitive* PT). The older children in Gopnick and Astington's study understood that John would not know something which *they did*.

 Lucy cried when her mother left and Peter ran to comfort her. Perceptual perspective-taking explains how Peter could perceive (Level 1 PT) Lucy's distress, but his behaviour indicated he was able, at 2½, to empathise with her.

Conservation

The ability to conserve also seems to occur earlier than Piaget believed. Rose and Blank (1974) showed that when the *pre-transformation question* (the question asked before one row of counters, say, is rearranged) was dropped, 6-year-olds often succeeded on the number conservation task. Importantly, they made fewer errors on the standard version of the task when tested a week later. These findings were replicated by Samuel and Bryant (1984) using conservation of number, liquid quantity and substance.

According to Donaldson (1978), the standard version of the task unwittingly 'forces' children to produce the wrong answer against their better judgement, by the mere fact that the same question is asked twice – before and after the transformation. Hence, children believe they are expected to give a different answer to the second question. On this explanation, *contextual cues* may override purely linguistic ones. Children may think the experimenter has rejected their first answer, so they feel they are required to give a *different* answer to the second question to please the adult questioner.

Bruner (1966) argues that children's attention is so captured by the transformed state that they disregard the pre-transformed state and fail to attend to it when asked the second question.

Isn't this another indication of centration? (And isn't 'pleasing the questioner' an example of 'demand characteristics' in research?)

Cross-cultural tests of the stages

The few cross-cultural studies of the sensorimotor stage have shown the sub-stages to be universal. Overall, it seems that ecological or cultural factors *do not* influence the sequence of stages, but *do* affect the rate at which they are attained (Segall et al., 1999).

Conservation experiments have been conducted with Aborigines in remote parts of the central Australian desert (Dasen, 1994), as well as Eskimo, African (Senegal and Rwande), Hong Kong and Papua New Guinea samples. Consistent with Dasen's findings, children from non-Western cultures often show a considerable lag in acquiring operational thought, but this applies mainly to those having minimal contact with white culture. Where Aborigines, for example, live in white communities and attend school there, they perform at a similar level to whites. Even where there is a lag in development compared with whites, the stages still appear in the same order. So (as with the sensorimotor sub-stages), cultural factors can affect the *rate* of attainment but not the developmental *sequence* (Schaffer, 2004).

This is, of course, why we provide appropriate learning experiences for children in nurseries and schools.

Perrin and Perrin (1983, in Taylor et al., 1999) concluded that physicians and nurses make little use of the notion of developmental stages, and approach all children as if they were in middle childhood or in the Piagetian stage of concrete operations whereas, as with adults, we should treat them as individuals.

The role of social factors in cognitive development

Meadows (1995) maintains that Piaget implicitly saw children as largely independent and isolated in their construction of knowledge and understanding of the physical world (children-as-scientists). This excluded the contribution of other people to children's cognitive development. The social nature of knowledge and thought is a basic proposition of Vygotsky's theory. According to Vygotsky (1987):

> The child [in Piaget's theory] is not seen as part of the social whole, as a subject of social relationships. He is not seen as a being who participates in the societal life of the social whole to which he belongs from the outset...

Vygotsky's theory: The child-as-apprentice

Vygotsky and Piaget agree that development does not occur in a vacuum: knowledge is constructed as a result of the child's active interaction with the environment. But, as we have seen, for Piaget that environment is essentially *asocial* (so, his account is described as *constructivist*). But for Vygotsky, cognitive development is a thoroughly *social* process (hence, he is a *social constructivist*). His aim was to spell out and explain how the higher mental functions (reasoning, understanding, planning, remembering and so on) arise out of children's social experiences. He did this by considering human development in terms of three levels: the *cultural, interpersonal* and *individual*. He had much more to say about the first two, so we will concentrate on these here.

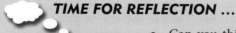 Vygotsky's theory that we understand the world (other people?) through interactive processes, justifies taking time to play with Ben at home and the children in the ward.

The cultural level

Children do not need to 'reinvent the world anew' (as Piaget seemed to believe): they cannot avoid benefiting from the accumulated wisdom of previous generations. So, each generation stands on the shoulders of the previous one, taking over the particular culture including its intellectual, material, scientific and artistic achievements – to develop it further before handing it on, in turn, to the next generation (Schaffer, 2004).

However, Piaget was exploring the **process** of cognitive development which helps explain, for example, how Lucy perceives the world differently from Peter.

TIME FOR REFLECTION ...

- Can you think of examples of cultural tools that might be especially important for children's cognitive development?

Cultural tools are what the child 'inherits'. These can be

- *Technological* (clocks, bicycles and other physical devices)
- *Psychological* (concepts and symbols, such as language, literacy, maths and scientific theories)
- *Values* (such as speed, efficiency and power)

Figure 15.5 The computer: a powerful and pervasive cultural tool.

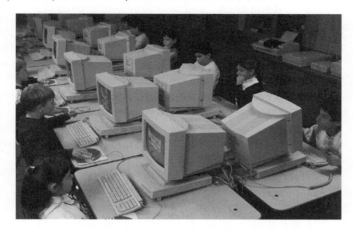

It is through such tools that children learn to conduct their lives in socially effective and acceptable ways, as well as understand how the world works. Schaffer (2004) gives the example of *computers* (Figure 15.5) as a major – and relatively recent – cultural tool:

> There are few instances in history where a new technical invention has assumed such a dominant role in virtually all spheres of human activity as the computer... in the space of just a few decades computing expertise is regarded as an essential skill for even quite young children to acquire …

 Jacob has his own laptop and there is a computer in the activities room. All the children love it – even Peter can locate his favourite programme!

The most essential cultural tool is *language*.

- It is the pre-eminent means of passing on society's accumulated knowledge.
- It enables children to regulate their own activities.
- At about age 7, speech becomes internalised to form internal thought: an essential *social* function thus becomes the major tool for *cognitive* functioning.

A reminder why we should be concerned about Ben's limited language skills (see page 353)

The interpersonal level

It is here that culture and the individual meet, and it is the level at which Vygotsky made his major contribution.

Internalisation and the social nature of thinking

The ability to think and reason by and for ourselves (inner speech or verbal thought) is the result of a fundamentally *social* process. At birth, we are social beings capable of interacting with others, but able to do little either practically or intellectually, by or for ourselves. But gradually, we move towards self-sufficiency and independence, and by participating in social activities, our abilities become transformed. For Vygotsky, cognitive development involves an active *internalisation* of problem-solving processes that takes place as a result of mutual interaction between children and those with whom they have regular social contact (initially the parents, but later friends, classmates and teachers).

I've frequently heard children 'talking themselves through' a solitary activity —articulating this problem-solving process.

This is the reverse of how Piaget (at least initially) saw things. Piaget's idea of 'the child as a scientist' is replaced by the idea of 'the *child as an apprentice*', who acquires the culture's knowledge and skills through graded collaboration with those who already possess them (Rogoff, 1990). According to Vygotsky (1981),

> any function in the child's cultural development appears twice, or on two planes. First it appears on the social plane, and then on the psychological plane.

So, cognitive development progresses from the *intermental* to the *intramental* (from joint regulation to self-regulation).

Scaffolding and the zone of proximal development

The *zone of proximal development* (ZPD) defines those functions that have not yet matured but are in the process of maturing (Vygotsky, 1978). These could be called the 'buds' or 'flowers' rather than the 'fruits' of development. The actual developmental level characterises mental development *retrospectively*, while the ZPD characterises mental development *prospectively*.

Scaffolding refers to the kind of guidance and support adults provide children in the ZPD by which children acquire their knowledge and skills (Wood et al., 1976; Wood and Wood, 1996). As a task becomes more familiar to the child and more within its competence, those who provide the scaffold leave more and more for the child to do until it can perform the task successfully. In this way, the developing thinker does not have to create cognition 'from scratch': there are others available who have already 'served' their own apprenticeship.

The internalised cognitive skills remain social in two senses. First, as mature learners we can 'scaffold' ourselves through difficult tasks (self-instruction), as others once scaffolded our earlier attempts. Second, the only skills practised to a high level of competence for most people are those offered by their culture: cognitive potential may be universal, but cognitive expertise is culturally determined (Meadows, 1995).

TIME FOR REFLECTION ...

- How does this distinction between cognitive potential and expertise relate to Dasen's (1994) assessment of Piaget's stages?

The English National Board (in Downie and Basford, 2003, pages 228 and 229) defines a mentor as 'an appropriately qualified and experienced first level nurse/midwife/health visitor who, by example and facilitation, guides, assists and supports the student in learning new skills, adopting new behaviour and acquiring new attitudes'. Which also seems an accurate definition of scaffolding!

An evaluation of Vygotsky's theory

TIME FOR REFLECTION ...

- What would you say is the key difference between Vygotsky's and Piaget's theories?

- Vygotsky's theory clearly 'compensates' for one of the central limitations of Piaget's theory. As Segall et al. (1999) put it, 'Piaget produced a theory of the development of an "epistemic subject", an idealised, non-existent individual, completely divorced from the social environment.' For Vygotsky, culture (and especially language) plays a key role in cognitive development: the development of the individual cannot be understood – and indeed cannot happen – outside the context of social interaction.
- While Vygotsky's theory has not been tested cross-culturally as Piaget's has, it has influenced cross-cultural psychology through the development of *cultural psychology* (e.g. Cole, 1990) according to which cognition is not necessarily situated 'within the head' but is *shared* among people and settings (Segall et al., 1999).
- In contrast with Piaget's theory, Vygotsky's is not truly developmental. His ideas are based on a 'prototype' child, who functions in the same way at age 2 or 12: nothing is said about changes in the processes underlying learning (such as attention, memory and intellectual capacities) and how these affect social interaction at different ages.
- He makes no reference to what *motivates* the child to achieve particular goals: 'While cognition was given a social appearance, Vygotsky's treatment of the child is as "cold" as Piaget's ...' (Schaffer, 2004).

I've so enjoyed my (unusual) feeling of self-confidence in this placement with the HV and on the children's ward as I could see how relevant the theoretical knowledge I had is to caring for children – well or sick. I also see that knowledge grows and develops because theorists disagree; we need both Piaget's constructivist and Vygotsky's **social** constructivist perspectives and critiques of both. Schaffer (2004) says we also need to consider emotion and motivation, which is a humanistic perspective.

In the future, I mustn't make assumptions about children based on their chronological age nor from a cultural point of view. Having worked with children I brought some useful (aesthetic) knowledge to this placement, but, having researched more empirical psychology I realise how much it has increased my understanding of children. An example of a 'stretched schema' I think!

CHAPTER SUMMARY

- Piaget sees *intelligence* as *adaptation to the environment,* and he was interested in how intelligence changes as children grow (*genetic epistemology*). Younger children's intelligence is *qualitatively different* from that of older children.

- *Cognitive development* occurs through the interaction between innate capacities and environmental events. It progresses through a series of *hierarchical, invariant and universal stages*: the *sensorimotor, preoperational, concrete operational* and *formal operational stages.*

- Underlying cognitive changes are *functional invariants,* the most important being *assimilation, accommodation* (which together constitute *adaptation*) and *equilibration.* The major cognitive structures that change are *schemas/schemata.*

- During the *sensorimotor stage,* frequent interaction with objects ultimately leads to *object permanence,* which is fully developed when the child can *infer invisible displacements.*

- By the end of the sensorimotor stage, schemas have become '*interiorised*'. *Representational/make-believe play,* like *deferred imitation,* reflects the *general symbolic function.*

- *Preoperational children* have difficulty in *seriation tasks* and also display *transductive reasoning* and *animism. Centration* is illustrated by the *inability to conserve.* Preoperational children are also *egocentric.*

- During the *concrete operational stage,* logical operations can be performed only in the presence of actual or observable objects.

- *Formal operational thinkers* can manipulate *ideas* and *propositions* ('second order' operations) and think *hypothetically.*

- Four- and five-year-olds are capable of perspective-taking (PT), enabling them to attribute false beliefs to other people. This is a crucial feature of the child's *theory of mind.*

- While basic cognitive processes may be *universal,* how these are brought to bear on specific contents is influenced by *culture.*

- According to Vygotsky, the initially helpless baby actively *internalises* problem-solving processes through interaction with parents. Vygotsky's *child apprentice* acquires cultural knowledge and skills through *graded collaboration* with those who already possess them (*scaffolding*).

- Vygotsky's zone of proximal development (ZPD) characterises development *prospectively.* It defines those functions that have not yet matured but are in the process of maturing.

16 Development of the self-concept

Introduction and overview

The self-concept (or simply 'self') is a *hypothetical construct*; it is a 'theory' each one of us develops about who we are and how we fit into society. It is repeatedly revised during childhood in the light of both cognitive development and social experience. On the one hand, as children get older they become more competent at self-awareness and more realistic; on the other hand, other people's perceptions and responses will come to play a more central role in shaping the nature of that awareness (Schaffer, 2004).

Although adolescence is a crucial period for its development (see Chapter 17), the formation of the self is never complete. At no time does the self function as a closed system, and it is always affected by others' evaluations of us (Schaffer, 2004). This is consistent with the view of the self as 'social to the core' (Fiske, 2004). Even when tracing how self-perception changes in the individual, this is an *inherently social process*, as reflected in the early theories of James, Cooley and Mead.

For many patients, the bodily self – or body image – is a crucial aspect of the self that undergoes revision as a result of their illness and the treatment they receive for it. This is especially true for cancer patients (including women with breast cancer who have a mastectomy, and anyone who undergoes facial surgery for their cancer), ostomy patients and those with HIV/AIDS, amputees and people who suffer severe burns or disability as a result of an accident.

 From my diary (9): Year 2/Surgical Ward

Clare is a 22-year-old with ulcerative colitis who had an ileostomy two days ago; today the stoma specialist nurse (Eulette) arrived to change her ileostomy bag for the first time. The link Staff Nurse between Eulette and our ward suggested I accompany her, partly to learn but also because I was a familiar presence to Clare who was very apprehensive. Although Clare had counselling and met other ileostomy patients and had been involved in choosing the ileostomy

site, she held my hand tightly as Eulette removed the dressing and when she saw the stoma became very distressed. Eulette reassured her that it would look much better in a few days as it was still bruised and swollen from the operation. She also reminded Clare that it was the means of 'getting her life back', which seemed to calm her a bit, but when Eulette had gone I sat with her as she'd started crying. 'I know it will make me better, but I hate it, it's disgusting; I don't feel I'm me any more,' she said.

Consciousness and self-consciousness

TIME FOR REFLECTION ...

- What do you think is the difference between consciousness and self-consciousness?

When you look in the mirror at your face, you are both the person who is looking and that which is looked at. Similarly, when you think about the kind of person you are or something you have done, you are both the person doing the thinking and what is being thought about. In other words, you are both *subject* (the thinker or looker) and *object* (what is being looked at or thought about). We use the personal pronoun 'I' to refer to ourselves as subject, and 'me' to refer to ourselves as object, and this represents a rather special relationship we have with ourselves, namely *self-consciousness/ self-awareness*.

Non-human species possess consciousness (they have sensations of cold, heat, hunger and thirst, and can feel pleasure, pain, fear, sexual arousal and so on – they are *sentient* creatures). But only humans possess self-consciousness. We often use the term 'self-conscious' to describe our response to situations where we are made to feel object-like or exposed in some way. But this is a *secondary* meaning: the *primary* meaning refers to this unique relationship in which the same person, the same self, is both subject and object.

Being ill and in hospital usually means regarding ourselves as objects to be 'treated'. This was so evident with Clare. The dramatic change in her 'bodily self' seems to have drastically affected her subjective self, her idea of who she is.

What is the self?

'*Self*' and '*self-concept*' are used interchangeably to refer to an individual's overall self-awareness. According to Murphy (1947), 'the self is the individual as known to the individual', and Burns (1980) defines it as 'the set of attitudes a person holds towards himself'.

A photo of herself and her boyfriend on Clare's locker showed her as a smiling, pretty, young woman. In spite of her illness, I'd have said she had a very positive, self-enhancing view of herself. Since her operation, this clearly isn't so.

Components of the self-concept

The self-concept is a general term that normally refers to three major components: *self-image, self-esteem* and *ideal self.*

Self-image

Self-image refers to how we describe ourselves, what we think we are like. One way of investigating self-image is to ask people the question 'Who are you?' 20 times (Kuhn and McPartland, 1954). This typically produces two main categories of answer.

> **TIME FOR REFLECTION ...**
>
> - Give 20 different answers to the question 'Who are you?'

1. *Social roles* are usually objective aspects of the self-image (e.g., daughter, son, sister and student). These are 'facts' that can be verified by others.
2. *Personality traits* are more a matter of opinion and judgement, and what we think we are like may be different from how others see us. But how others behave towards us has an important influence on our self-perception (see Gross, 2010).

As well as social roles and personality traits, people's answers often refer to their *physical characteristics* (such as tall, short, fat, thin, blue-eyed and brown-haired). These are part of our *body image/bodily self*, the 'bodily me', which also includes bodily sensations, such as pain, cold and hunger. A more permanent feature of our body image relates to what we count as part of our body (and hence belonging to us) and what we do not.

According to Blackmore (1989), the concept of body image has been well defined in nursing literature. For example, Smitherman (1981), while acknowledging that body image is only part of our total self-concept, sees it as occupying

> ... a very prominent position. Our society is very concerned with physical appearance ... the ideal body image ... has been said to represent youth, beauty, vigour, intactness and health. There is likely to be a resulting reduced self-esteem, insecurity and anxiety among those who deviate significantly from this ideal.

Clare's job is an integral part of her self-concept; she sells a well-known (expensive) brand of make-up in a large store. She's very concerned about her physical appearance, likes to wash her hair every day and is always beautifully made up.

Fawcett and Fry (1980) recognise that body image is a complex concept and that 'body perception' (direct mental experience of physical appearance) is not the whole picture. They identify 'body attitude' as 'the broad spectrum of feelings, attitudes and emotional reactions towards the body'.

Changes in body image as a result of disease and accidents

This complex concept of body image is not static. Whenever our body changes in some way, so our body image changes (altered body image [ABI]; Price, 1986). Price (1990) defines ABI as 'any significant alteration to body image occurring outside the realms of expected human development'. It can arise from either the *external* environment (e.g., major surgery, including mastectomy; burns; or medical interventions, such as intravenous (IV) lines or naso-gastric tubes) or the *internal* environment (e.g., congenital defects such as Down's syndrome; malignant tumours; psychiatric illness such as anorexia nervosa; or HIV-related diseases). In extreme cases, we would expect a correspondingly dramatic change in body image.

As a result of her operation, the image Clare had of herself as having (in spite of her illness) an 'ideal body' is destroyed and her emotional reaction to it changed from pleasure to distaste.

According to Price (1986), ABI affects patients in all the usual clinical divisions of the modern hospital, such as dermatology, accident and emergency, surgery, medicine and psychiatry. Some areas, notably oncology, will have a preponderance of ABI problems to deal with (see Box 16.1).

Price believes that *hidden* and *open* ABIs may cross many of these categories. Hidden ABIs are not necessarily any easier for the patient to deal with. For example, a woman who has undergone a total hysterectomy may not appear to have a body image problem. Other examples include epilepsy, colostomy/ileostomy and renal failure that requires haemodialysis or continuous ambulatory peritoneal dialysis. As far as the outside world is concerned, the problem is hidden (and so appears not to exist), but to the spouse the problem may be open. Equally, if a patient denies having a problem with a new body shape or form, the problem becomes hidden for them too (Price, 1986)

While Clare's public body image needn't necessarily change, her private body image has changed drastically; a previously hidden part of her body is now visible and she is only too aware of all the implications. She was so upset at first and said she was going to finish with her boyfriend and give up her job, but Eulette persuaded her to postpone any such decisions until she felt better from her operation.

Box 16.1 Categories of patients with altered body images

- *Those with congenital/hereditary conditions:* These include a range of paediatric problems, such as cleft lip and palate, spina bifida, Down's syndrome and orthopaedic deformities. Although such altered images affect and persist in adult patients, they have a more acute impact in childhood, when body image has not fully developed and is fragile. It may become increasingly negative through peer criticism and ostracism, especially if the child and its family are not helped to develop adequate coping strategies.

- *Those who have suffered a traumatic alteration of their body image:* These include those with facial scarring following a road traffic accident or children who have scalded themselves. In these cases, the change in body image is rapid and there is no time to prepare the individual psychologically (Figure 16.1). Another example is surgical amputation (see discussion in pages 377 and 378).

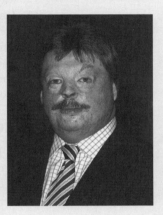

Figure 16.1 Simon Weston, survivor – and casualty – of the Falklands War in 1982.

- *Developmental ABIs:* These include psychiatric disorders such as anorexia nervosa (see Gross, 2010). This is developmental to the extent that it is a potentially progressive disorder, and because it affects individuals as they move through the complex changes of body and self-image in puberty (see Chapter 17).

- *Pathological ABIs:* These include some potentially life-threatening conditions, such as cancers, dermatological conditions and infections. They may develop very slowly, appear to go into remission, or even disappear altogether. There may be time to adapt, but the patient is never certain how the ABI will develop and this causes great insecurity.

- *Sexual body image problems:* These include actual changes in sexual appearance and function, or experience of our sexuality and its appropriateness to our self-image. The surgical amputation of the penis for cancer, or the lack of well-developed masculine characteristics in a young adult male, may both be traumatic in their own ways.

Source: Price, B., *Nursing Times*, 58–61, 1986.

In the context of testicular cancer and its treatment, Blackmore (1989) describes three kinds of loss that occur:

1. *Loss of psychological self* relates to a man's feelings about his masculinity. Many patients who have had a testicle removed (orchidectomy) describe themselves as no longer being a 'real man' or only 'half a man'. The patient may feel he is less virile and less able to perform sexually than before.

Related to these feelings about masculinity are feelings about overall self-worth/esteem (see discussion in pages 378 and 379).

2. *Loss of sociocultural self* results from the stigma attached not just to the diagnosis of cancer but to disease of the genital organs. Although fears of sexual performance and fertility may be very real or completely unfounded, either way the disease will affect intimate sexual relationships.

3. *Loss of physical self* occurs in many ways after diagnosis and treatment. First, there is the loss of a testicle and a surgical scar from an inguinal incision. If the remaining testicle is not functioning, testosterone production may be reduced, leading to reduced libido, hot flushes and a slowing of growth of facial hair. There is also likely to be a reduction in fertility. Both radiotherapy and chemotherapy will have similar effects to their use for any other form of cancer.

TIME FOR REFLECTION …

- Try to identify similarities and differences between men who have undergone an orchidectomy and women who have had a mastectomy, in terms of the three kinds of loss described by Blackmore (1989).

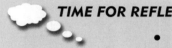 Clare's intention to finish with her boyfriend must indicate, I believe, that she is thinking about their sexual relationship.

Patients with breast cancer and mastectomy

Survival rates for breast cancer have been improving for more than 20 years and women can now reduce the risk of a genetic predisposition by opting for *prophylactic mastectomy*. The number of women with altered appearance resulting from the surgical removal of a section (*lumpectomy*) or the whole breast (*mastectomy*) will continue to rise as our population ages and as advances in cancer detection and treatment continue (Williamson and Wallace, 2012).

According to Willis (1998), dealing with a life-threatening condition is made all the more difficult by the permanent change in body image that breast removal entails. For some women, the psychological impact of losing a breast casts a shadow that remains even if the cancer is treated successfully (see Box 16.2).

Trying to help, I did say to Clare that mastectomy patients probably felt the same as her and she said, in a way that clearly indicated the self-disgust she was feeling, 'Yes, but at least theirs is clean; they don't smell!'

Breast reconstruction (BR) can offer solace to some women, but it is not a choice that is automatically extended to everyone who would benefit or is suitable. Women referred to specialist breast care units are most likely to be offered BR, where they have access to plastic surgeons or general surgeons who have sub-specialised in breast cancer surgery and reconstruction. It is often the advocacy of the patient's breast care nurse that ensures women are offered this treatment (Willis, 1998). Developments in treatments to conserve breast tissues (e.g., lumpectomy plus radiotherapy rather than mastectomy) and in BR reflect greater recognition by healthcare providers of the negative impact of breast loss (Williamson and Wallace, 2012).

Box 16.2 Mastectomy and sexual identity

- The loss of a part of the body invested with the significance of feminine identity and functioning is especially difficult (Dunn, 1988).
- Breasts have always been associated with femininity, motherhood and sexuality (Khan et al., 2000). Media pressure further promotes the unrealistic expectation that for women to feel feminine, attractive and sexy, they must not only be beautiful and thin but have large and perfect breasts. Any appearance concerns a woman has prior to diagnosis are likely to be exacerbated by breast loss and disfigurement (Williamson and Wallace, 2012). If the woman thinks her sexual partner will find the mastectomy mutilating, it can result in avoidance of sexual contact and intimacy (Dunn, 1988; Williamson and Wallace, 2012).
- Viewing the physical space caused by mastectomy and comparing their changed body to their former healthy ('intact') self can trigger feelings of emptiness and grief (Williamson and Wallace, 2012). Some fear the stigma of looking 'monstrous' and shocking. The distress caused by visual and physical asymmetry and postural imbalance has led some women to consider bilateral mastectomy (Piot-Ziegler et al., 2010).

Patients with HIV/AIDS

In a focused interview study, Firn and Norman (1995) attempted to describe how patients with AIDS and their nurses perceived the emotional and psychological issues faced by people with AIDS and the nurse's role in responding to these issues (see Chapter 3).

Changes in body image were identified by patients as a source of great emotional distress. An instrument designed to identify people at risk of developing a seriously ABI (Price, 1990) identifies three major components:

1. *Body reality* refers to our body as it really is and to the areas of the body that are altered in appearance, with changes in the face, hands and sexual organs potentially causing the greatest distress. These seem to be the areas most affected in HIV disease. For example, *Kaposi's sarcoma* is a type of skin cancer that commonly affects the face and is the most common primary tumour found in HIV disease. Although make-up can disguise many of the lesions and scars, the psychological implications have a massive impact on the patient's mental health (Jamieson, 1996). Some of Firn and Norman's participants described the very visible effects of weight loss and the distressing effects of repeated infections in the genital area, such as herpes and thrush.

2. *Body presentation* is how we present our body to the world (including how we dress, pose and move). Firn and Norman's participants repeatedly mentioned incontinence as being a particularly distressing loss of bodily control.

3. *Body ideal* refers to our perceptions of how we expect our body to appear and function. As some people with AIDS are relatively young, it is reasonable to assume that they have high expectations from life and so are less prepared for debilitating illness than people with other potentially life-threatening conditions.

Firn and Norman found that nurses tended to underestimate the extent of the distress experienced by AIDS patients as a result of their ABIs. This is reflected in the AIDS literature (Firn and Norman, 1995).

Highly active antiretroviral therapy (HAART) refers to treatments which suppress viral replication in HIV-positive patients. Although not curative, the evident and lasting benefits of HAART are such that this condition has been reinterpreted as chronic rather than terminal. However, the treatment itself produces distinctive appearance changes, most commonly

1. *Lipodystrophy* (changes in fat distribution across the body), including *lipoatrophy* (peripheral fat loss) in the legs, face and buttocks, or *lipoaccumulation* (fat gain) in the abdomen and breasts, and the characteristic 'buffalo hump' at the back of the neck
2. *Facial lipoatrophy* (fat loss, causing protruding facial bones and visible musculature)
3. Jaundice, scleral icterus (yellowing of the whites of the eye) and hair loss

The psychosocial impact of these appearance-related side-effects can be far-reaching (Williamson and Wallace, 2012).

Patients with a stoma

Stomas are surgically constructed openings made in the wall of the abdomen to eliminate faeces or urine, when obstruction or disease make it necessary to remove part of the normal elimination route (Pullen, 1998). An estimated 100,000 people in the United Kingdom have bowel or urinary stomas, with ileostomies, colostomies and urostomies being the most common.

Stomas inevitably change a patient's lifestyle. They must come to terms with altered physical control over their elimination processes, as well as the practicalities of wearing a bag and dealing with problems such as leakage or odour. They often feel frustrated, helpless, embarrassed or disgusted, but the loss of a positive body image can be the most significant difficulty (Pullen, 1998).

Clare is a fastidious young woman who carefully controlled the image she presented to the world; this was something she can't control and it did so obviously distress her.

The fact that the stoma excretes urine or faeces at will, rendering the patient incontinent, can have a devastating effect on self-esteem. A bodily function that is usually tucked away out of sight and can be dealt with discreetly is suddenly the focus of attention (Taylor, 1994). Also, a lack of control over elimination can be perceived as returning (regressing) to childhood (Topping, 1990).

Pullen (1998) notes that body image and sexuality are interrelated and both are important factors in the recovery of an ostomy patient. According to Topping (1990), research has consistently found that GPs, surgeons and nurses are unwilling or unable to help them with sexual difficulties (see Box 16.3).

Box 16.3 Sexual difficulties faced by stoma patients

- Some male patients become impotent but there can be a return of erectile function over time and the less a man focuses on having hard erections, the less anxiety will impair what function remains. Treatment options include intercavernosal self-injection of papaverine, penile prostheses and vacuum devices. Careful counselling of both the patient and his partner is essential.
- Dry orgasm (ejaculation) occurs because of damage to the parasympathetic nerves in the presacral area, or surgical trauma to the prostate, seminal vesicles or the bladder neck. So, some men do not actually ejaculate, while others ejaculate backwards into the bladder.
- Dyspareunia (painful intercourse) can result from anatomical changes such as shortening of the vaginal vault, damage to the posterior vaginal wall, or from changes in the volume of vaginal secretions.

Source: Topping, A., *Nursing Standard*, 4(41), 24–26, 1990.

These studies sum up the things Clare had been expressing and also adds an interesting point about threatening her 'grown-up' status. Eulette had told me that prior to the operation they had discussed the 'incontinence' issue but Clare had avoided her effort to discuss her relationship with her boyfriend and I confessed to Eulette I don't find it easy to discuss sexual relationships. Eulette said immediately that we should take opportunities to convince Clare she could have a healthy sexual relationship; we could suggest alternative positions to avoid the bag and provide access to attractive coverings to keep the bag in place. It was so helpful to have practical and positive advice and afterwards I felt much more confident I could encourage Clare to discuss it.

Human beings are sexual beings, so sexuality should be an important aspect of nursing care (Taylor, 1994). However, sex still remains a subject that is avoided when patients are interviewed. Taylor quotes (1982), who claims that, 'Nurses who are comfortable with their own sexuality and the sexuality of others, who have a sexual health knowledge base and who cultivate sensitive and perceptive communication skills, can effectively integrate sex into the nursing process'.

I regret that I too have avoided discussing the subject with patients. But I also realise my reluctance sprang predominantly (and typically) from worrying I had an inadequate 'knowledge base' to instigate discussion. So, learning from Eulette's pragmatic attitude and her expertise was invaluable; I'm confident I'll be able to talk to Clare positively about it now.

Patients with a facial disfigurement

According to Kelly (1990), particular attention has been paid to the effects of breast and bowel cancer and the resultant devastation on the body. But rather less attention (or certainly less publicity) has been given to the effects of a totally *visible* ABI. Surely it is reasonable to assume that a visible change (such as involved in maxillofacial surgery or facial disfigurement caused by

Box 16.4 Psychological impact of visible difference

- According to the charity Changing Faces, there are over 2,300,000 people in the United Kingdom with a significant disfigurement of the face, caused by accidents, surgery (such as for cancer), strokes (such as facial paralysis), skin conditions (such as psoriasis or acne) or some congenital or birth conditions (such as birthmarks, cleft lips/palates).
- The term 'disfigurement' is widely understood by the general public and is enshrined in the 1995 Disability and Discrimination Act. Changing Faces uses the word primarily as a noun ('a person *has* a disfigurement', not '*is* disfigured') but some people prefer to talk about 'visible differences' or 'unusual appearance'. Changing Faces also encourages spelling out the cause of the disfigurement.
- There is remarkable consensus concerning the 'headline' difficulties reported by people with a visible difference, namely (1) the experience of negative emotions (e.g., self-consciousness, anxiety and depression); (2) detrimental effects on self-evaluations (negative self-perceptions and self-esteem: see discussion in pages 378 and 379); (3) difficult encounters with others (e.g., intrusive questioning and staring); and (4) behavioural consequences (e.g., social avoidance).

Source: Harcourt, D. and Rumsey, N., *The Psychologist*, 21(6), 486–489, 2008.

accidents) would cause even more anxiety than one that can be hidden, at least for some of the time, from a partner, and, if one chooses, nearly always from the casual observer (see Box 16.4).

At least Clare is able to keep her 'altered body' mostly hidden; if she had a visible disfigurement, I think the task of adjusting would be even harder for her.

Surprisingly, oral cancer has not been a major focus for psychological research despite the great personal and social significance of the oral cavity and the high mortality rate with more advanced tumours (McEleney, 1992). Surgery for facial cancer results in a permanent, visible alteration of the face that is difficult to disguise (David and Barrit, 1982) – only after surgery do patients seem to realise that part of their face is missing (Dropkin, 1981). If the face is regarded as the outward expression of our inner selves, what happens to the person whose expression is permanently dictated by external factors, regardless of how s/he might be feeling (Griffiths, 1989)?

Because of its unexpected occurrence, a facial malformation at an advanced age causes a violent mental shock (David and Barrit, 1977). Facially disfigured people have more difficulties accepting and adjusting to a new self-image than those who have been deformed since birth (Wellisch et al., 1983). A case in point is Adam Pearson, who was born with the genetic condition Type 1 neurofibromatosis (see Figure 16.2); this involves the growth of excess tissue on nerve endings, causing growths (fibromas) to grow all over the body. In his case, most of the growths are in his face and head. As he says, 'I have always had it and didn't have to make lifestyle adjustments suddenly' (in Partridge and Pearson, 2008).

Figure 16.2 Neurofibromatosis is the condition suffered by the 'Elephant Man', Joseph Merrick. (From NYPL/ Science Source/Science Photo Library.)

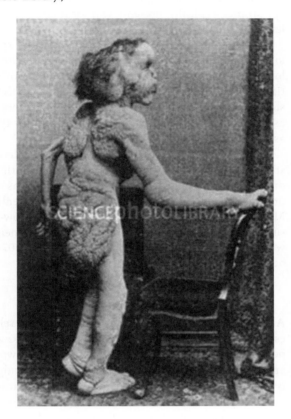

Nurses are in a unique position to support a patient's decision whether to go ahead with radical surgery, which is often the treatment of choice for head and neck cancer (Koster and Bergsma, 1990). They can help the patient to understand the planned surgery, giving further information and discussing the care involved. However, nurses must maintain a positive and supportive attitude if the patients and their family are to be reassured about the surgery being the right course, however radical it may be (McEleney, 1992).

Tschudin (2003) reminds us that informed consent can mean saying no as well as yes. But she also says that full explanations of the details of what, why and how something is being done have to be offered, not given only if patients ask for them, which encourages a proactive approach to a difficult subject. So, maybe I should bring up the question of sexual relationships with Clare?

Amputation

Often as a last resort, after other medical and surgical interventions have failed, conditions such as cancer, vascular disease and meningitis can result in the amputation of one or more limbs. Relief from pain and illness can lead some to view amputation in a positive way, especially those who regard the procedure as life-saving; however, such a rapid and highly visible change in appearance typically presents extraordinary psychological and social challenges (Williamson and Wallace, 2012).

Immediately after amputation, patients can experience feelings of shock, loss and mutilation (they have become an 'amputee') and many try to avoid looking at their stump. Initial meeting with family and friends can be particularly difficult, and patients have to manage reactions of alarm or distress, staring and curiosity (Sjodahl et al., 2004). Patients often describe themselves as being hypervigilant to these reactions, but this typically subsides over time as they adjust to their ABI.

Horgan and MacLachlan (2004) report considerable evidence of the social stigma associated with lower limb amputation; this reflects both the visible difference and the associated physical disability as many rely on a wheelchair or walking aids, either temporarily or permanently. However, Horgan and MacLachlan also report how individuals with low-limb amputation develop successful strategies for managing other people's negative reactions (as do men with upper limb amputation: Saradjian et al., 2007). These strategies include both humour and wearing a prosthesis.

Self-esteem

Although the self-image is essentially *descriptive*, self-esteem (or *self-regard*) is essentially *evaluative*. It refers to how much we like and approve of the kind of person we think we are (our self-image) and how worthy a person we think we are. Coopersmith (1967) defined it as 'a personal judgement of worthiness, that is expressed in the attitudes the individual holds towards himself'.

Clearly, certain characteristics or abilities have a greater value in society generally, and so are likely to influence our self-esteem accordingly – for example, being physically attractive as opposed to unattractive. The value attached to particular characteristics will also depend on culture, gender, age and social background (see Gross, 2010).

Part of Clare's recovery may depend on her ability to derive self-esteem from qualities she has apart from her physical appearance. She has a friendly, open and bubbly personality, and takes pleasure from making others feel good about themselves.

The ideal self

Self-esteem is also partly determined by how much the self-image differs from the *ideal self* (*ego-ideal* or *idealised self-image*) – the kind of person we would *like to be*. This can vary in extent and degree. We may want to be different in certain aspects, or we may want to be a totally different person. (We may even wish we were someone else!) Generally, the greater the gap between our self-image and our ideal self, the lower our self-esteem (see Rogers' *self theory*, Chapter 2).

Most people have a complex self-concept with a relatively large number of *self-schemata* (complex and clear information relating to various aspects of ourselves). These include an array of *possible* selves, *future-orientated* schemata of what we would like to become (ideal self) (Markus and Nurius, 1986). Visions of future possible selves may influence how we make important life decisions, such as career choice.

Before her surgery Clare's self-image and her ideal self were much closer together; now her altered self-image falls short of her ideal self and threatens at least one future schema – to have a lasting sexual relationship.

Developmental changes in the self-concept

How do we get to know ourselves?

Achieving identity (in the sense of acquiring a set of *self-schemas*) is one of the central developmental tasks of a social being (Lewis, 1990). It progresses through several levels of complexity and continues to develop through the lifespan (see Chapters 17 through 19).

During the first few months, the baby gradually distinguishes itself from its environment and from other people, and develops a sense of *continuity through time* (the *existential self*). But at this stage, the infant's self-knowledge is comparable to that of other species (such as monkeys). What makes human self-knowledge distinctive is becoming aware that we have it – we are conscious of our existence and uniqueness (Buss, 1992).

According to Maccoby (1980), babies are able to distinguish between themselves and others on two counts:

1. Their own fingers hurt when bitten (but they do not have any such sensations when they are biting their rattle or their mother's fingers)
2. Probably quite early in life, they begin to associate feelings from their own body movements with the sight of their own limbs and the sounds of their own cries. These sense impressions are bound together into a cluster that defines the *bodily self*, so this is probably the first aspect of the self-concept to develop (see Figure 16.3).

Other aspects of the self-concept develop by degrees, but there seem to be fairly clearly defined stages of development. Young children may know their own names and understand the limits of their own bodies and yet be unable to think about themselves as coherent entities. So, self-awareness/self-consciousness develops very gradually.

According to Piaget, an awareness of self comes through the gradual process of *adaptation to the environment* (see Chapter 15). As the child explores objects and accommodates to them (thus developing new *sensorimotor schemas*), it simultaneously discovers aspects of its self. For example, trying to put a large block into its mouth and finding that it would not fit is a lesson in selfhood, as well as a lesson about the world of objects.

Figure 16.3 A baby acquiring its bodily self.

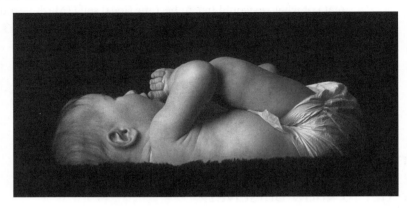

Self-recognition

One way in which the development of bodily self has been studied is through *self-recognition*. Although other kinds of self-recognition are possible (e.g., one's voice or feelings), only *visual* self-recognition has been studied extensively, both in humans and non-humans.

A number of researchers (e.g., Lewis and Brooks-Gunn, 1979) have used modified forms of a technique (first used by Gallup (1970) with chimpanzees) with 6–24-month-old children. The mother applies a dot of rouge (blusher) to the child's nose (while pretending to wipe its face) and the child is observed to see how often it touches its nose. It is then placed in front of a mirror and again the number of times it touches its nose is recorded. At about 18 months, there is a significant change. While touching the dot was never seen before 15 months, between 15 and 18 months, 5%–25% of infants touched it and 75% of the 18–20-month-olds did.

To use the mirror image to touch the dot on its nose, the baby must also have built up a schema of how its face should look in the mirror before (otherwise, it would not notice the discrepancy created by the dot). This does not develop before about 18 months – about the time when, according to Piaget, *object permanence* is completed; so object permanence seems necessary condition for the development of self-recognition (see Chapter 15).

Ben recognised himself in the TV 'mirror' at 22 months (Ch 15 P x). I've also seen photos of Clare as a child; in all of them she has pretty clothes and looks attractive, so she has grown up with that image of herself.

Self-definition

Several researchers, including Piaget, have pointed to the importance of language in consolidating the early development of self-awareness, by providing labels that permit distinctions between self and not-self ('I', 'you', 'me', 'it'). The toddler can then use these labels to communicate notions of selfhood to others. One important kind of label is the child's *name*. Names are not usually chosen randomly and are not neutral labels in terms of how people respond to them and what they associate with them. Indeed, they can be used as the basis for *stereotyping* (see Chapter 7).

The psychological self

Maccoby (1980) asks what children mean when they refer to themselves as 'I' or 'me'. Are they referring to anything more than a physical entity enclosed by an envelope of skin? (See Key Study 16.1.)

These answers suggest that by 3½ to 4 years, a child has a rudimentary concept of a private, thinking self that is not visible even to someone looking directly into its eyes. The child can distinguish this from the bodily self, which it knows is visible to others. In other words, by about age 4, children begin to develop a *theory of mind*, the awareness that they – and other people – have mental processes (e.g., Leekam, 1993; Shatz, 1994; Wellman, 1990).

Categorical self

Age and *gender* are both parts of the central core of the self-image. They represent two of the categories regarding the self that are also used to perceive and interpret the behaviour of others.

KEY STUDY 16.1

There is more to children than meets the eye

- Flavell et al. (1978) investigated development of the psychological self in 2½- to 5-year-olds.
- In one study, a doll was placed on the table in front of the child, and it was explained that dolls are like people in some ways – they have arms, legs, hands and so on (which were pointed to). Then the child was asked how dolls are different from people, whether they know their names and think about things and so on. Most children said a doll does not know its name and cannot think about things, but people can.
- They were then asked, 'Where is the part of you that knows your name and thinks about things?' and 'Where do you do your thinking and knowing?' A total of 14 out of 22 children gave fairly clear localisation for the thinking self, namely 'in their heads', while others found it very difficult. The experimenter then looked directly into the child's eyes and asked, 'Can I see you thinking in there?' Most children thought not.

Source: Flavell, J.H. et al., *What Young Children Think You See When Their Eyes Are Closed*, Unpublished report, Stanford University, 1978.

Age is probably the first social category to be acquired by the child (and is so even before a concept of number develops). Lewis and Brooks-Gunn (1979) found that 6- to 12-month-olds can distinguish between photographs, slides and papier-mâché heads of adults and babies. By 12 months, they prefer interacting with unfamiliar babies to unfamiliar adults. Also, as soon as they have acquired labels like 'mummy', 'daddy' and 'baby', they almost never make age-related mistakes.

Before age 7, children tend to define the self in *physical* terms: hair colour, height, favourite activities and possessions. During middle childhood through to adolescence, self-descriptions now include many more references to internal, psychological characteristics, such as competencies, knowledge, emotions, values and personality traits (Damon and Hart, 1988).

School highlights others' expectations about how the self should develop. It also provides a social context in which new goals are set and comparisons with others (peers) are prompted. This makes evaluation of the self all the more important (Durkin, 1995). This comparison becomes more important still during adolescence (see Chapter 17).

Reflecting on caring for Clare, I found Carper's types of knowledge (see case study 3, page 304) relevant. The psychology of the self-concept enlightened my theoretical (empirical) understanding of Clare's feelings about her 'altered body image from an external source' (Price, 1990, above) while Blackmore's (1989) three dimensions of loss – physical, psychological and socio-cultural-help me understand the many changes Clare has to adapt to. However, Chris Bulman (in Bulman and Schutz 2008, page 9) suggests 'nurses are interested in reflection because it provides a vehicle through which they can communicate and justify the importance of practice and practice knowledge,' (Carper's aesthetic knowledge) so the 'resource' of the specialist stoma nurse was invaluable. She provided Clare (and me) with practical suggestions, which added to my ability to communicate with Clare (personal knowledge). Eulette arranged visits from successfully adjusted ileostomy patients of Clare's age and shared her expertise with all the ward staff; her sensitive and comprehensive methods to help Clare's physical and psychological recovery showed me how such care should be managed (ethical knowledge).

If Clare is to adapt successfully to her new condition, her attitude to her self-concept has to change as, until now, an 'idealised' body image seems to have been the main source of her self-esteem. Hopefully, with support from her family and her boyfriend, she will soon regain a positive, if altered, self-concept.

CHAPTER SUMMARY

- An important distinction is that between *consciousness* and *self-consciousness/awareness*. Self-awareness allows us to see ourselves as others see us.
- Our *self-concept* refers to our perception of our personality, and comprises the *self-image* (which includes *body image/bodily self*), *self-esteem* (or *self-regard*) and *ideal self* (or *ego-ideal/idealised self-image*).
- Whenever our body changes in some way, our body image changes *altered body image* (ABI). ABI affects patients across all the main clinical hospital departments, but some areas, notably oncology, will face the most problems.

- Major categories of patients with ABIs are those with *congenital/heredity conditions* or who have suffered a *traumatic* ABI, *developmental* ABIs, *pathological* ABIs and *sexual body image problems*.
- Women undergoing mastectomy have to come to terms with the loss of a part of themselves traditionally associated with femininity, motherhood and sexuality.
- An instrument designed to identify people at risk of developing a seriously ABI distinguishes between *body reality*, *body presentation* and body ideal.
- *Highly-active antiretroviral therapy* (HAART) produces distinctive appearance changes, most commonly *lipodystrophy* (including *facial lipoatrophy* and *lipoaccumualtion*).
- Stoma patients' incontinence can have devastating effects on self-esteem. They also face sexual difficulties, including impotence in males, dry orgasm and dyspareunia.
- The effects of facial disfigurement and other totally visible ABIs have been relatively neglected compared with those of breast and bowel cancer.
- People who become facially disfigured through oral cancer or radical surgery for head and neck cancer have more difficulties accepting and adjusting to a new self-image than those who have been deformed since birth and who have regarded this from the beginning as part of themselves.
- Considerable social stigma is associated with lower limb amputation, reflecting both the visible difference and the associated physical disability.
- The self-concept develops in fairly regular, predictable ways. During the first few months, the *existential self* emerges, but the *bodily self* is probably the first aspect of the self-concept to develop.
- The bodily self has been studied through (mainly visual) *self-recognition* in mirrors. Self-recognition appears at about 18 months in children, and is also found in chimps.
- *Self-definition* is related to the use of language, including the use of labels, such as names. By 3½ to 4 years, children seem to have a basic understanding of a psychological self (or '*theory of mind*').
- *Age* and *gender* are two basic features of the *categorical self*. The categorical self changes from being described in *physical* to more *psychological* terms during middle childhood through to adolescence.

17 Adolescence

Introduction and overview

The word 'adolescence' comes from the Latin *adolescere* meaning 'to grow into maturity'. As well as being a time of enormous physiological change, adolescence is marked by changes in behaviour, expectations and relationships with both parents and peers. In Western, industrialised societies, there is generally no single initiation rite signalling the passage into adulthood. This makes the transition more difficult than it appears to be in more traditional, non-industrialised societies. Relationships with adults in general and parents in particular must be renegotiated in a way that allows the adolescent to achieve greater independence. This process is aided by changing relationships with peers.

Historically, adolescence has been seen as a period of transition between childhood and adulthood. But writers today are more likely to describe it as one of *multiple transitions*, involving education, training, employment and unemployment, as well as transitions from one set of living circumstances to another (Coleman and Roker, 1998).

This change in perspective in many ways reflects changes in the adolescent experience compared with those of previous generations: it starts 5 years earlier; marriage takes place 6–7 years later than it did; and cohabitation, perhaps as a prelude to marriage, is rapidly increasing (Coleman and Hendry, 1990).

Coupled with these 'adulthood-postponing' changes, in recent years adolescents have enjoyed greater self-determination at steadily younger ages. Yet this greater freedom carries with it more risks and greater costs when errors of judgement are made. As Hendry (1999) says,

> … 'dropping out' of school, being out of work, teenage pregnancy, sexually transmitted diseases, being homeless, drug addiction and suicide, are powerful examples of the price that some young people pay for their extended freedom …

From my diary (8): Year 2/Surgical Ward

This morning I helped look after Josh, a tall, well-built 16-year-old who was admitted last night from A&E after being found drunk in a doorway. He had a left temporal contusion and his neurological observations showed a Glasgow Coma Score (GCS) of 13 (he responded to speech and was a bit confused), but he had been drunk when admitted. I went with him for his computed tomogram (CT) scan to exclude neural trauma. In X-ray, the radiographer (Winston) explained what was going to happen, telling Josh he'd be in the scanner a very short time. However, after the initial lateral picture, Winston suggested that, while he set up for the main picture, I should keep Josh company as he seemed apprehensive; he said some people found the scanner claustrophobic. I was a bit surprised as I regarded Josh as a young man and I suppose I expected 'manly' behaviour! Anyway, I chatted to him, trying to reassure him, and it seemed to work, so I was dismayed when we returned to the ward and Josh saw his mother (Anna), who'd just arrived, and burst into tears. I quickly pulled the curtains round the bed and left them to talk. When I told Caroline (the ward manager), she said she'd ask Anna to let me sit in later when they discussed Josh.

Normative and non-normative shifts

 **TIME FOR REFLECTION …**

- What kinds of transition do adolescents in Western societies experience?
- Are they necessarily the same for all adolescents?

One way of categorising the various transitions involved in adolescence is in terms of *normative* and *non-normative* shifts (Hendry and Kloep, 1999; Kloep and Hendry, 1999).

- *Normative, maturational shifts* include the growth spurt (both sexes), menarche (first menstruation), first nocturnal emissions ('wet dreams'), voice breaking (boys), changes in sexual organs, beginning of sexual arousal, changed romantic relationships, gender-role identity, changed relationships with adults and increasing autonomy and responsibility.
- *Normative, society-dependent shifts* include the change from primary to secondary school, leaving school, getting started in an occupation, acquiring legal rights for voting, sex, purchasing alcohol, driving licence, military service and cohabitation.
- *Non-normative shifts* include parental divorce, family bereavement, illness, natural disasters, war, incest, emigration, risk-taking behaviours, 'disadvantage' (because of gender, class, regional or ethnic discrimination) and physical and/or mental handicap.

A normative shift may become non-normative if, say, there are other circumstances that cause a normal developmental 'task' to become more difficult. An example would be the unusually early or late onset of puberty.

Anna told us that Josh is a bright boy; he doesn't know what he wants to do yet but intends to go into the sixth form and to university; these would be normative shifts for Josh. She also said his father had died (in an accident at work) two years ago, so this was a tragic, non-normative shift for Josh.

Puberty: Social and psychological meaning of biological changes

Puberty and body image

Adjusting to puberty is one of the most important adjustments that adolescents have to make (Coleman and Hendry, 1990). Even as a purely biological phenomenon, puberty is far from being a simple, straightforward process. Although all adolescents experience the same bodily changes (see Box 17.1 and Figure 17.1), the sequence of changes may vary within individuals (*intra-individual asynchronies*: Alsaker, 1996). For example, for some girls menstruation may occur very early on in puberty, whereas for others it may occur after most other changes have taken place.

Major changes in puberty

Physiologically, puberty begins when the seminal vesicles and prostate gland enlarge in the male and the ovaries enlarge in the female. Both males and

---

Box 17.1 Adolescents' brains

- According to some neuroscientists, the brain undergoes some fundamental restructuring during adolescence, just as it does during the earliest years of childhood. While the 'plasticity' of the infant's and young child's brain is widely accepted (see Gross, 2010, 2012a), this has traditionally been seen as stopping at puberty. However, recent research suggests otherwise.
- Areas of the cortex that deal with more basic functions, such as sensory and motor processing, do indeed stabilise in early childhood. But the parietal and frontal lobes, which are specialised for visuospatial and *executive functions* (e.g., planning and self-control), respectively, show a growth surge between the ages of 10 and 12.
- This sudden 'bulking up' is then followed by an equally dramatic *reduction* in size (cerebral 'pruning'), which continues right through the teenage years and into the early 20s. This reduction in the number of synaptic connections between neurons is a measure of the brain's maturity and occurs earlier in certain brain regions than others.
- Among the last to mature is the *dorsolateral prefrontal cortex* (DPFC) (at the very front of the frontal lobe); this is involved in impulse control, judgement and decision-making. The DPFC also controls and processes emotional information sent from the amygdala (Gogtay et al., 2009).
- This lack of impulse control may produce risk-taking behaviours, such as drug and alcohol abuse, smoking and unprotected sex. According to Gosline (2009), imaging studies suggest that the motivation and reward circuitry in teenage brains makes them almost hard-wired for addiction (see Chapter 12).
- These research findings suggest that the neural basis of *theory of mind* continues to develop well past early childhood (Blakemore, 2007) (see Chapter 15).

Figure 17.1 Development of secondary sex characteristics: the curved lines represent the average increase in height from 8 to 18 years of age. The characteristics shown may occur earlier or later in a person's development, but they usually occur in the order shown. (From Tanner, J.M., Foetus into Man; Physical Growth from Conception to Maturity, Cambridge, MA, Harvard University Press, 1978; Tanner, J.M. and Whitehouse, R.H., Archives of Disease in Childhood, 51, 170–179, 1976. Reproduced with permission of the copyright holders, Castlemead Publications.)

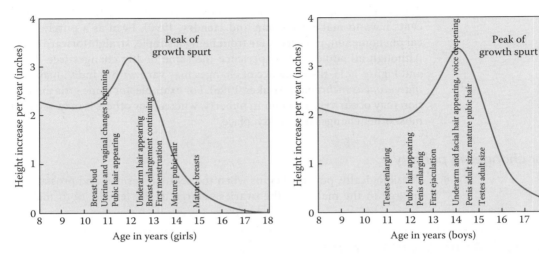

females experience the adolescent growth spurt. Male secondary sex characteristics include growth of pubic and then chest and facial hair, and sperm production. In females, breast size increases, pubic hair grows and menstruation begins (see Critical Discussion 17.1).

Anna said Josh is 6'2" and that he 'shot up' between the ages of 12 and 14 (which is average). The difficulty in adjusting spatially to his new body could explain her grumble that Josh is clumsy, and 'always breaking things'.

These physiological changes (I had no idea of them until now) help explain Josh's behaviour. Anna said that over the last year, he'd come home very late at night and when he was at home was anti-social and uncooperative. Recently he'd become subject to unpredictable mood swings and she was terrified he's taking drugs.

According to Davies and Furnham (1986), the average adolescent is not only sensitive to but also critical of his or her changing physical self. Because of gender and sexual development, young people are inevitably confronted, perhaps for the first time, by cultural standards of beauty in evaluating their own body images (via the media and the reactions of others). This may produce a non-normative shift in the form of dieting practices, leading to eating disorders (see the study by Gross [2010]). Young people may be especially vulnerable to teasing and exclusion if they are perceived by their peers as over- or underweight (Kloep and Hendry, 1999) (see Figure 17.2).

CRITICAL DISCUSSION 17.1

Adolescents in hospital: Do they have special needs?

- Young people who need hospital care may find themselves admitted to either adult or children's wards. According to Gillies (1992), this is despite recommendations by the Platt Report (1959), the British Paediatric Association (1985) and the WHO (1986) to provide specialised wards designed to meet the needs of teenagers.

- Part of the nurse's role is to help patients settle into the often unfamiliar and potentially threatening environment of a hospital ward. However, there is no special training in caring for adolescents, so health professionals tend to be less aware of their needs and their rights as individuals (Gillies, 1992).

- Acute or chronic illness, hospitalisation and terminal admission all affect adolescent developmental issues (Kuykendall, 1989). Kuykendall gives the example of a 14-year-old girl with spina bifida and hydrocephalus who had had her shunt revised throughout her life without any complications. Everyone assumed that this very sophisticated patient would be able to handle the latest lengthening of the catheter perfectly well, because she had had it done so many times before. But in hospital she became hysterical, and at home she became reclusive.

- Adolescents are highly sensitive about their appearance, and any deformity or imperfection can cause feelings of shame and disgust (Tait et al., 1982). Those with cancer may be particularly vulnerable to the effects of a disrupted body image. In addition, nurses may be reluctant to discuss sexual matters with the adolescent patient and may contribute to adolescents with cancer being ignored as sexual beings (Burt, 1995) (see also Chapter 16).

- Adolescents' formal operational intelligence (see Chapter 15) can induce anxiety and depression. For example, they can imagine what might happen in their lives as a result of hospitalisation, such as missing school and having to make up the missed work (Denholm, 1987); this can induce significant anxiety. It can be acutely distressing if hospitalisation disrupts exams (Muller et al., 1988) (see Chapter 3).

Figure 17.2 The need to not be different.

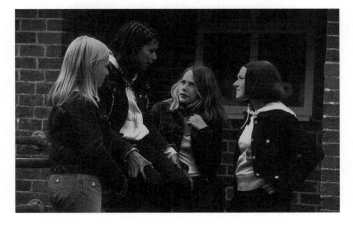

Gender differences

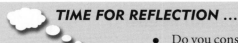
Although puberty may be a normative, maturational shift, it may be a more difficult transition for girls than boys. This is because of the *subjective meaning* of bodily change (what it means for the individual), which mirrors the *socio-cultural significance* of puberty (its significance for society). According to the *cultural ideal hypothesis* (CIH) (Simmons and Blyth, 1987), puberty will bring boys closer to their physical ideal (an increase in muscle distribution and lung capacity produces greater stamina, strength and athletic capacities), whereas girls move further away from theirs.

For girls, who begin puberty on average 2 years ahead of boys, it is normal to experience an increase in body fat and rapid weight gain, thus making their bodies less like the Western cultural ideal of the thin, sylph-like supermodel. In addition, they have to deal with menstruation, which is negatively associated with blood and physical discomfort (Crawford and Unger, 1995) (see Figure 17.3).

Figure 17.3 Pre-teens are growing up faster than ever before, and early-maturing girls are most at risk of mental disorder and delinquency.

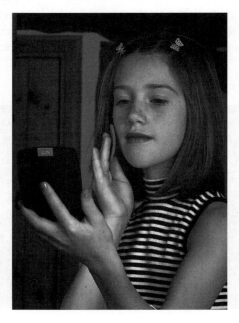

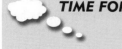 I'd noticed Josh has quite bad acne and asked Anna how it affected him. She said he was very self-conscious about it and has tried 'every acne skin preparation advertised'. It seems boys have 'cultural beauty sensitivity' too.

Importance of timing

If the CIH is valid, it follows that *early-maturing boys* will be at an *advantage* relative to their 'on-time' and late-maturing peers (they will be moving faster towards the male ideal). By the same token, *early-maturing girls* will be at a *disadvantage* (they will be moving faster away from the female ideal).

Indeed, according to Alsaker (1996), '… pubertal timing is generally regarded as a more crucial aspect of pubertal development than pubertal maturation itself'. In other words, it is not the fact of puberty that matters as much as *when* it occurs, and it matters mainly in relation to body image and self-esteem.

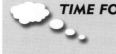 Although Josh's puberty timing was 'normal' it brought with it clumsiness and acne, which wasn't good for Josh's self-esteem.

TIME FOR REFLECTION …

- A common finding is that early-maturing girls and late-maturing boys suffer lower self-esteem. Why do you think this might be?

- One popular explanation is the *deviancy hypothesis* (DH), according to which those who are 'off-time' in physical maturation are socially deviant compared with peers of the same age and gender (Wichstrom, 1998). Since girls begin puberty on average 2 years before boys, early-maturing girls are the first to enter this deviant position, followed by late-maturing boys.
- An alternative explanation is the *developmental readiness hypothesis* (DRH) (Simmons and Blyth, 1987). In the case of early or sudden puberty, too little time will have been spent on ego development during latency, with early-maturing girls once more being the most affected. (This explanation is consistent with Coleman's focal theory; see pages 399 and 400.)
- As far as CIH is concerned, the suggestion that the pubertal girl moves further away from the Western stereotyped female ideal may not be true. Both boys and girls move closer to their ideals, provided they do not put on excessive weight (Wichstrom, 1998).

Adolescents in hospital

TIME FOR REFLECTION …

- What are some of the major problems that adolescent patients are likely to experience compared with children on the one hand and adults on the other? (You may find it useful to look at Piaget's theory [Chapter 15] and research into altered body image [Chapter 16].)

Similarly, adolescents understand that an amputation has implications for the future, often inducing depression. In contrast, a young child who has a leg amputated goes home and still talks about becoming a firefighter when he or she grows up (Kuykendall, 1989).

- Although they may find it difficult to discuss, adolescents who are seriously ill will be thinking about death (MacKenzie, 1988). They may display a great deal of anger at the prospect of dying before achieving their ambitions, which may prove a barrier to communication (Brook, 1986) (see Chapter 13).
- Wards often provide little privacy, which, together with physical examinations, treatments and maintaining hygiene, can embarrass young people, who are already acutely aware of their bodies.

I knew that Section 8 of the Family Law and Reform Act 1969 says that, at 16, minors can give valid consent to treatment – treatment covers all nursing care (Dimond, 2008). However, I'd not known of the proposal about specialised wards for them and here we have none. But it's obvious now the company of two middle-aged men and an elderly one who is confused and incontinent is not suitable for Josh.

Hospitalisation can threaten adolescents' developing sense of independence role by 'infanticising' teenagers: they can revert from being increasingly independent at home to being dependent in hospital. Many inpatients have chronic conditions that may result in readmission. Some often take medicines at home or need special care, such as stoma care or regular physiotherapy. Having become used to performing self-care at home, readmission to hospital restricts that independence for adolescents, especially in relation to medication. Relaxing the regulations and guidelines could mean more continuity for those adolescents considered to be responsible (Gillies, 1992).

Josh's behaviour at home indicates clearly he's trying to assert his independence, so although his mother may want to take charge, while he's here we should, as far as possible, defer to him.

Theories of adolescence

Hall's theory: Adolescence as storm and stress

Hall (1904) saw adolescence as a time of 'storm and stress' (or *Sturm* und *Drang*), and there is some evidence suggesting that emotional reactions are more intense and volatile during adolescence compared with other periods of life (see Gross [2010]). However, a more important indicator of storm and stress is mental disorder.

Studies of mental disorder

Several studies have found that early-maturing girls score higher on measures of depressive feelings and sadness (e.g., Alsaker [1992] and Stattin and Magnusson [1990]), although this was true only when the measures were taken before or simultaneously with changing schools (Petersen et al., 1991). They have also been reported to have more psychosomatic (psychophysiological) symptoms (e.g., Stattin and Magnusson [1990]), to display greater concerns about eating (e.g., Brooks-Gunn et al. [1989]) and to score higher on measures of emotional disturbance (e.g., Brooks-Gunn and Warren [1985]).

As far as early-maturing boys are concerned, the evidence is much more mixed (Alsaker, 1996). Although early maturation is usually found to be advantageous, it has also been found to be associated with more psychopathology (e.g., Petersen and Crockett [1985]), depressive tendencies and anxiety (e.g., Alsaker [1992]).

Based on their study of over two thousand 14–15-year-olds, Rutter et al. (1976) concluded that:

- There is a rather modest peak in psychiatric disorders in adolescence.
- Although severe clinical depression is rare, some degree of *inner turmoil* may characterise a sizeable minority of adolescents; it is not a myth, neither should it be exaggerated.
- A substantial proportion of adolescents with psychiatric problems had had them since childhood. Also, when problems did first appear during adolescence, they were mainly associated with stressful situations (such as parents' marital discord): 'adolescent turmoil is fact, not fiction, but its psychiatric importance has probably been overestimated in the past' (Rutter et al., 1976).

In Western societies, only a relatively small minority show clinical depression or report inner turmoil (Compas et al., 1995). Instead, the majority worry about everyday issues, such as school and examination performance, finding work, family and social relationships, self-image, conflicts with authority and the future generally (Gallagher et al., 1992).

Anna's concerns about Josh support Gallagher et al.'s (1992) findings (above). She said Josh is 'the anxious type' – he worried a great deal about his recent GCSE exams. Since his father died, Josh constantly challenges her authority and seems angry and resentful towards her; it's almost as though he blames her for his death.

Erikson's theory: Identity crisis

Erikson (1963) believed that it is human nature to pass through a genetically determined sequence of *psychosocial stages*, covering the whole life span. Each stage involves a struggle between two conflicting personality outcomes, one of which is positive (or *adaptive*) and the other is negative (or *maladaptive*). Healthy development involves the adaptive outweighing the maladaptive.

The major challenge of adolescence is to establish a strong sense of *personal identity*. The dramatic onset of puberty – combined with more sophisticated intellectual abilities (see Chapter 15) – makes adolescents particularly concerned with finding their own personal place in adult society.

In Western societies adolescence is a *moratorium*, an authorised delay of adulthood, which frees adolescents from most responsibilities and helps them make the difficult transition from childhood to adulthood. Although this is meant to make the transition easier, it can also have the opposite effect. Most of the societies studied by cultural anthropologists have important public ceremonies to mark the transition from childhood to adulthood. This is in stark contrast to Western, industrialised nations, which leave children to their own devices in finding their identity. Without a clearly defined procedure to follow, this process can be difficult, both for adolescents and for their parents (see the section *Sociological approaches: Generation gap*, page 397).

Does society create an identity crisis?

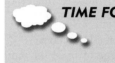

TIME FOR REFLECTION …

- Can you think of any inconsistencies or contradictions that adolescents face between different aspects of their development?
- How do they perceive their social status?

As well as the perceived absence of 'rites of passage' in Western society, a problem for both adolescents and their parents is the related lack of consensus as to where adolescence begins and ends and precisely what adolescent rights, privileges and responsibilities are. For example, the question 'when do I become an adult?' elicits a different response from a teacher, doctor, parent or police officer (Coleman, 1995).

For girls, isn't the onset of menstruation regarded as a clear delineation of girls' **physical** sexual maturity – almost a rite of passage? In contrast, if girls and boys (like Josh) go to university, their 'adolescence' could be prolonged until 21 or 22.

The *maturity gap* refers to the incongruity of achieving biological maturity at adolescence without simultaneously being awarded adult status (Curry, 1998). According to Hendry and Kloep (1999):

> … young people, as they grow up, find themselves in the trap of having to respond more and more to society's demands in a 'responsible' adult way while being treated as immature and not capable of holding sound opinions on a wide range of social matters.

One possible escape route from this trap is *risk-taking behaviour*. As well as having to deal with the question 'who am I?', the adolescent must also ask 'who will I be?'. Erikson saw the creation of an adult personality as achieved mainly through choosing and developing a commitment to an occupation or role in life. The development of *ego identity* (a firm sense of who one is and what one stands for) is positive and can carry people through difficult times.

When working with psychiatrically disturbed soldiers in the Second World War, Erikson coined the term *identity crisis* to describe the loss of personal identity that the stress of combat seemed to have caused. Some years later, he extended the use of the term to include 'severely conflicted young people whose sense of confusion is due … to a war within themselves'.

Role confusion

The failure to integrate perceptions of the self into a coherent whole results in *role confusion*, which, according to Erikson, can affect several areas of life:

Intimacy: a fear of commitment to, or involvement in, close relationships arises from a fear of losing one's identity.

Time perspective: the adolescent is unable to plan for the future or retain any sense of time.

Industry: difficulty in channelling resources in a realistic way into work or study, both of which require commitment.

Negative identity: engaging in abnormal or delinquent behaviour (such as taking drugs or even suicide) as an attempt to resolve the identity crisis ('a negative identity is better than no identity').

Related to Erikson's claims about negative identity is risk-taking behaviour. Hendry (1999) asks if risk-taking is '… part of the psychological make-up of youth – a thrill-seeking stage in a developmental transition – a necessary rite of passage en route to the acquisition of adult skills and self-esteem …'.

Many teenagers seek out excitement, thrills and risks as earnestly as in childhood, perhaps to escape a drab existence or to exert some control over their own lives and to achieve something (see Figure 17.4). Two ways of achieving this are drugs and sex. Traditionally, what parents of teenagers have most feared is that their children will engage in (particularly unprotected) sex and (especially hard) drugs (see Chapter 12).

Figure 17.4 Thrill seeking: a rite of passage into adulthood?

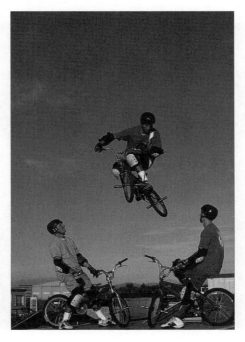

Anna is frantically worried about both of these and when they searched Josh's pockets for some identification, they found cigarettes and a packet of condoms (so at least he's aware of the need for protection), but no drugs were found on him. Anna seemed relieved when Sister told her Josh would be referred to the School Nurse. With the prospect of my own adolescent child in view, I later managed to arrange a visit to her!

For some, delinquency may be the solution to role confusion: it could actually be adaptive as a way of facilitating self-definition and expressing autonomy (Compas et al., 1995).

According to Bergevin et al. (2003),

> … One of the challenges of the self in adolescence is with identifying the ways that one is unique and how one is similar to others. Maintaining a sense of individuality while trying to fit into the group is an important task for adolescents. Emphasising differences can lead to loneliness and alienation, while emphasising similarities may impede the development of autonomy.

Such conflict seems to be largely absent in societies where the complete transition to adulthood is officially approved and celebrated at a specific age, often through a particular ceremony. This enables both the individual and the society to adjust to the change and enjoy a sense of continuity (Price and Crapo, 1999) (see Figure 17.5).

Figure 17.5 The Jewish bar mitzvah marks a 13-year-old boy's entry into manhood. But to the rest of the society, he is still just a teenager.

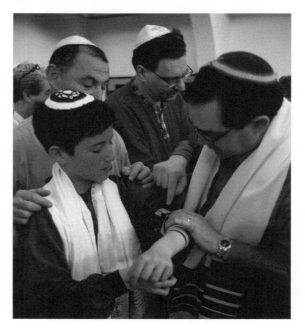

Sociological approaches: Generation gap

Sociologists see *role change* as an integral aspect of adolescent development (Coleman, 1995). Changing school or college, leaving home and beginning a job all involve new sets of relationships, producing different and often greater expectations. These expectations themselves demand a substantial reassessment of the self-concept and speed up the socialisation process. Some adolescents find this problematic because of the wide variety of competing socialising agencies (such as the family, mass media and peer group), which often present conflicting values and demands (see the earlier discussion on identity crisis).

Sociologists also see socialisation as being more dependent on the adolescent's *own generation* than on the family or other social institutions (*auto-socialisation*: Marsland, 1987). As Marsland says, 'The crucial meaning of youth is withdrawal from adult control and influence compared with childhood … .' Young people withdraw into their peer groups, and this withdrawal is (within limits) accepted by adults. What Marsland is describing is the *generation gap*.

Josh's withdrawal into his peer group was a source of conflict with Anna; she disapproved of the fact they all seemed to demand 'too much freedom for their age'.

Parent–adolescent relationships

Adolescence as a transition from childhood to adulthood requires changes from child–parent relationships to young adult–parent relationships (Hendry, 1999). Failure to negotiate new relationships with parents, or having highly critical or rejecting parents, is likely to make adolescents adopt a negative identity (Curry, 1998). Also, parents who rate their own adolescence negatively report more conflict in their relationships with adolescent children and less satisfaction with their family (Scheer and Unger, 1995). Parents of adolescents in general are often going through a time of transition themselves, reappraising their life goals, career and family ambitions and assessing whether they have fulfilled their expectations as parents (see Chapter 18).

Anna understandably found it hard to cope with Josh's mood swings and open defiance; as well as coping with her own and Josh's grief, she has had to establish a new identity for herself as a single mother resuming a career.

TIME FOR REFLECTION …

- While adolescents and their parents are, by definition, different generations, does this necessarily and inevitably mean that there is a generation gap, that is, that there will be conflict between them because they occupy 'different worlds'?

For most adolescents, relationships with parents become more equal and reciprocal and parental authority comes to be seen as open to discussion and negotiation (e.g., Hendry et al. [1993]). The study by Hendry et al. (1993) also suggests that relationships with mothers and fathers do not necessarily change in the same ways and to the same extent.

Studies conducted in several countries have found that young people get along well with their parents (e.g., Hendry et al. [1993] and Kloep and Tarifa [1993]), adopt their views and values and perceive family members as the most important 'significant others' in their lives (McGlone et al., 1996). Furthermore, most adolescents who had conflicts with their parents already had poor relationships with them before puberty (Stattin and Klackenberg, 1992).

Disagreements between young people and their parents are similar everywhere in Europe. According to Jackson et al. (1996), disagreements can arise because:

- Parents expect greater independence of action from their teenagers.
- Parents do not wish to grant as much autonomy as the adolescent demands (with young women having more conflict than young men over independence).
- Parents and adolescents have different personal tastes and preferences.

Despite this potential for conflict, evidence suggests that competence as an independent adult can best be achieved within the context of a secure family environment, where exploration of alternative ideas, identities and behaviour is allowed and actively encouraged (Barber and Buehler, 1996). So, although detachment and separation from the family are necessary and desirable, young people do not have to reject their parents to become adults in their own right (Hill, 1993; Ryan and Lynch, 1989) (see Chapter 14) (see Figure 17.6).

Figure 17.6 Generational harmony, not generation gap.

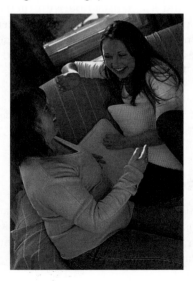

📃 It was reassuring that, when upset, Josh turned to his mother for comfort, reaffirming his close relationship with her.

Peer relationships

Adolescent *friendship groups* (established around mutual interests) are normally embedded within the wider network of *peer groups* (which set 'norms' and provide comparisons and pressures to conform to 'expected' behaviours). Friendship groups reaffirm self-image, and enable the young person to experience a new form of intimacy and learn social skills (such as discussing and solving conflicts, sharing and self-assertion). They also offer the opportunity to expand knowledge, develop a new identity and experiment away from the watchful eyes of adults and family (Coleman and Hendry, 1990).

Generally, peers become more important as providers of advice and companionship, as models for behaviour and as sources of comparison with respect to personal qualities and skills. But while peer groups and friendship groups become important points of reference in social development and provide social contexts for shaping day-to-day values, they often support traditional parental attitudes and beliefs. Hence, peer and friendship groups can work *in concert* with, rather than in opposition to, adult goals and achievements (Hendry, 1999).

Coleman's focal theory: Managing one change at a time

According to Coleman and Hendry (1990), the picture that emerges from the research as a whole is that while adolescence is a difficult time for some, for the majority it appears to be a period of relative stability. Coleman's (1980) *focal theory* is an attempt to explain how this is achieved.

The theory is based on a study of eight hundred 6-, 11-, 13-, 15- and 17-year-old boys and girls. Attitudes towards self-image, being alone, heterosexual and parental relationships, friendships and large-group situations all changed as a function of age. More importantly, concerns about different issues reached a peak at different ages for both sexes (Figure 17.7).

Figure 17.7 Peak ages of the expression of different themes: these data are for boys only. (From Coleman, J.C. and Hendry, L.B., *The Nature of Adolescence* (2nd edn.), Routledge, London, 1990.)

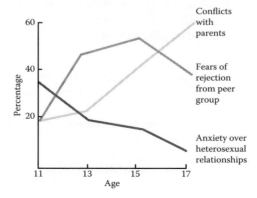

Particular sorts of relationship patterns come into *focus* (are most prominent) at different ages, although no pattern is specific to one age. The patterns overlap and there are wide individual differences.

Coleman believes that adolescents are able to cope with the potentially stressful changes as well as they do by dealing with one issue at a time. They spread the process of adaptation over a span of years, attempting to resolve one issue first before addressing the next. It is those adolescents who, for whatever reason, must deal with more than one issue (or normative shift) at a time who are most likely to experience difficulties. If normative shifts coincide with non-normative ones, the situation is even more problematic (Hendry and Kloep, 1999).

This is so pertinent to Josh and I am filled with sympathy for him now. He's had to cope with his new body, his acne, his role confusion and the shock of his father's death within a short time span. Being focused on his GCSEs probably helped him cope with his grief, but with that goal achieved and no clear substitute it's not surprising he lost direction.

Conclusions

Adolescence involves a number of important transitions from childhood to adulthood, including puberty. The potential for storm and stress in Western societies is increased by the lack of clear definitions regarding when adulthood is reached. This makes the task of attaining an adult identity, as well as relationships with parents, more difficult compared with non-industrialised societies.

However, adolescence in Western societies is not as problem-ridden as the popular stereotype would have it. If any serious problems do arise, they are directly linked to rapid social change (Dasen, 1999) and with the associated extension of adolescence and youth. Young people are not given a productive role to play when entering adult society (Segall et al., 1999).

Although most of the major theories of adolescence paint a picture of adolescence as an inherently difficult developmental stage, the evidence suggests that this is not necessarily so. Certain groups may be more vulnerable than others (such as early-maturing girls), but the majority seem to cope well. According to Coleman's theory, it is not adolescence itself that is stressful but the timing and combination of the transitions faced by young people.

My experience with Josh in hospital showed me that to care sensitively for adolescent young people at a time of crisis I needed to learn a great deal more about the complexity of their needs. Researching theories of adolescence has reinforced how closely the physical, psychological and social elements affecting teenagers are integrated.

I'm pleased that later, I did visit Josh's school. Nadine, the specialist nurse heading the health team, explained they have a comprehensive health education programme and run a drop-in centre for advice and counselling. As unplanned pregnancy is a significant problem, they provide free condoms and run a programme which emphasises peer support called 'A PAUSE – Added Power And Understanding in Sex Education' (projects.exeter.ac.uk/europeeruk/DHguide.pdf).

I was pleased to learn Josh is involved in this. However, health issues usually need to include economic and political analysis (see Goodman 1984 , case study 2, page 230); in hospitals, although we recognise adolescents' special status, it isn't always possible to provide ideal facilities for their care.

CHAPTER SUMMARY

- Adolescence involves *multiple transitions*. Compared with previous generations, it begins sooner and ends later. Various *adulthood-postponing* changes have coincided with increased freedom at earlier ages.

- These transitions or shifts can be categorised as *normative maturational*, *normative society-dependent* and *non-normative*. Normative shifts can become non-normative, as when puberty begins unusually early or late.

- Puberty involves the *adolescent growth spurt* and the development of *secondary sex characteristics* (both sexes). Although girls typically enter puberty 2 years before boys, there are important individual differences within each sex (such as *intra-individual asynchronies*).

- The adolescent brain appears to undergo some fundamental restructuring (bulking up followed by pruning). Among the last brain regions to mature is the dorsolateral prefrontal cortex (DPFC), which is involved in impulse control, judgement and decision-making.

- This lack of impulse control may produce the stereotypical adolescent risk-taking behaviour.

- Adolescents evaluate their changing body images in terms of cultural standards of beauty, especially as these relate to weight. According to the cultural ideal hypothesis (CIH), girls move further away from their physical ideal and early-maturing girls will face a double disadvantage. Early-maturing boys will move fastest towards their physical ideal.

- Some of the particular problems faced by adolescents in hospital include lack of privacy and a renewed dependence on adults for the care and management of their illness.

- Hall's *recapitulation theory* saw adolescence as a time of *storm and stress*. While mood swings are more common during adolescence, rates of mental disorder are higher only in early-maturing girls and adolescents with problems prior to puberty. The evidence for off-time maturation in boys is more mixed.

- According to Erikson, adolescence involves a conflict between *ego identity* and *role confusion*. In Western societies, adolescence is a *moratorium*, intended to help ease the transition to adulthood. However, the lack of clear definitions of adulthood may contribute to the adolescent *identity crisis*.

- Role confusion can take the form of *negative identity*, related to which is *risk-taking behaviour*. These problems are largely absent in societies that mark the transition to adulthood by *initiation ceremonies*.

- *Sociological approaches* stress *role change*; the conflicting values and demands of different socialising agencies; and *auto-socialisation*, which produces a *generation gap*.

- Renegotiating relationships with parents is necessary and, although there are inevitable disagreements, adult status is probably best achieved within the context of a secure family environment.
- *Friendship groups* (as sub-groups of the wider *peer group*) assume much greater significance during adolescence, such as helping to shape basic values. But these values are often consistent with parents' values, goals and achievements.
- According to Coleman's *focal theory*, most adolescents cope as well as they do by spreading the process of adaptation over several years. Having to deal with more than one issue at a time is stressful, especially if changes occur too early or suddenly.

18 Adulthood

Introduction and overview

Assuming that we enjoy a normal lifespan, the longest phase of the life cycle will be spent in adulthood. Until recently, however, personality changes in adulthood attracted little psychological research interest. Indeed, as Levinson et al. (1978) have observed, adulthood is 'one of the best-kept secrets in our society and probably in human history generally'.

This chapter attempts to reveal some of these secrets by examining what theory and research have told us about personality change in adulthood, including the occurrence of crises and transitions.

Many theorists believe that adult concerns and involvements are patterned in such a way that we can speak about *stages* of adult development. However, evidence concerning the predictability of changes in adult life (or what Levinson, 1986, calls *psychobiosocial transitions*) is conflicting. The following three kinds of influence can affect the way we develop in adulthood (Hetherington and Baltes, 1988):

1. *Normative age-graded influences* are biological (such as the menopause) and social changes (such as marriage and parenting) that normally occur at fairly predictable ages.
2. *Normative history-graded influences* are historical events that affect whole generations or *cohorts* at about the same time (examples include wars, recessions and epidemics).
3. *Non-normative influences* are idiosyncratic transitions, such as divorce, unemployment and illness.

Levinson's (1986) term *marker events* refers to age-graded and non-normative influences. Others prefer the term *critical life events* to describe such influences, although it is probably more accurate to describe them as *processes*. Some critical life events, such as divorce, unemployment and bereavement, can occur at any time during adulthood (bereavement is discussed in Chapter 13).

Others occur late in adulthood, such as retirement (see Chapter 19). Yet others tend to happen early in adulthood, such as marriage (or partnering) and parenting.

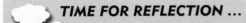

TIME FOR REFLECTION …

- What do you understand by the term 'adulthood'?
- What does it mean to be an adult?

From my diary (13): Year 2/Medical Ward

Mr Briggs (Frank), a 49-year-old police officer who had a myocardial infarction (MI) two days ago was transferred to us from the Coronary Care Unit (CCU) as they needed the bed. His wife, Denise accompanied him and appeared very anxious. He went into a high-dependency bed and at hand over, Helen (the ward manager) said we should be sensitive to their need for reassurance and attention as the transfer was at short notice and they would be suffering from what she called 'CCU blues' (feelings of fear and vulnerability at losing the one-to-one attention they received in intensive care situations). Apparently Frank's father died of a heart attack at 62, which scared Frank into giving up smoking and watching his weight and cholesterol levels, although he was still a fairly heavy social drinker.

As I arrived to do his observations, his wife was trying to arrange his pillows more comfortably and obviously hadn't succeeded because I heard him say irritably, 'Oh, you're hopeless!' Denise, looking tearful, left; Frank looked embarrassed so I chose not to have heard. I tried to be cheerful and reassuring, thinking that later I'd try to talk to Denise.

Erikson's theory: Achieving intimacy and generativity

Erikson believes that human development occurs through a sequence of *psychosocial stages*. As far as early and middle adulthood are concerned, Erikson described two primary developmental crises (see Table 18.1).

The first involves the establishment of *intimacy*, which is a criterion of having attained the psychosocial state of adulthood. By intimacy, Erikson means the ability to form close, meaningful relationships with others without 'the fear of losing oneself in the process' (Elkind, 1970). Erikson believed that a prerequisite for intimacy is the attainment of *identity* (see Chapter 17). We cannot know what it means to love someone and seek to share our life with them until we know who we are and what we want to do with our lives.

Intimacy need not involve sexuality. Since intimacy refers to the essential ability to relate our deepest hopes and fears to another person, and in turn to accept another's need for intimacy, it describes the relationship between friends just as much as that between sexual partners (Dacey, 1982). By sharing ourselves with others, our personal identity becomes fully realised and consolidated. The negative outcome of young adulthood is *isolation*: a sense of being alone without anyone to share with or care for.

We normally achieve intimacy in young adulthood (our 20s and 30s), after which we enter middle age (our 40s and 50s). This involves the attainment of *generativity*, the positive outcome of the second developmental crisis (see Box 18.1).

Table 18.1 Comparison between Erikson's and Freud's stages of development

No. of stage	Name of stage (psychosocial crisis)	Psychosocial modalities (dominant modes of being and acting)	Radius of significant relationships	Human virtues (qualities of strength)	Freud's psychosexual stages	Approximate ages
1	Basic trust vs basic mistrust	To get. To give in return	Mother or mother figure	Hope	Oral	0–1
2	Autonomy vs shame and doubt	To hold on. To let go	Parents	Willpower	Anal	1–3
3	Initiative vs guilt	To make (going after). To 'make like' (playing)	Basic family	Purpose	Phallic	3–6
4	Industry vs inferiority	To make things (completing). To make things together	Neighbourhood and school	Competence	Latency	6–12
5	Identity vs role confusion	To be oneself (or not to be). To share being oneself	Peer groups and outgroups. Models of leadership	Fidelity	Genital	12–18
6	Intimacy vs isolation	To lose and find oneself in another	Partners in friendship, sex, competition, cooperation	Love		20s
7	Generativity vs stagnation	To make be. To take care of	Divided labour and shared household	Care		Late 20s–50s
8	Ego integrity vs despair	To be, through having been. To face not being	'Humankind', 'my kind'	Wisdom		50s and beyond

Source: Erikson, E.H., *Childhood and Society*, New York: Norton, 1950; Thomas, R.M., *Comparing Theories of Child Development* (2nd edn.), Belmont, CA, Wadsworth Publishing Company, 1985.

> ## Box 18.1 Generativity
>
> - The central task of the middle years of adulthood is to determine life's purpose, and to focus on achieving aims and contributing to the well-being of others (particularly children).
> - *Generativity* means being concerned with others beyond the immediate family, such as future generations and the nature of the society and world in which those future generations will live. Generativity is shown by anyone actively concerned with the welfare of young people and in making the world a better place for them to live and work.
> - Failure to attain generativity leads to *stagnation*, in which people become preoccupied with their personal needs and comforts. They indulge themselves as if they were their own (or another's) only child.

I found Denise in the corridor and was relieved to be able to talk. Between her concerns about Frank's illness I gathered he's a 'workaholic', they'd been married for 25 years and have 2 children. Tom is 24 and also a policeman; Chloe is 20 and at university; both visited later in the day and clearly showed loving concern for their father, indicating a mutual caring relationship. Denise is a teacher, so both parents have socially responsible jobs and appear to have successfully completed the stages of intimacy and generativity

Evaluation of Erikson's theory

The sequence from identity to intimacy may not accurately reflect present-day realities. In recent years, the trend has been for adults to live together before marrying, so they tend to marry later in life than people did in the past (see below). Many people struggle with identity issues (such as career choice) at the same time as dealing with intimacy issues.

Erikson's psychosocial stages were meant to be *universal*, applying to both genders in all cultures. However, he acknowledged that the sequence of stages is different for a woman, who suspends her identity as she prepares to attract the man who will marry her. Men achieve identity before achieving intimacy with sexual partners, whereas, for women, Erikson's developmental crises appear to be fused. As Gilligan (1982) has observed, 'The female comes to know herself as she is known, through relationships with others'.

Denise said she'd happily given up her secretarial work (her words, not mine!) when she married Frank. In contrast, her son Tom and Ellie (his partner) are living together, both working full time, and have no intention of getting married or having a family yet. However, the developmental task of achieving intimacy is the same.

Levenson et al.'s *The Season's of a Man's Life*

Perhaps the most systematic study of personality and life changes in adulthood began in 1969, when Levinson et al. (1978) interviewed 40 men aged 35 to 45 years. Transcripts were made of the 5 to 10 tape-recorded interviews that each participant gave over several months. Levinson et al. looked at how adulthood is actually experienced.

In *The Seasons of a Man's Life*, Levinson et al. (1978) advanced a *life-structure theory*, defining life structure as the underlying pattern or design of a person's life at any given time. Life structure allows us to 'see how the self is in the world and how the world is in the self', and evolves through a series of *phases* or *periods* that give overall shape to the course of adult development. Adult development comprises a sequence of *eras* which overlap in the form of *cross-era transitions*; these last about 5 years, ending the outgoing era and initiating the upcoming one. The four eras are pre-adulthood (age 0–22 years), early adulthood (17–45 years), middle adulthood (40–65 years) and late adulthood (60 years onwards) (see Figure 18.1).

The phases or periods alternate between those that are stable (or *structure-building*) and transitional (or *structure-changing*). Although each phase involves biological, psychological and social adjustments, family and work roles are seen as central to the life structure at any time, and individual development is interwoven with changes in these roles.

According to Levinson et al.'s (1978) theory, Frank spent his early adulthood stage 'structure building' his career, as well as being married with a family. At 49, he's moved into middle adulthood.

Figure 18.1 Levinson et al.'s theory of adult development. The life cycle is divided into four major eras that overlap in the form of cross-era transitions. (From D.J. Levinson et al., 1978, The Seasons of a Man's Life. New York: A.A. Knopf, a division of Random House, Inc. Reprinted by permission of SLL/Sterling Lord Literistic, Inc. © 1975 by Daniel J. Levinson.)

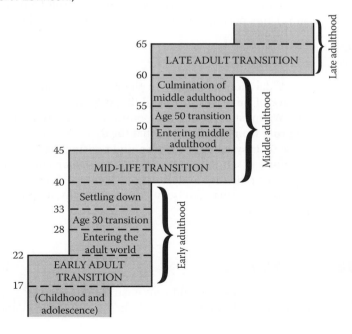

The era of early adulthood

Early adult transition (17–22) is a developmental 'bridge' between adolescence and adulthood. Two key themes are *separation* and the *formation of attachments* to the adult world.

- *External separation* involves moving out of the family home, increasing financial independence, and entering more independent and responsible roles and living arrangements.
- *Internal separation* involves greater psychological distance from the family, less emotional dependence on the parents, and greater differentiation between the self and family. However, this process of separation continues throughout life.
- *Attachment* involves exploring the world's possibilities, imagining ourselves as part of it, and identifying and establishing changes for living in the world before we become 'full members' of it.

 Both Ellie and Chloe are in the early adult transition stage; Chloe is living in a student house with friends and independent – except financially, Denise says! Ellie may still be developing her identity as well as trying to achieve 'intimacy' with Tom.

Between the ages of 22 and 28 years, we *enter the adult world*. This is the first *structure-building* phase (the *entry life structure for early adulthood*).

In the *novice phase*, we try to define ourselves as adults and live with the initial choices we make concerning jobs, relationships, lifestyles and values. However, we need to create a balance between 'keeping our options open' (which allows us to explore possibilities without being committed to a given course) and 'putting down roots' (or creating stable life structures).

Tom is in the novice phase – and this is just what he's doing, it seems!

Our decisions are made in the context of our *dreams*: the 'vague sense' we have of ourselves in the adult world and what we want to do with our lives. We must overcome disappointments and setbacks, and learn to accept and profit from successes, so that the dream's 'thread' does not get lost in the course of 'moving up the ladder' and revising the life structure. To help us in our efforts at self-definition, we look to *mentors*, older and more experienced others, for guidance and direction. Mentors can take a formal teaching role or a more informal, advisory and emotionally supportive function role (as a parent does).

TIME FOR REFLECTION ...

- What qualities would your ideal mentor possess?
- What qualities do you think she/he would like to find in a mentee?

Figure 18.2 Learning from a mentor.

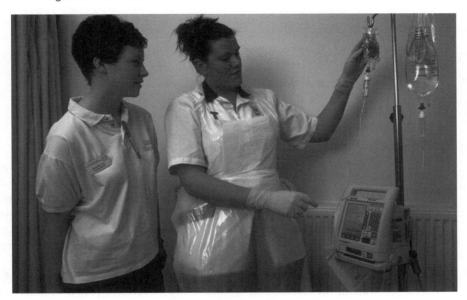

Frank was no doubt an informal mentor to Tom during his police training. However, formal mentoring is finding its place in the police service as well as in teaching and nursing (Morton-Cooper and Palmer, 2003, in Downie and Basford, 2003). These authors suggest the characteristics of an effective mentor can be drawn together under a framework of three important personal attributes: competence, personal confidence and a commitment to the development of others. These all apply to Adam, my mentor; he's highly skilled, decisive and is always challenging and encouraging me.

The age-30 transition (28–33) provides an opportunity to work on the flaws and limitations of the first life structure, and to create the basis for a more satisfactory structure that will complete the era of young adulthood. Most of Levinson et al.'s participants experienced *age-30 crises* which involved stress, self-doubt, feelings that life was losing its 'provisional quality' and becoming more serious, and time pressure. Thus, the participants saw this as being the time for change, if change was needed. However, for a minority, the age-30 transition was crisis free (Figure 18.2).

Settling down

- The *settling down* (or *culminating life structure for early adulthood*) (33–40) *phase* represents consolidation of the second life structure. This involves a shift away from tentative choices regarding family and career towards a strong sense of commitment to a personal, familial and occupational future: we see ourselves as responsible adults.
- *Early settling down* (33–36) is followed by *becoming one's own man* (BOOM), in which men strive to advance and succeed in building better lives, improve and use their skills, be creative, and in general contribute to society.

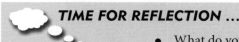 Adam is in this 'BOOM' phase, which may explain his commitment and enthusiasm for his mentoring role.

> ### TIME FOR REFLECTION …
> - What do you think is meant by the 'mid-life crisis'?
> - Do you think it is a real phenomenon?

The era of middle adulthood

The *mid-life transition* (40–45) involves terminating one life structure, initiating another and continuing the process of *individuation* started during the BOOM sub-stage. This is a time of soul-searching, questioning and assessing the real meaning of the life structure's achievement. It is sometimes referred to as the *mid-life crisis*, although Levinson et al. did not actually use this term. For some people, the change is gradual and fairly painless; for others, it is full of uncertainties.

The crisis stems from unconscious tensions between attachment and separation, the resurfacing of the need to be creative (which is often repressed in order to achieve a career), and retrospective comparisons between dreams and life's reality.

Most participants in Levinson et al.'s study had not reached the age of 45 years. Following interviews 2 years after the main study was concluded, some were chosen for more extensive study. But the evidence for the remaining phases is much less detailed than for the earlier ones.

Denise said Frank missed the children when they left home (a normative shift) and had 'thrown himself into work'; he was hoping for promotion to chief inspector. His illness – what Levinson calls a 'marker event' – has severely disrupted his plans.

Is there a 'mid-life crisis'?

Just as the 'identity crisis' is part of the popular stereotype of adolescence (see Chapter 17), Levinson et al. have helped to make the 'mid-life crisis' part of the common sense understanding of adult development. Like Erikson, Levinson et al. see crisis as both inevitable and necessary (*normative* to use Erikson's term).

However, this view is controversial. People of all ages suffer occasional depression, self-doubt, sexual uncertainty and concerns about the future. According to Tredre (1996), the concept of a mid-life crisis is too narrow: we need to think in terms of early-, mid- and late-life crises (see Box 18.2).

According to Bainbridge (2012), middle age (a resilient, healthy, energy-efficient and productive phase of life which has laid the foundations for our species' success) is unique to human beings. One of its key roles is to provide an 'elite caste of skilled, experienced 'super-providers' on which everyone else depends'; a second is the propagation of information (i.e., culture) (see Vygotsky's theory, Chapter 15, pages 362 through 365).

I would think mentors of all kinds should be included in this category.

Box 18.2 Identity crisis, the life cycle and human evolution

- Marcia (1998) also believes that the concept of a mid-life crisis is misleading and too narrow. He argues that 'adolescing' (making decisions about one's identity) occurs *throughout* the lifespan, whenever we review or reorganise our lives. At the very least, we might expect identity crises to accompany (in Erikson's terms) intimacy–isolation, generativity–stagnation and integrity–despair (see Chapter 19).

- Just as puberty and other changes in early adolescence disrupt the partial identities of childhood, so the demands of intimacy require a reformulation of the initial identity achieved at late adolescence. Similarly, the generative, care-giving requirements of middle age differ from those of being with an intimate partner. The virtues of fidelity, love and care (see Table 18.1), which derive from positive resolution of young and middle adulthood, do not emerge without a struggle. According to Marcia (1998), 'Periods of adolescing are normal, expectable components of life cycle growth'. However, the crises associated with middle (and old) age are especially difficult.

The Seasons of a Woman's Life

In *The Seasons of a Woman's Life* (1997), Levinson and Levinson presented their findings for 45 women (aged 35 to 45 years), comprising 15 homemakers (full-time housewives/mothers), 15 business women and 15 academics. The broad pattern of developmental periods based on the original all-male sample was confirmed. But men and women differ in terms of their dreams.

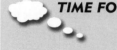 *Both Denise and I put our careers second to caring for children. Denise's change of role, when her children left home, was normative; mine, at 28, was triggered by divorce and non-normative. Or did my age-30 transition contribute to my divorce?*

Gender splitting is relevant to discussion of marriage/partnering and parenthood (see pages 413 and 414).

The validity of stage theories of adult development

TIME FOR REFLECTION ...

- Do you think it is appropriate to describe adulthood in terms of distinct stages?

The view of adult development as 'stage-like' has been criticised on the grounds that it underestimates the degree of *individual variability* (Rutter and Rutter, 1992).

Stage theories also imply a *discontinuity* of development. But many psychologists believe that there is also considerable *continuity* of personality during adult life.

From what I've seen and been told, I think Frank is ambitious, tetchy and driven. This describes what is known as a 'Type A behaviour pattern personality'; such people appear to respond physiologically more to stress than other 'types' (Fletcher, 1995; see Chapter 5).

Current views of adult development stress the transitions and milestones that mark adult life, rather than a rigid developmental sequence (Baltes, 1983; Schlossberg, 1984). This is commonly referred to as the *life-events approach*. Yet, despite the growing unpredictability of changes in adult life, most people still unconsciously evaluate their transitions according to a *social clock*, which determines whether they are 'on time' with respect to particular life events – such as getting married (see Schlossberg et al., 1978). If they are 'off time', either early or late, they are *age deviant*. Like other types of deviancy, this can result in social penalties, such as amusement, pity or rejection.

While all cultures have social clocks that define the 'right' time to marry, begin work, have children, and so on, these clocks vary greatly *between* cultures (Wade and Tavris, 1999). Because of the sheer diversity of experiences in an adult's life, Craig (1992) does not believe it is possible to describe major 'milestones' that will apply to nearly everyone (Critical Discussion 18.1).

Both Denise and I might be seen as 'age-deviant' regarding our late career development, but in our culture, the social clock for this particular life event (Wade and Tavris, 1999) is changing; there are so many mature students in nursing now I don't feel deviant!

CRITICAL DISCUSSION 18.1

What is an adult? Re-setting the social clock

- Just as social clocks are 'set' at different times in different cultures for different life changes, in Western societies, the clock becomes 're-set' over time.
- For example, 40–50 years ago, a stable job and income could be achieved (by men) by the age of 21 years, so this was seen as the time to 'settle down'. If a woman was not married by the time she was 25, she was 'on the shelf', and if still single by 29, she was an 'old maid'.
- Common beliefs about the appropriate age for child-bearing put pressure on women to become mothers by their early 20s, and pregnancy after 26 was seen as 'late' (Apter, 2001). These patterns are drastically different now.
- In *The Myth of Maturity* (2001), Apter argues that it is taking young people far longer to achieve adult status than it used to. She refers to 18- to 24-year-olds as 'thresholders', because they are only *on the brink* of achieving self-sufficiency and autonomy (commonly cited adult qualities). They are like 'apprentices to adulthood'.
- Maturity is a myth, in two senses: (1) maturity *is not* achieved as soon as adolescence comes to an end (for males or females) and (2) independence from one's family *is not* necessary to achieve adult competence (Apter, 2001). Indeed, Apter's research found that thresholders benefited from parental support (emotional, practical and financial); this finding has been replicated by other large-scale studies (Catan, 2004).

> With support from their families, young people were better placed to acquire the experience, training and confidence to thrive as adults

(Apter, 2010).

TIME FOR REFLECTION ...

- Would you describe yourself as a thresholder?
- Are many of your peers thresholders?

Marriage

Since over 90 per cent of adults in Western countries marry at least once, marriage is an example of a *normative age-graded influence* (see *Introduction and Overview*). Marriage is an important transition for young adults, because it involves a lasting personal commitment to another person (and so is a means of achieving Erikson's *intimacy*), financial responsibilities and, perhaps, family responsibilities.

*But social norms too are changing; marriage now frequently **follows** living together, like Tom and Ellie, and often having children.*

It has long been recognised that mortality is affected by marital status. Married people tend to live longer than unmarried people, and are happier, healthier and have lower rates of various mental disorders than the single, widowed or divorced. The greater mortality of the unmarried relative to the married has generally been increasing over the past two to three decades, and it seems that divorced (and widowed) people in their 20s and 30s have particularly high risks of dying compared with other people of the same age (Cramer, 1995).

TIME FOR REFLECTION ...

- Why – or how – might marriage be beneficial?

It's worrying the incidence of coronary heart disease (CHD) in women is increasing. Hayes et al. (1980 in Ogden, 2004) found that having a higher number of children increased the risk of CHD in working women, but not in non-working women; evidence of the stress of gender splitting?

For most people, parenthood and child-rearing represent key transitions. While most people become parents, this may occur at any time from adolescence to middle age, and for some men – and a growing number of women – may even occur in late adulthood. Parenthood may also be planned or unplanned, wanted or unwanted, and there are many motives for having children.

Traditionally, parenthood is the domain of the married couple. However, it may involve a single woman, a homosexual couple (see pages 413 through 417), a cohabiting couple or couples who adopt or foster children. In recent decades, there has been a marked rise in the number of teenage pregnancies, and even more recently, the phenomenon of 'minimal parenting' (as in donor insemination; see Chapter 14).

Equally, though, the increasing importance of careers for women has also led to more and more couples postponing starting a family, so that the woman can become better established in her career (see Box 18.3). For example, women's average age at the birth of their first child was almost 30 in 2003 – compared with 23 in the 1960s (Groskop, 2004). Consequently, there is a new class of middle-aged parents with young children (Turnbull, 1995).

Pregnancy and childbirth

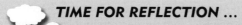

TIME FOR REFLECTION …

- Assuming that they are planned, why do people have children? What are their motives?
- Is it 'natural' (at least for women) to want children?

Oakley (1980) found that the most normal of births can involve elements of loss for the mother: of self-confidence, body image (see Chapter 16) and previous employment. Many women worry that their baby may be abnormal, and about how well they'll cope with motherhood.

Box 18.3 Women's dreams and 'gender splitting'

- Levinson (1986) argued that a *'gender splitting'* phenomenon occurs in adult development. Men have fairly unified visions of their futures, which tend to be focused on their careers. But women's 'dreams' are more likely to be split between a career and marriage.
- This was certainly true of academics and business women, although the former were less ambitious and more likely to forego a career, whereas the latter wanted to maintain their careers but at a reduced level. Only the homemakers had unified dreams (to be full-time wives and mothers, as their own mothers had been).
- Women's dreams were constructed around their relationships with their husbands and families, which subordinated their personal needs. So, part of *her* dream is *his* success. Women who give marriage and motherhood top priority in their 20s tend to develop more individualistic goals for their 30s. However, those who are career-oriented early on in adulthood tend to focus on marriage and family concerns later.
- Generally, the transitory instability of the early 30s lasts longer for women than for men, and 'settling down' is much less clear cut. Trying to integrate career and marriage/family responsibilities is very difficult for most women, who experience greater conflicts than their husbands are likely to.

In addition to these 'normal' stressors, the woman who has had a Caesarean section (CS) has to cope with the physical and psychological impact of anaesthesia and major surgery, which may have occurred on top of a long and exhausting labour (Hillan, 1991). The very use of 'section' distinguishes a Caesarean from other types of abdominal surgery (Oakley, 1983). For example, a common consequence of major surgery is depression, yet the same assumption is not made about a CS. At the same time, the woman who has undergone a Caesarean delivery is often expected to cope with the demands of her new baby, and this may involve activities that are normally forbidden to patients who have had abdominal surgery.

Hillan cites several studies that show a range of negative responses to delivery by CS, including the following:

- A sense of failure, anger and disappointment at not being able to deliver the baby normally
- A sense of guilt at putting the baby in danger and depriving her partner of the shared experience of birth (Figure 18.3)

She also cites studies which suggest that three factors in particular may moderate some of these negative responses, namely:

1. Being prepared for the CS (i.e., it is planned)
2. Having an epidural (and so remaining conscious throughout)
3. The presence of a partner during the procedure

Figure 18.3 Being at the birth of his child can help counteract a father's feelings of being excluded during the pregnancy – and afterwards. It can also help him to form an emotional bond with the baby.

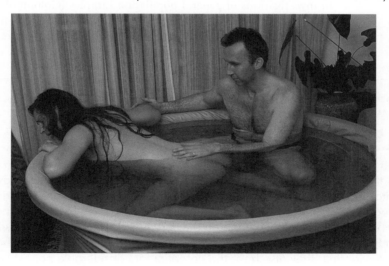

Nicky, a young single mother failing to bond with her second baby who I met in the community (see case study 4, page 26) had all these negative experiences: a Caesarean section under general anaesthetic, her baby in intensive care for 24 hours and the father absent (from choice). It's not surprising she needed help to develop mothering skills.

Lesbian and gay parenting

In the context of advocating that psychologists should study homosexual relationships in their own terms (and not by comparison with heterosexual ones), Kitzinger and Coyle (1995) suggested that we might want to ask how the children of lesbian/gay couples understand and talk about their parents' relationships, and how they can develop positive views about homosexuality in a heterosexual culture. Homosexual couples have always been involved in parenting through partners' previous heterosexual relationships. The recent increase in fostering/adoption of children by gay men, and the ongoing 'lesbian baby boom', means that many more homosexual couples are parents than used to be the case.

According to Kitzinger et al. (1998), research into lesbian/gay parenting was initially concerned with whether or how far the children of lesbians and (to a lesser extent) gay men could be distinguished psychologically from those of heterosexuals. On balance, this research suggested that these children were no more 'at risk' than children raised in heterosexual families.

For example, Taylor (1993) found no evidence that children reared in gay/lesbian families were more disturbed or had greater gender identity confusion than those reared in heterosexual families. Comparisons between children in lesbian families and their counterparts from heterosexual families have found no differences in psychological well-being or in the gender-role behaviour of boys or girls (Tasker and Golombok, 1995; Golombok and Tasker, 1996). These findings have been replicated in studies of children raised in lesbian families from birth (Golombok et al., 1997; MacCallum and Golombok, 2004) and in investigations of general population samples (Golombok et al., 2003). The only clear difference found between family types is that co-mothers in lesbian families are more involved with the children than are fathers in heterosexual homes (Golombok, 2010) (Critical Discussion 18.2).

CRITICAL DISCUSSION 18.2

Impact of gay parenting

- Barrett and Robinson (1994) reviewed the impact of gay fathering on children. They stress the need to take into account that these children are likely to have experienced parental divorce and to show the psychological distress that often accompanies it. Although these children may be isolated, angry and in need of help sorting out their feelings about homosexuality in general, they are in little danger of being sexually abused, and adjust well to their family situations. While the relationships with their fathers may be stormy at first, they also have the potential for considerable honesty and openness.

- As Golombok (2010) observes, the circumstances of children in gay father families are more unusual than those of children raised by lesbian mothers. Not only are they being raised by same-sex parents, but it is also rare for fathers, whether heterosexual or gay, to be the primary caretaker. Research on the development of children in gay father families is just beginning.

Increasingly, psychologists are researching areas directly rooted in the concerns of lesbian/gay parents themselves, including coming out to one's children, and managing different co-parenting arrangements (such as a lesbian mother with her female lover, her ex-husband, a gay male sperm donor, or a gay male co-parent) (Kitzinger et al., 1998).

Conclusions

Although some of the most influential and popular explanations of personality change in early and middle adulthood have adopted *stage approaches*, critics argue that adult development does not occur in predictable and ordered ways. An alternative, yet *complementary*, approach is to assess the impact of *critical life events*. These include two major normative age-graded influences, marriage/partnering and parenthood.

Levinson's theory of development explains how our roles change 'normally' at different ages (although the life experiences of Frank's family show that what is considered 'normal' can change over a generation). It also helps me understand the significance of Frank's MI as a life-changing event for him, or what Moos and Schaefer (1984) call a 'crisis' – an illness or hospitalisation that may represent a turning point in an individual's life. Stress may well have played a significant role in causing his illness and given his anxiety must still be a factor; his emotional care could affect his recovery (see Chapter 4). Frank may have to become less ambitious – or even take early retirement as policing is (like nursing) a high-stress occupation.

Denise now has her own satisfying career but this could lead to conflict between her own goals and her investment in her husband's future needs (Durkin, 1995). Although Frank's life-threatening physical condition must take immediate priority, his future care must take account of the psychosocial factors that make up his unique lived experience.

CHAPTER SUMMARY

- In Erikson's *psychosocial theory*, the task of *young adulthood* is to achieve *intimacy* and to avoid *isolation*. The central task of *middle adulthood* is the attainment of *generativity* and avoidance of *stagnation*.
- Many people struggle with issues of identity and intimacy *at the same time*, and women tend to achieve intimacy *before* 'occupational identity', submerging their identity into those of their partners.
- Levinson et al. were concerned with how adulthood is actually *experienced*. Their *life-structure theory* identifies *phases/periods* that are either stable (*structure-building*) or transitional (*structure-changing*). A sequence of *eras* overlaps in the form of *cross-era transitions*.
- *Early adult transition* is a developmental bridge between adolescence and adulthood, and *entry life structure for early adulthood* is the first structure-building phase.

- Levinson et al. see *crisis* as both inevitable and necessary (*normative*). But people of all ages suffer crises (*'adolescing'*), both earlier and later than 'mid-life'.
- According to Bainbridge, far from being a time of crisis, mid-life represents a uniquely human, resilient, productive phase of life which has been crucial for the evolutionary success of human beings.
- While men have fairly unified, career-focused visions of the future, women's *dreams* are split between career and marriage/family responsibilities (*gender splitting*).
- The *age-30 transition* generally lasts longer for women than for men, and *'settling down'* is much less clear cut. Trying to integrate career and marriage and family responsibilities is very difficult for most women.
- The view that adult development is *'stage like'* has been criticised on the grounds that it underestimates *individual variability*. Stage theories also imply a *discontinuity* of development.
- *Social clocks* are 'set' at different times in different cultures and 're-set' over time within Western societies. According to Apter, *thresholders* are only on the brink of achieving adult qualities, demonstrating the *myth of maturity*.
- *Marriage* and *parenting* are *normative, age-graded influences*. These are also called *marker events* or *critical life events*.
- *Married people* tend to live longer, and are happier, healthier and have lower rates of mental disorder than unmarried people. *Parenthood* has greater variability in meaning and impact than any other life transition.
- It is vital that women receive sufficient information about *childbirth* so that they are able to participate fully in the process. This applies especially in the case of birth by Caesarean Section (CS).
- Early research found no evidence that the children of *gay/lesbian* parents were more 'at risk' than those raised in heterosexual families.
- More recently, the emphasis has shifted to issues such as co-parenting arrangements, and research into the development of children in *gay* father families is just beginning.

19 Late adulthood

Introduction and overview

While 'growing up' is normally seen as desirable, 'growing old' has far more negative connotations. This negative view is based on the *decrement model*, which sees ageing as a process of decay or decline in physical and mental health, intellectual abilities and social relationships.

An alternative to the decrement model is the *personal growth model*, which stresses the potential advantages of late adulthood (or 'old age'), such as increased leisure time, reduced responsibilities and the ability to concentrate only on matters of high priority (Kalish, 1982). This much more positive view is how ageing has been studied within the *lifespan approach*.

In this chapter, we consider some of the theories and research concerned with *adjustment to late adulthood*. It begins by looking at what is meant by the term 'old', which turns out to be more complex than it might seem. *Stereotyped beliefs* about what elderly people are like are an inherent part of prejudiced attitudes towards them. Research into some of the cognitive and social changes that occur in late adulthood brings these stereotypes and prejudice into sharp focus. *Retirement* (a *normative, age-graded influence*) is often taken to mark the 'official' start of old age.

According to Brown (2007),

> It is tempting to think that ageing is 'natural', but the opposite is the case. Ageing is an artefact of culture. It … was rare in humans until 200 years ago. As the population inexorably ages, maladies that were formerly rare or non-existent become commonplace … Death is not the enemy; it is an integral part of life. It is ageing and its diseases that we should be fighting.

One of the major 'enemies', Alzheimer's disease, is discussed in detail in Chapter 11.

 From my diary (17): Year 2/Teaching Block

Today I went to the Arthritis Club to see Alfred Green, the subject of my case study of an elderly person showing client-led assessment of needs. I met Alfred (he'd asked me to call him that) during my community placement; he was caring for his wife who'd had a stroke two years previously and has since died. The osteoarthritis of his left hip has worsened recently and he's waiting for surgery. He leaned heavily on his stick as he hobbled painfully to the tea table, where Joan, the regular Health Care Assistant (HCA), was serving tea.

As Alfred sat down, Joan took his stick and put it in the corner 'out of the way', she said, but also out of his reach. She was chatting to everyone as she offered the biscuits to Alfred which he refused, indicating his waistline. Joan patted him on the head and told him he was a 'very good boy' and moved on, oblivious to his reaction. Alfred became suddenly angry, pushed back his chair and struggled to get up. He shook my hand away as I tried to help him so I quickly fetched his stick and suggested we go to a quiet corner for our chat. I felt anxious about his anger as it seemed out of character.

The meaning of 'old'

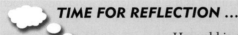 **TIME FOR REFLECTION ...**

- How old is old?
- Is 'old' simply a matter of chronological age? (Not the same question.)

Since the industrial revolution in the mid-nineteenth century, average female life expectancy in Western societies has increased from about 45 to currently more than 80 (corresponding to an increase of 2.3 years per decade). Men's life expectancy has also risen, although more slowly: the gap between females and males has widened from 2 to 6 years (Westendorp and Kirkwood, 2007).

For the first time in 2009, the percentage of the U.K. population aged under 16 fell below the percentage of the population over 60. The fastest-growing age group is now the over-80s (McVeigh, 2009). If current trends continue, the number of people over 65 will triple from 4.6 million (2007) to 15.5 million (2074); the number of centenarians (people of 100 or more) will increase 100 times, from 10,000 to 1 million (Brown, 2007) (see Figure 19.1).

Because of this *demographic imperative* (Swensen, 1983), developmental psychologists have become increasingly interested in our later years. But what do we mean by 'old'? Kastenbaum's (1979) *The ages of me* questionnaire assesses how people see themselves at the present moment in relation to their ages (see Box 19.1 and Figure 19.1).

Few people, irrespective of their chronological ages, describe themselves *consistently* (i.e., they tend to give *different* responses to the different questionnaire items). For example, people over 20 (including those in their 70s and 80s)

Figure 19.1 The oldest person who has ever lived: Jeanne Calment died in 1997 at the age of 122.

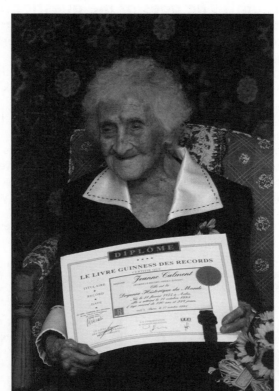

usually describe themselves as feeling younger than their chronological age. We also generally consider ourselves to be *too* old.

Alfred is 75 and looks younger; he's very trim, energetic and is usually affable. His osteoarthritic hip indicates bodily ageing (i.e. his biological age); this limits his activity, which affects his functional, and no doubt his social, age. His condition is painful, which may affect his subjective age. When he was settled with his tea I asked how he was feeling and he said, 'Fine, except when I'm treated as if I'm in my second childhood'. So although the age perceptions seem interrelated, Alfred's negative feelings seemed to stem more from his functional age and the attitude of others.

TIME FOR REFLECTION ...

- How old are you according to Kastenbaum's questionnaire?
- Which measure of age is most significant in defining current health-care policy?

Box 19.1 Kastenbaum's *The ages of me* questionnaire

- My *chronological age* is my actual or official age, dated from my time of birth. My chronological age is …
- My *biological age* refers to the state of my face and body. In other people's eyes, I look as though I am about … years of age. In my own eyes, I look like someone of about … years of age.
- My *subjective age* is indicated by how I feel. Deep down inside, I really feel like a person of about … years of age.
- My *functional age*, which is closely related to my *social age*, refers to the kind of life I lead, what I am able to do, the status I believe I have, whether I work, have dependent children and live in my own home. My thoughts and interests are like those of a person of about … years of age, and my position in society is like that of a person of about … years of age (Figure 19.2).

Figure 19.2 While (c) might depict someone's chronological age, (a) might correspond to his biological age and (b) might represent his subjective age.

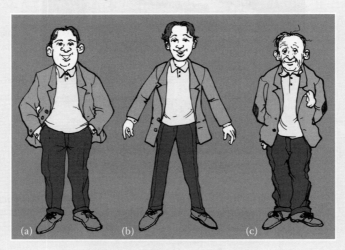

Source: Adapted from Kastenbaum, R., *Growing Old – Years of Fulfilment*, Harper & Row, London, 1979.

Ageism

It seems, then, that knowing a person's chronological age tells us little about the sort of life that person leads or what she/he is like. However, one of the dangerous aspects of ageism is that chronological age is assumed to be an accurate indicator of all the other ages.

According to Bromley (1977), most people react adversely to 'the elderly' because they seem to deviate from our concept of 'normal' human beings. As part of the 'welfarist approach' to understanding the problems of an ageing society (Fennell et al., 1988), 'they' (i.e., elderly people) are designated as different, occupying another world from 'us' – a process that for all perceived minorities tends to be dehumanising and sets lower or different standards of social value or individual worth (Manthorpe, 1994).

According to Penedo et al. (2010),

> Older adults are often stereotyped as a critically limited subgroup of the population that suffers from severe limitations in social, physical and functional capacity. While this perception likely represents our own fears of ageing, it significantly misrepresents the realities for a considerable majority of older adults.

Using a collective term, whatever it is, for a particular group of people indicates stereotyping, a way of thinking, **which may lead to discrimination**– in this case, 'ageism'.

Effects of stereotyping

It is not stereotypes themselves that are dangerous or objectionable, but how they affect behaviour (Key Study 19.1) (see Chapter 7). While Bargh et al.'s (1996) study shows that anyone can be affected by negative stereotypes, under normal circumstances it is elderly people who are affected by negative stereotypes of the elderly. The same applies, of course, to ethnic minority groups and race stereotypes and to women and gender stereotypes (again see Chapter 7) (see Box 19.2).

Reading all this makes me uncomfortably aware of how easy it is to make stereotypical assumptions about patients.

KEY STUDY 19.1

How stereotypes can slow you down

- Under the guise of a language proficiency experiment, 30 male and female college students were asked to unscramble sentences scattered with either negative age-related words (such as 'grey'/'bingo'/wrinkle') or neutral, non-age-specific words. This represented the *priming phase*, making attributes of the elderly (the 'elderly stereotype') more accessible in participants' minds. Words relating to slowness (a common part of the elderly stereotype) were *excluded*.

- Students who had sorted sentences containing negative words walked down the corridor at the end of the experiment significantly more slowly and remembered less about the experiment than students who had sorted neutral words.

Box 19.2 Can stereotypes make you ill?

- In April 2000, the charity Age Concern highlighted the plight of Jill Baker, a cancer patient in her 60s. She was shocked to discover that, despite still being in a generally good state of health, a junior doctor she had never met had put 'not for resuscitation' on her records.
- According to Ebrahim (in Payne, 2000), 'Medical students still rejoice in their stereotypes of "geriatric crumbly" and "GOMER" (get out of my emergency room) patients.'
- Ebrahim cites U.S. evidence showing that 'do not resuscitate' orders are commonly used for people with HIV, blacks, alcohol misusers and non-English speakers, suggesting that doctors have stereotypes of who is not worth saving.
- In the United Kingdom, 1 in 20 people aged over 65 had been refused treatment by the National Health Service, with 1 in 10 over-50s believing they were treated differently (i.e., worse) because of their age (based on an Age Concern survey).

Adler (2000) cites American research by Levy and her colleagues showing that stereotypes can affect how elderly people think about themselves in ways that can be detrimental to their mental and physical health. In one study, elderly participants spent a few minutes concentrating on a computer-based reaction-time test. Age-related words were subliminally presented on the screen (too quickly to be consciously registered) and were either negative (e.g., 'senile, 'forgetful', diseased'), or positive (e.g., 'wise', 'astute', 'accomplished').

The participants were subsequently asked if they would request an expensive but potentially life-saving medical treatment, without which they would die within a month. Most of those who had 'seen' the positive words (evoking a positive stereotype) chose the life-saving treatment, but most of those who were exposed to negative words declined.

In another study, participants were challenged with a series of math problems following 10-minute exposure to positive or negative words. The latter showed signs of stress – heart rate, blood pressure and skin conductance all increased, and stayed high for over 30 minutes. In contrast, those exposed to positive words sailed through the challenge stress-free.

Since many studies have linked chronic stress to disease (see Chapter 5), Levy suspects that repeated triggering of negative stereotypes over a period of several years may be making elderly people ill (Adler, 2000).

Stereotypes of older people – 'the elderly' – are more deeply entrenched than (mis)conceptions of gender differences. It is therefore not surprising that people are overwhelmingly unenthusiastic about becoming 'old' (Stuart-Hamilton, 1997).

TIME FOR REFLECTION ...

- If you are being honest, do you stereotype elderly people?
- If so, what characteristics do you attribute to them?

Joan's remark obviously caused Alfred stress; I could almost see his BP rising!

 Basing treatment on chronological age makes no sense; no age groups are all equally healthy. Alfred was a talented tennis player when young and worked as a tennis coach and manager of a large sports shop. He conscientiously watches his weight, follows a recommended 'arthritis' diet and exercises daily, although he finds weight-bearing ones painful now. 'I've resorted to playing computer games and Sudoku instead,' he said, sounding apologetic.

Bodily changes and advanced old age

According to Coleman and O'Hanlon (2004), the lack of research interest in *advanced old age* (AOA) has produced an imbalance in theories of ageing. A major focus of recent developmental accounts has been on the concept of '*successful ageing*' (Rowe and Kahn, 1998).

Successful ageing

 TIME FOR REFLECTION …

- What do you understand by the term '*successful ageing*'?

Successful ageing is typically measured in terms of health, finances and social relationships. More adults are reaching age 65 in better physical and mental health than ever before, as a consequence of improved diet, physical fitness and health care (Penedo et al., 2010). However, 'normal' or primary ageing involves some physical decline, such as decreased mobility and sensory abilities, slower reaction time and mild memory deficits and decreased pulmonary and immune function (Rowe and Kahn, 1987).

Some researchers have proposed a *continuum perspective* of successful ageing: at one extreme, we can eliminate ageing through specific treatments or interventions, while at the other we face inevitable ageing with few opportunities to postpone or stop the negative effects. In the middle of this continuum, we find successful ageing: here we can improve the disease and disability associated with ageing through lifestyle choices (Penedo et al., 2010).

A more balanced view is the McArthur Model of Successful Ageing (Rowe and Kahn, 1998). This is described in (Box 19.3).

Strawbridge et al. (1998) have proposed that *frailty* (a functional loss in at least two of physical and nutritional status, cognitive functioning and sensory functioning) is much more useful than *disability* in relation to late life. They found that only 20% in the 65–74 age group were frail, compared with 32% of 75–84-year-olds and 49% of the over-85s. This is consistent with the clinical observation that half of the 'very old' (i.e., 85 and over) need practical help. So,

Box 19.3 The McArthur model of successful ageing

This proposes three interactive components:

1. Absence of disabling disease and the disability associated with the disease or no significant physical impairment
2. Maintaining high cognitive and physical function, thus allowing the individual to be active and competent (see *Activity (or re-engagement) theory*, pages 431 and 432)
3. Engagement with life as reflected by involvement in productive activities and involvement with others (again, Activity (or re-engagement) theory)

Research shows that, for most of us, growing old is not filled with despair and depression; the few personality changes that do take place in late life are typically positive ones and older adults maintain relatively high levels of psychological well-being (Costa et al., 2008). This 'paradox of well-being' suggests that despite difficult circumstances, people in later life feel good about themselves and their situations. Therefore, successful ageing is the *norm*. But despite these findings, we typically view successful ageing as the exception rather than the rule.

According to Coleman and O'Hanlon (2004), one effect of this emphasis on successful ageing has been to stigmatise further *very* old people. If successful ageing includes the avoidance of disease and disability, preservation of cognitive abilities and an active life, then sooner or later many people will fail the test. As Tobin (1999) puts it, 'What comes after successful ageing?' Towards the end of his long life, Erikson questioned whether there might be a stage beyond *ego integrity* (versus *despair* – see page 434).

Source: Rowe, J.W., Kahn, R.L., *Successful Ageing*, Plenum Press, New York, 1998.

85 seems to be a convenient age to define late life (AOA) at the present time in most Western societies. It is also worth noting that this age group are 'survivors': they represent just 25% of their original birth cohort (while those over 95 represent a mere 3%) (Smith and Baltes, 1997).

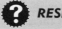 *Frail is the last word I'd use to describe Alfred; he's at the early end (the intervention stage) of the ageing continuum. When his hip replacement is done I'm sure he'll be back to 'successfully ageing' status.*

Cognitive changes in late adulthood

Until recently, and consistent with the *decrement model* (see *Introduction and overview*), it was commonly believed that intellectual capacity peaked in the late teens or early 20s, levelled off and then began to decline fairly steadily during middle age and more rapidly in old age.

? RESEARCH QUESTION
- Why cannot we generalise from cross-sectional studies?

The evidence on which this claim was based came from *cross-sectional studies* (studying different age groups at the same time).

We cannot draw firm conclusions from such studies, because the age groups compared represent different generations with different experiences (the *cohort effect*). Unless we know how 60-year-olds, say, performed when they were 40 and 20, it is impossible to say whether or not intelligence declines with age.

An alternative methodology is the *longitudinal study*, in which the same people are tested and retested at various times during their lives. Several such studies have produced data contradicting the results of cross-sectional studies, indicating that at least some people retain their intellect well into middle age and beyond (Holahan and Sears, 1995). However, the evidence suggests that there are some age-related changes in different kinds of intelligence and aspects of memory.

Alfred **seems** as mentally alert as he ever was, but this highlights the difficulty in establishing individual baseline measures for psychological, as well as physiological, observations.

Changes in intelligence

Although psychologists have always disagreed about the definition of intelligence, there is general acceptance that it is *multidimensional* (composed of several different abilities). An important – and very relevant – distinction is that between crystallised and fluid intelligence.

- *Crystallised intelligence* results from accumulated knowledge, including a knowledge of how to reason, language skills and an understanding of technology. This type of intelligence is linked to education, experience and cultural background and is measured by tests of general information.
- *Fluid intelligence* is the ability to solve novel and unusual problems (those not experienced before). It allows us to perceive and draw inferences about relationships among patterns of stimuli and to conceptualise abstract information, which aids problem-solving. Fluid intelligence is measured by tests using novel and unusual problems not based on specific knowledge or particular previous learning.

Crystallised intelligence *increases* with age, and people tend to continue improving their performance until near the end of their lives (Horn, 1982). Using the *cross-longitudinal method* (in which *different* age groups are *retested* over a long period of time), Schaie and Hertzog (1983) reported that fluid intelligence *declines* for all age groups over time, peaking between 20 and 30.

TIME FOR REFLECTION ...

- Does slower necessarily mean less intelligent?
- Why should Alfred be encouraged to pursue his latest hobbies?

Explaining changes in intelligence

Intelligence (IQ) tests are typically heavily loaded with *fluid* intelligence questions at the expense of crystallised, and they are also usually *timed*. This implies that tests of general intelligence are biased against older people. But tests of crystallised intelligence are, arguably, biased *in favour* of older people (there is usually *no* time limit). However, removing the time limit from tests of fluid intelligence does not remove the age difference – but it does reduce it. So, the preservation of crystallised intelligence in later life is, in part, illusory (Stuart-Hamilton, 2000).

Physiological changes (such as cardiovascular and metabolic dysfunction) can have serious effects on physiological processes in the brain; in turn, these can lower intellectual performance. For example, *response times* (RTs) are a good indicator of how efficiently the nervous system operates. Not only do we get slower as we get older, but this slowing is strongly correlated with IQ test scores: the slower the RTs, the lower the test score (the *general slowing hypothesis* – Stuart-Hamilton, 2003).

The prime cause of the decline in intelligence in elderly people is a slowing of nervous system processes (Stuart-Hamilton, 2003). Some argue that an even better indication of change is the state of the *sensory systems* (as measured by vision and hearing). A composite index composed of measures of sensory efficiency correlates impressively with IQ test scores (Baltes and Lindenberger, 1997). Alternative measures of intellectual activity (such as problem-solving or memory) are highly correlated with IQ (Rabbitt, 1993).

Alfred no longer has to meet the demands of a work environment so if he takes a bit longer to solve his puzzles or complete his games, does it matter? And does it prove he has less 'fluid intelligence'?

Changes in memory

- Some aspects of memory appear to decline with age, possibly because we become less effective at processing information (which may underlie cognitive changes in general) (Stuart-Hamilton, 1994).
- On *recall* tests, older adults generally perform more poorly than younger adults.
- On *recognition* tests, the differences between younger and older people are less apparent and may even disappear.
- As far as everyday memory is concerned, the evidence indicates that elderly people do have trouble recalling events from their youth and early lives (Miller and Morris, 1993).
- Significant memory deficits are one feature of *dementia* (mental frailty) (see Chapter 11).

Alfred complains his short-term memory has deteriorated, which I expected. But I thought older people enjoyed talking about their past because they had little to look forward to; I fear that was another stereotypical assumption.

Social changes in late adulthood

Social disengagement theory

According to Manthorpe (1994), Cumming and Henry's (1961) *social disengagement theory* (SDT) represented the first major attempt to produce a theory about individuals' relationships with society. It is based on a 5-year study of 275 50–90-year-olds in Kansas City. SDT claims that social disengagement involves the *mutual withdrawal* of society from the individual (through compulsory retirement, children growing up and leaving home, the death of a spouse and so on) and of the individual from society (Cumming, 1975).

Cumming sees disengagement as having three components:

1. *Shrinkage of life space*: The tendency to interact with fewer other people as we grow older and to occupy fewer roles.
2. *Increased individuality*: In the roles that remain, older people are much less governed by strict rules and expectations.
3. *Acceptance* (even embrace) *of these changes*: Withdrawal is a voluntary, natural and inevitable process and represents the most appropriate and successful way of growing old.

As far as society is concerned, the individual's withdrawal is part of an inevitable move towards death – the ultimate disengagement (Manthorpe, 1994). By replacing older individuals with younger people, society renews itself and the elderly are free to die (Bromley, 1988).

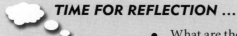 Manthorpe's (1994) view of old age predominantly as a progression towards death is so pessimistic! Disengagement may be welcome for some, but his present disability stops Alfred from socialising as much as he would like. I know he has plans!

An evaluation of social disengagement theory

> **TIME FOR REFLECTION …**
>
> - What are the implications of SDT for the current emphasis on caring for elderly people in the community?

- While the first two components are difficult to dispute, the third is more controversial because of its view of disengagement as a natural, voluntary and inevitable process, rather than an imposed one (Bee, 1994).
- Bromley (1988) argues that such a view of ageing has detrimental *practical* consequences for the elderly, such as encouraging a policy of segregation, even indifference, and the very destructive belief that old age has no value. An even more serious criticism concerns whether everyone actually does disengage.

Havighurst *et al's* (1968) and Bromley's (1988) *comments are convincing and confirm that Alfred may not have voluntarily 'disengaged'. I think he's a reorganiser; he has an outgoing personality and been involved in raising funds for the Stroke Association since his wife died. And recently he joined the local U3A which he said has lots of activities that interest him.*

Importance of friendships

Although many of these losses are beyond the older person's control (Rosnow, 1985), such as retirement, *friendships* are voluntary, non-institutionalised and relatively enduring relationships that offer comfort and stability. Informal support from friends (and other primary relationships) also reduces dependency on social security agencies, the helping professions and other formal organisations (Duck, 1991; Rainey, 1998) (Key Study 19.2). It is the choice element that differentiates

---

KEY STUDY 19.2

Do all older people disengage?

- Havighurst et al. followed up about half the sample originally studied by Cumming and Henry (1961).
- Although increasing age was accompanied by increasing disengagement, at least some remained active and engaged, and they tended to be the happiest have the highest morale and live the longest; this contradicts SDT's view that withdrawal from mainstream society is a natural and inherent part of the ageing process (Bee, 1994).
- While some people may choose to lead socially isolated lives and find contentment in them, such disengagement does not appear to be necessary for overall mental health in old age.
- Havighurst et al. also identified several different *personality types*. These included the following:
  a. *Reorganisers*, who were involved in a wide range of activities and reorganised their lives to compensate for lost activities
  b. The *disengaged*, who voluntarily moved away from role commitments
- Consistent with SDT, the disengaged reported low levels of activity but high 'life satisfaction'. However, the disposition to disengage is a *personality dimension* as well as a characteristic of ageing (Bromley, 1988).
- SDT focuses on *quantitative* changes, such as the reduced number of relationships and roles in old age. But for Carstensen (1996), it is the *qualitative* changes that are crucial:

  Although age is associated with many losses, including loss of power, social partners, physical health, cognitive efficiency, and, eventually, life itself – and although this list of losses encompasses the very things that younger people typically equate with happiness – research suggests that older people are at least as satisfied with their lives as their younger counterparts.

Source: Havighurst, R.J. et al. *Middle Age and Ageing*, University of Chicago Press, Chicago, 1968.

friendships from other types of relationships (Baltes and Baltes, 1986), providing older people with control over at least one life domain (Rainey, 1998).

These findings regarding the role of friendships and other relationships are consistent with *socio-emotional selectivity theory* (see pages 432 through 434).

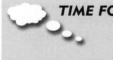 *When I asked Alfred if he enjoyed the weekly meetings at the Arthritis Club he laughed and said, 'Not a lot, but it gets me out.' As he seems to have little physical contact with his family, he may well be lonely.*

Activity (or re-engagement) theory

The major alternative to SDT is *activity* (or *re-engagement*) *theory* (AT) (Havighurst, 1964; Maddox, 1964). Except for inevitable biological and health changes, older people are essentially the same as middle-aged people, with the same psychological and social needs. Decreased social interaction in old age is the result of the withdrawal of an inherently ageist society from the ageing person and happens against the wishes of most elderly people. The withdrawal *is not* mutual.

Optimal ageing involves staying active and managing to resist the 'shrink-age' of the social world. This can be achieved by maintaining the activities of middle age for as long as possible and then finding substitutes for work or retirement (such as leisure or hobbies) and for spouses and friends upon their death (such as grandchildren). It is important for older adults to maintain their role counts, to ensure they always have several different roles to play.

This makes me feel sad for Alfred; his roles changed dramatically in retirement. He lost his work role of manager, but became secretary of the bowling club. He gave that up to become a carer; he admitted learning to be a housekeeper and nurse had been hard but now he's also lost that role – along with the most significant one of husband.

An evaluation of activity theory

> **TIME FOR REFLECTION ...**
>
> - Can you think of any objections to activity theory?
> - Is it realistic?
> - Does it repeat any of the mistakes of SDT?

According to Bond et al. (1993), AT can be criticised for being

> ... unrealistic because the economic, political and social structure of society prevents the older worker from maintaining a major activity of middle age, namely, 'productive' employment.

The implication seems to be that there really is no substitute for paid employment (at least for men). According to Dex and Phillipson (1986), society appears to measure people's worth by their ability to undertake paid labour, and the more autonomous people are in their working practices, the more respect they seem to deserve. When someone retires, they not only lose their autonomy and right to work for money, but they also lose their *identity*: they cease to be a participant in society and their status is reduced to 'pensioner/senior citizen' or simply 'old person'.

- Just as disengagement may be involuntary (as in the case of poor health), so we may face involuntarily high levels of activity (as in looking after grandchildren). Both disengagement and activity may, therefore, be equally maladaptive. SDT might actually *under*estimate, and AT *over*estimate, the degree of control people have over the 'reconstruction' of their lives.
- Additionally, both theories represent *options* (Hayslip and Panek, 1989) and people will select the styles of ageing best suited to their personalities and past experience or lifestyle. There is no single 'best way' to age (Neugarten and Neugarten, 1987). For Turner and Helms (1989), personality is the key factor, and neither theory can adequately explain successful ageing.

As a manager Alfred was used to being in control and was very active but now his arthritis prevents him from choosing a way of ageing that fits his personality. He also confided that paying for help and extra treats for his wife had been costly so he is less well off; that too could limit his social activities.

Socio-emotional selectivity theory

According to *socio-emotional selectivity theory* (SST) (Carstensen, 1992, 1993, 1995; Carstensen and Turk-Charles, 1994; Lang and Cartsensen, 2002), social contact is motivated by various goals, including basic survival, information-seeking, development of self-concept and the regulation of emotion. While these all operate throughout life, the importance of specific goals varies, depending on one's place in the life cycle. For example, when *emotional regulation* (how we determine which emotions we have, when we have them and how we experience and express them) is the major goal, people are highly selective in their choice of social partners, preferring familiar others. This selectivity is at its peak in infancy (see Chapter 14) and old age: elderly people turn increasingly to friends and adult children for emotional support (see Figure 19.3).

- According to SST, a major factor contributing to these changes in social motives is *construal of the future*. When the future is perceived as largely open-ended, long-term goals assume great significance. But when the future is perceived as limited, attention shifts to the *present*. Immediate needs, such as emotional states, become more salient. So, contrary to SDT (which sees reduced social contact as being caused by emotional states becoming diluted), SST predicts that emotional concerns will become *more* important in old age. Health is the other major factor that accounts for these changes. In many cases, healthy older people *do not* show these patterns of social activity (Carstensen, 1991).

When his wife died, Alfred lost his most significant emotional role and support; that, and the loss of his work role must affect his self-concept (see Chapter 6, page 248) His family don't live near, so he may well come to the Arthritis Club simply for company. I'm convinced when Alfred's functional ability (health) is restored he'll be socially active again.

An evaluation of SST

If SST is correct, it would follow that when younger people hold expectations about the future that are similar to those of elderly people, they should make the same kinds of social choices as those typically made by the latter (Key Study 19.3).

Figure 19.3 Idealised illustration of the lifespan trajectory. (From Carstensen, L.L., *The Developmental Psychologists: Research Adventures across the Life Span*, McGraw-Hill, New York, Copyright 1996, reproduced with permission of the McGraw-Hill Companies.)

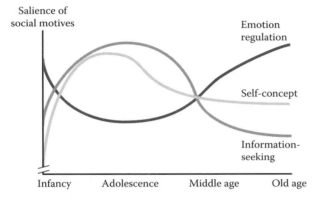

KEY STUDY 19.3

How a limited future can influence current concerns

- Carstensen describes a study involving a group of healthy gay men, a group of HIV-positive, asymptomatic gay men and a group of HIV-positive, symptomatic gay men. A group of young, middle-aged and old men representing the general population served as a control group.
- The social preferences of the healthy gay men were similar to those of the young men from the control group. Those of the asymptomatic group mimicked those of the middle-aged controls, while those of the symptomatic group were strikingly similar to those of the oldest control participants. In other words,

  The closer the men were to the end of their lives, the greater weight they placed on affective qualities of prospective social partners … changes in social preferences appear to be altered in much the same way when futures are limited by age as when futures are limited by disease …. (Carstensen, 1996)

Source: Carstensen, L.L., *The Developmental Psychologists: Research Adventures across the Life Span*, McGraw-Hill, New York, 1996.

- Lang and Carstensen (2002) found that older individuals perceived their time as more limited than younger adults and thus prioritised emotionally meaningful goals, such as being with close friends and family, rather than meeting new people. Adult children not only stay in contact with their elderly parents but also continue to share close emotional relationships with them (Lang and Carstensen, 1998).

- Age-related reduction in social contact appears to be highly selective (rather than reflecting a reduced capacity), such that interaction is limited to those people who are most familiar and can provide the greatest emotional security and comfort. This is an excellent strategy when time and social energy need to be invested wisely (Carstensen, 1996).

- However, this optimism may reflect a context in which the older person is dealing with familiar situations and can rely on well-rehearsed solutions to emotional problems. But where they are having to deal with novel and demanding situations, older people may experience greater levels of disturbance (Labouvie-Vief, 2005)

Alfred is resourceful – he told me (proudly) he's set up Skype on his computer so he can see and talk to his grandchildren. I said I was very impressed (which on reflection, I fear may be patronising!).

Psychosocial theory

Another alternative to SDT and AT is Erikson's *psychosocial theory* (see Chapters 17 and 18). A more valid and useful way of looking at what all elderly people have in common might be to examine the importance of old age as a stage of development, albeit the last (which is where its importance lies).

Erikson's theory suggests that in old age, there is a conflict between *ego integrity* (the positive force) and *despair* (the negative force). As with the other psychosocial stages, we cannot avoid the conflict altogether, which occurs as a result of biological, psychological and social forces. The task is to end this stage, and hence life, with greater ego integrity than despair, and this requires us to take stock of our life, reflect on it and assess how worthwhile and fulfilling it has been.

Characteristics of ego integrity

- We believe that life does have a purpose and makes sense.
- We accept that, within the context of our lives as a whole, what happened was somehow inevitable and could only have happened when and how it did.
- We believe that all life's experiences offer something of value and that we can learn from everything that happens to us. Looking back, we can see how we have grown psychologically as a result of life's ups and downs. We see our parents in a new light and understand them better, because we have lived through our own adulthood and have probably raised children of our own.
- We realise that we share with all other human beings, past, present and future, the inevitable cycle of birth and death. Whatever the historical,

cultural and other differences, we all have this much in common. In the light of this, death 'loses its sting'.

In *The Life Cycle Completed* (1997), Erikson detailed some of the issues involved in the challenge of old age by pointing to the struggle for finding a sense of *integration* in one's identity: this occurs through such means as *reviewing* one's life to find threads of continuity and attempting to reconcile those elements that may have long been denied or abandoned. It also involves coming to terms with the many changes and losses that each one of us is likely to encounter.

Just as integrity's ultimate demand is facing death (ideally, with some degree of acceptance), so *fear of death* is the most conspicuous symptom of despair. In despair, we express the belief that it is too late to undo the past and turn the clock back to right wrongs or do what has not been done. Life is not a 'rehearsal'; this is the only chance we get.

That's what Alfred used to say about his wife's 'treats'; he didn't want there to be anything to regret. I believe he intends to apply that philosophy to his own life now.

Reminiscence and the life review

According to Coleman and O'Hanlon (2004), *reminiscence* is the process of recalling past events and experiences. It illustrates the practical relevance of developmental theory, especially Erikson's concept of ego integrity. Encouraging older people to reminisce is now seen as a natural activity and very much part of care work (which was not so 30 years ago). But it owes an even greater debt to Butler's (1963) *Life Review* (LR), which refers to a more focused consideration of one's past life as a whole.

Butler proposed that LR is a normative process that all people undergo as they realise their lives are coming to an end. While this may be beneficial, a failure to resolve troublesome memories may produce feelings of despair and LR requires high levels of inner skills that most older people may not possess. Reminiscence in adulthood seems to be more often used to reassert previous patterns of self-understanding than to create the new understanding arising from LR (Coleman and O'Hanlon, 2004).

Butler's LR implies the search for meaning through reflection on one's life experience. A longitudinal study begun in the late 1920s showed that although LR was not associated with self-ratings of life satisfaction in those in their late 60s to mid-70s, it was positively related to ratings of creativity, spirituality and generativity (Wink, 1999). Coleman and O'Hanlon (2004) consider these to be much more socially relevant than subjective well-being.

Wink and Schiff (2002) believe that LR is an adaptive response to ageing in those who have encountered marked difficulties in their lives; for the majority, it is *not* a necessary adaptation. Indeed, Butler originally described LR as a means of achieving self-change, but this is a difficult and anxiety-provoking task, especially for those (the majority) who are reasonably satisfied with their lives and are not seeking self-growth.

In recording this incident I used the stages of Gibbs' reflective framework.

Because I knew some of Alfred's history already my overall feelings were respect for him; he'd adapted to changed circumstances and learned new roles very successfully. He cared well for his wife, respecting her dignity and independence and I think it's right he should feel entitled to the same kind of health care for himself.

The good things about this experience for me were learning the importance of older people's individuality and experiencing how easy it is to stereotype them.

Reading this chapter has shown we shouldn't make assumptions about what older people think and want; while the theories conflict at times, they all add to understanding the complexities of caring for them. There is no single 'best way' to age (Neugarten and Neugarten, 1987), people will select styles of ageing to suit them (Hayslip and Panek 1989). Turner and Helms (1989) suggest personality is the key factor in how people age, but Alfred's beliefs, life events, financial situation and, perhaps most of all, his present health status are relevant. This again shows the importance of considering physical, psychological and social factors in providing care. I regret I didn't say anything to Joan about how Alfred felt; another time I would make her aware of her unintentional (and my unconscious) patronising attitude; it might have led to a beneficial discussion of stereotyping!

Conclusions

According to Voss (2002),

> Older people may not feel old; they may not feel any different than they did during their younger years. They simply face life from an angle that bears the shadow of death more acutely than before. This provides them with an insight unavailable to others and the wisdom not yet achieved by those trying to help them. Acknowledging this is an invaluable part of promoting the respect that older people deserve as fellow human beings ... we should ... help older adults to welcome integrity and wisdom, in whatever form, at the conclusion of their winter years.

CHAPTER SUMMARY

- While 'growing up' has positive connotations, 'growing old' has negative ones, reflecting the *decrement model*. An alternative, more positive view is the *personal growth model*.
- Far from being natural, ageing is an artefact of culture and was rare in humans until 200 years ago. Average life expectancy for males and females has been steadily increasing during that time.
- One feature of *ageism* is the assumption that *chronological age* is an accurate indicator of *biological*, *subjective*, *functional* and *social age*. *Stereotypes* of the elderly are deeply rooted in rapidly changing Western societies, where their experience and wisdom are no longer valued.

- An alternative view of successful ageing to a continuum perspective is the McArthur Model.
- Research suggests that for most people, growing old is not filled with despair and depression: personality changes are mostly positive and relatively high levels of psychological well-being are maintained.
- The claim that intelligence declines fairly rapidly in old age is based on *cross-sectional studies*, which suffer from the problem of the *cohort effect*. *Longitudinal studies* indicate that while *crystallised intelligence* increases with age, *fluid intelligence* declines for all age groups over time.
- Some aspects of *memory* decline with age, perhaps due to less effective *information-processing*. Older adults generally perform more poorly than younger adults on *recall* tests, but the differences are much smaller when *recognition* tests are used.
- *Negative cultural stereotypes* of ageing actually cause memory decline in the elderly and may become *self-fulfilling prophecies*.
- The most controversial claim made by *social disengagement theory* (*SDT*) is that the elderly accept and even welcome disengagement and that this is a natural and inevitable process.
- SDT emphasises the *quantitative* changes to the exclusion of *qualitative* changes, which may become more important with age. The latter includes *friendships*, which are under the older person's control and provide essential informal support.
- *Activity theory* (*AT*) claims that older people are psychologically and socially essentially the same as middle-aged people. The withdrawal of society and the individual is not mutual, and optimal ageing involves maintaining the activities of middle age for as long as possible.
- Socio-emotional selectivity theory (*SST*) maintains that for the elderly, *emotional regulation* assumes major importance, making them highly selective as regards social partners. This change in social motives is largely determined by *construal of the future*.
- According to Erikson's *psychosocial theory*, old age involves a conflict between *ego integrity* and *despair*. The task of ageing is to assess and evaluate life's value and meaning. Despair is characterised by a fear of death.
- The process of *reminiscing* has been influenced both by Erikson's concept of ego integrity and by Butler's *Life Review*.

Glossary

Note: In most cases, terms in italics are defined in bold.

Acceptance and commitment therapy (ACT): An approach to pain management that aims to help individuals identify their priorities and achieve their goals by focusing on the present moment without struggling to eliminate the distress caused by their pain. Assumes that pain is partially uncontrollable and is essential in evolutionary terms.

Accommodation: In Piaget's theory, the modification of the child's existing schemas to match new environmental demands. Complementary to *assimilation*.

Accommodative coping: An attempt to adjust to the problem (e.g., pain) rather than change the problem itself (as in *assimilative coping*).

Addiction: Traditionally used to denote a physiological compulsion to keep taking a particular drug (including alcohol), despite the awful physical and psychological symptoms produced when trying to stop. More recently, it refers to a field of study covering *substance abuse* and *dependence*.

Adherence: Taking medication in the way that it was prescribed. There are various ways in which patients can deviate from doctors' recommendations, and non-adherence can be both intentional and unintentional.

Adoption studies: A way of overcoming family resemblance studies' confusion of genetic and environmental influences, as when the rates of a trait (such as schizophrenia) among separated identical twins (MZs) are compared with those for MZs reared together.

Affectionless psychopathy: The inability to have deep feelings for other people and the consequent lack of meaningful relationships, plus the inability to experience guilt – a major effect of *privation* (as in an institutional upbringing).

Agentic state: Seeing oneself as an instrument of an authority figure's will. According to Milgram, this is the essence of obedience and involves surrendering all responsibility for one's actions (the *autonomous state*).

Aggregation principle: The claim that only by sampling several instances of the attitude-relevant behaviour will the influence of specific factors (in addition to the attitude) 'cancel out'.

Alcohol dependence syndrome (ADS): A modified, more flexible version of the *disease model of alcohol dependence*; it takes account of psychological, rather than exclusively physiological, processes.

Allodynia: Tenderness in response to the nine paired 'tender points' on either side of the body being touched; a major symptom of fibromyalgia.

Allostatic load (or allostatis): Maintenance of physiological parameters outside the normal range to match chronic demands (either physical or psychological). Maintaining an allostatic load in the long term may cause pathology. Contrasted with *homeostasis*.

Analogy: Comparing something that is less well understood with something else that is better understood to make sense of the former. Often something complex is compared with something more simple. Since the 1950s and the development of computer science, the *computer analogy* has become very popular as a way of trying to understand how the mind works.

Animism: The belief that inanimate objects are alive.

Anterograde amnesia: The inability to store new memories.

Anticipatory grief: Grief that begins before someone has died, including grieving for their own death in the case of terminally ill patients.

Anticonformity: Refusing to conform as an attempt to remain independent as a matter of principle.

Aphasia (or dysphasia): Can be *receptive* (difficulty understanding what others are saying), *expressive* (difficulty expressing what you want to say) or *mixed/global*.

Artificialism: According to Piaget, young children's perception of the natural world as existing exclusively to solve human problems.

Asch paradigm: An experimental method for testing conformity, involving a single naive participant and a number of stooges/confederates, who give the wrong answer on an unambiguous perceptual task. Conformity is measured as the number of critical trials on which the naive participant gives the same wrong answer as the stooges.

Assimilation: In Piaget's theory, the process by which the child incorporates new information into existing *schemas*. Complementary to *accommodation*.

Assimilative coping: An attempt to cure or reduce pain through medical or non-medical methods.

Attachment: An intense emotional relationship specific to two people, that endures over time and in which prolonged separation from the attachment figure induces distress (*separation anxiety*).

Attachment process: According to Schaffer, a series of phases/stages the infant goes through from 6 weeks up to 9 months and beyond: *pre-attachment, indiscriminate attachment, discriminate attachment* and *multiple attachment*.

Attachment styles: Based on the *Strange Situation* (Ainsworth et al.), the classification of children as displaying either *secure* attachment or one of two types of *insecure* attachment (*anxious-avoidant/detached* and *anxious-resistant/ambivalent*).

Authoritarian personality: According to Adorno et al., someone who is prejudiced by virtue of a set of characteristics, including intolerance of ambiguity and upholding traditional values and life styles; these combine to make minorities 'them' (=bad).

Autistic hostility: Ignorance of those from whom we are segregated, resulting in a failure to understand the reasons for their actions.

Automatic intelligence: The ability to apply the intelligence we have acquired during our lifetime without having to think about it.

Autosomal recessive disease: A disease that requires the child to inherit two copies of the *mutant* gene (one from each parent) if the disease is to develop.

Aversion therapy: A form of *behaviour therapy* in which some undesirable behavioural response (e.g., drinking alcohol) to a particular stimulus (e.g., a whisky bottle) is removed by pairing the stimulus with an aversive stimulus (e.g., antabuse or some other emetic).

Behaviour genetics: The scientific study of the extent to which the variability of any given trait can be attributed to *heritability, shared environments* and *non-shared environments.*

Behaviour modification: The application of operant conditioning principles to the treatment of abnormal behaviour. An important example is the *token economy.*

Behaviour therapy: The application of classical conditioning principles to the treatment of abnormal behaviour. An important example is *systematic desensitisation.*

Behavioural neuroscience: An interdisciplinary discipline that uses behavioural techniques to understand brain function and neuroscientific techniques to throw light on behavioural processes.

Behavioural pharmacology: The use of *schedules of reinforcement/reinforcement contingencies* to assess the behavioural effects of new drugs that modify brain activity.

Biofeedback: A non-medical treatment for pain and stress-related symptoms, in which the patient learns to control normally involuntary autonomic activity (such as heart rate and blood pressure).

Biological age: How old the individual feels his/her body and face look to others – and him/herelf.

Biomedical model: The view that disease can be fully explained in terms of deviations from the norm of biological (somatic) factors; mind and body function independently and illness may have psychological consequences – but not psychological causes.

Biopsychosocial (BPS) model: In opposition to the *biomedical model*, the view that illness is often the product of a combination of biological, psychological and social factors. This is the model underpinning *health psychology.*

Bodily rhythm: A cyclical variation over some period of time (from less than 24 hours to 1 year) in physiological and/or psychological processes.

Catastrophisation: A distressed response to pain in which pain is viewed horrifically and the individual worries about its effects on his/her body.

Categorical self: How we classify ourselves in terms of age, gender and social roles.

Centration: Focusing on only a single perceptual quality at a time. Associated with the inability to *conserve.*

Chromosome: A highly folded and compressed stretch of *DNA*; every *gene* has a specific location on one of the 23 pairs of chromosomes (22 *autosomes* – non-sex chromosome – and one pair of *sex chromosomes*).

Circadian rhythm: Fluctuations in physiological and/or psychological processes that occur within a 24-hour cycle (circa = about, diem = a day).

Classical conditioning: A form of associative learning in which, following the repeated pairing of two previously unrelated stimuli, one comes to elicit an involuntary response previously only elicited by the other. Also known as *Pavlovian* or *respondent* conditioning.

Closed awareness: The dying patient's failure to recognise that s/he is dying, when everyone else does.

Cognition models: According to Ogden, models such as the health belief model (HBM), protection activation theory (PMT) and health action process approach (HAPA), which are specifically health models.

Cognitive behaviour therapy (CBT): The application of a variety of techniques designed to modify the person's dysfunctional beliefs and faulty information processing (cognitive restructuring). Derived from *behaviour therapy* and *psychoanalysis*, cognitive restructuring is, in turn, aimed at changing target emotions and behaviour. Major forms of CBT include Beck's treatment of automatic thoughts and Ellis's rational emotive therapy.

Cognitive consistency: A characteristic of human beings, who sort through and modify a large number of cognitions to achieve some degree of cognitive coherence.

Cognitive dissonance: According to Festinger, a state of 'psychological discomfort or tension' that arises when two simultaneously held cognitions are psychologically inconsistent; this motivates us to reduce it by achieving consonance.

Cognitive miser: A view of *stereotypes* as resource-saving devices that simplify the processing of information about other people.

Cognitive psychology: The scientific study of attention, memory, perception, language, reasoning and other 'higher-order' mental activities.

Cognitive science: The scientific study of cognition, involving a number of disciplines, including cognitive psychology and neuroscience.

Collectivism: One pole of one of the major *cultural syndromes* (individualism-collectivism), in which one's identity is defined by characteristics of the collective group one is permanently attached to (family, tribal or religious group, or country). Prevalent in Eastern and socialist societies.

Compliance: As a type of *conformity*, agreeing with others publicly while disagreeing with them privately. More generally, doing what others ask of us (a more active form of social influence); this includes *obeying* authority figures (such as doctors).

Conformity: Yielding to group pressure, both *membership* groups (such as family or peers) and *reference* groups (those whose values we aspire to but do not actually belong to); they can also have a *majority* or *minority* status.

Conformity bias: According to Moscovici, the tendency to regard all social influence as serving the need to adapt to the status quo for the sake of uniformity and stability.

Congenital analgesia: An extremely rare, genetically determined inability to perceive pain. Also known as *chronic indifference to pain*.

Conservation: Understanding that any quality (e.g., number, length, substance) remains the same despite physical changes in the arrangement of objects.

Constructivist: A way of describing Piaget's *asocial* theory of cognitive development (*the child-as-scientist*).

Contralateral hemiparesis: Muscle weakness in the *opposite* side of the body to the brain lesion caused by a stroke/*cerebrovascular accident* (CVA); usually affects the face, arm or leg.

Correlational study: Research method in which two or more variables are measured to see how they are *related*. Neither is manipulated and neither can logically be thought of as the cause of the other. Correlations can be positive or negative and can range from zero to one.

Cortical dementias: Those (such as Alzheimer's disease [AD]) that produce the classic neuropsychological deficit syndromes of symptoms of *amnesia* (memory loss), *aphasia/dysphasia* (loss of language function), *agnosia* (loss of perceptual – predominantly visual – function) and *apraxia/dyspraxia* (loss of simple motor skills).

Cross-cultural health psychology: The study of how cultural factors influence various aspects of health and the health of individuals and groups as they adapt to new 'host' cultural circumstances (*acculturation*).

Cross-longitudinal study: A study of different age groups retested over a long period.

Cross-sectional study: A study of different age groups at the same point in time.

Crystallised intelligence: Accumulated knowledge of how to reason, language and technology, linked to education, experience and cultural background. Tends to go on increasing with age.

Cupboard love theories (of attachment): Accounts of how attachments develop towards caregivers who satisfy the baby's basic needs for food. Examples include both Freud's psychoanalytic theory and behaviourist accounts based on conditioning.

Cultural syndrome: As defined by Triandis, a pattern of values, attitudes, beliefs, norms and behaviours that can be used to contrast one group of cultures with another group.

Deferred imitation: The ability to reproduce a previously witnessed action when the model is no longer present.

Demand characteristics: The sum total of the cues – explicit and implicit – within the experimental situation that convey to participants the hypothesis being tested. This is one feature of the experiment as a social situation.

Despair: In Erikson's theory, the negative outcome of old age – the major feature is fear of death.

Dignity therapy (DT): An individualised therapy that involves interviewing the dying patient regarding significant aspects of his/her life, recording and transcribing the interview, thus producing a lasting paper legacy that can be of benefit to both the patient and loved ones.

Disinhibited attachment (DA): A lack of close, confiding relationships, indiscriminate friendliness, a tendency to respond to all adults in the same way and go off with strangers; one form of *reactive attachment disorder* (RAD).

Divided attention: The ability to do two or more things at the same time (e.g., multi-tasking).

Dominant gene: A mutant gene, only one of which is required to produce the associated phenotype. In *autosomal dominant disease*, each individual has a 50% chance of passing the mutant gene to his/her children and also has the disease.

Dorsolateral prefrontal cortex (DPFC): One of the last brain regions to mature in the adolescent; involved in impulse control, judgement and decision-making and the processing of emotional information from the amygdala.

Dysarthria: Weakness to the muscles involved in speech.

Egocentrism: Seeing the world exclusively from one's own standpoint, hence failing to appreciate that others might see things differently. Children under seven are subject to the *egocentric illusion* – they fail to understand that what they see is relative to their own position. Related to *perspective-taking* (PT) ability.

Ego defence mechanisms: Unconscious ways of dealing with threats, either external or those that arise from within the individual; they involve some degree of self-deception and/or distortion of reality. For Freud, the critical defence was *repression*, a form of forgetting that involves forcing a threat out of consciousness and making it unconscious.

Ego identity: Erikson's term for a firm sense of who one is and what one stands for. This is the positive outcome of adolescence.

Ego integrity: According to Erikson, the positive outcome of old age; this includes the belief that life is meaningful, that we share certain basic experiences with all other human beings, and that death is not to be feared.

Ego psychology: A theoretical approach, promoted by Anna Freud, that focuses on the rational, decision-making ego, including the ego defence mechanisms, in contrast with Freud's emphasis on the id's innate drives.

Emotion-focused coping: According to Lazarus and Folkman, trying to reduce the negative emotions that are part of the experience of stress. Contrasted with *problem-focused coping*.

Emotional intelligence: A form of social intelligence that involves the ability to monitor one's own and others' emotions and to use this information to guide one's thoughts and actions.

Emotional labour: According to Hochschild, 'The induction or suppression of feeling in order to sustain an outward appearance that produces in others a sense of being cared for in a convivial safe place', that is, putting on a professional 'front' despite stressful working conditions.

Emotional regulation: Carstensen's term for the processes used to adjust our emotions: which ones we have, when we have them and how we experience and express them.

Emotionalism: How stroke patients become more emotional than before and/or have difficulty controlling their emotions.

Endorphins: The body's natural painkillers; they are pharmacologically identical to morphine.

Episodic analgesia: The experience of pain only minutes or hours after the injury that causes it.

Episodic memory: A form of autobiographical memory that stores a record of our past personal experiences.

Equilibration: In Piaget's theory, the process by which *equilibrium* (mental balance) is achieved – equilibrium is reached when the child can deal with most/all new experiences through *assimilation*.

Ethnocentrism: Judging all other groups as inferior compared with the superiority of one's own membership group.

Executive functioning: Decision-making, concentrating, planning, making judgements, and thinking under pressure.

Exhaustion: The final stage of the *general adaptation syndrome* (GAS), in which psychophysiological disorders develop, including high BP, CAD and CHD; Selye called these the *diseases of adaptation*.

Existential self: Our sense of continuity through time.

Experiment: A research method in which the researcher *manipulates* (deliberately changes) one variable (the *independent variable/IV*) to see its influence on another (the *dependent variable/DV*). These correspond, roughly, to cause and effect respectively. While most *true experiments* are conducted under controlled conditions in the laboratory, they can also occur in real-life (*naturalistic*) settings.

Experimenter bias: The unconscious influence an experimenter has on the outcome of an experiment over-and-above the 'formal', explicit features of the experimental situation (such as the hypothesis being tested and the measurement of variables).

External validity: In the context of an experiment, the degree to which the experimental situation resembles real-life situations and, thereby, the extent to which the results can be generalised to real-life situations. Also known as *ecological* validity or *mundane realism*.

Familial aggregation: The most basic method used to determine the *heritability* of a disease, in which the relatives of patients with a particular disorder are studied to determine if they are at greater risk of developing the disorder than would be expected by chance.

Family resemblance study: Similar to *familial aggregation*, a commonly used method of studying individual differences in intelligence and schizophrenia.

Fight-or-flight syndrome: Sympathetic nervous changes representing the individual's instinctive, biological preparation for confronting danger or escaping it. Occurs as part of the General adaptation syndrome (GAS)'s *alarm reaction* and involves the ANS-adrenal-medulla system (or sympatho-adrenomedullary [SAM] axis). Also known as the *fight-or-flight response* (FOFR).

Fluid intelligence: The ability to solve novel problems (those not previously experienced) using inference and abstract information. Declines for all age groups over time, peaking between 20 and 30.

Foetal alcohol syndrome (FAS): A set of physical and psychological characteristics, including *microcephaly* (unusually small head and brain), heart defects, short nose and low nasal bridge, learning difficulties and/or academic and attentional deficits.

Formication: The sensation experienced by cocaine users that 'insects' are crawling beneath their skin.

Functional age: The kind of lifestyle the individual has, including work, children, home, and interest; closely related to *social age*.

Functional invariants: In Piaget's theory, fundamental aspects of the developmental process that work in the same way throughout all the stages; most importantly, *assimilation, accommodation* and *equilibration*.

Gender-splitting: According to Levenson et al., the conflict within women's dreams between career and marriage; this contrasts with men's focus largely on their future career.

Gene: A strand of deoxyribonucleic acid (DNA), the basic unit of heredity/hereditary transmission. A DNA chain is composed of four chemical bases: adenine (A), cytosine (C), guanine (G) and thymine (T); these are arranged in the form of a double helix. The estimated 23,500 human genes are strung along the 23 pairs of chromosomes, one member of each pair being inherited from each parent.

General adaptation syndrome (GAS): Selye's term for a non-specific response to illness that represents the body's defence against stress; it comprises the *alarm reaction, resistance* and *exhaustion stages*.

General symbolic function: Piaget's term for a range of cognitive structures that have developed by age 2, including *self-recognition, symbolic thought* (such as *language*), *deferred imitation* and *representational* (make-believe) *play*.

Generation gap: A sociological view of adolescents as occupying a different world from that of their parents and other adults; young people withdraw from adult control into their peer groups who assume a socialising role (*auto-socialisation*).

Generativity: According to Erikson, concern for future generations and the society and world in which they might live. Not confined to parents, but applies to anyone concerned with the welfare of the young. The positive outcome of middle age.

Genetics: The scientific study of the inheritance of both physical and behavioural traits.

Genome: The total set of biological information needed to build and maintain a living individual of any particular species. The biological information is encoded in the form of *genes*.

Genotype: (1) An individual's unique set of *genes*; (2) the *gene* or *genes* associated with particular characteristics or conditions (i.e., observable traits or characteristics).

Gestalt psychology: An approach that advocates the application of 'laws' or principles of organisation (such as 'the whole is greater than the sum of its parts') to study perception and problem-solving.

Habituation: In relation to drug abuse, another term for *psychological dependence*: it describes the repeated use of a drug because of the pleasurable feelings it produces or its reduction of unpleasant feelings.

Health psychology: The use of psychological principles to promote changes in people's attitudes, behaviour and thinking in relation to health and illness.

Heritability: The extent to which differences in particular traits or abilities between individuals can be attributed to genetic differences.

High availability factor: In the context of attitude change, the greater the effectiveness of messages designed to frighten people into changing their behaviour when they contain specific and precise instructions.

Hippocampus: Located in the *medial temporal lobe* (MTL), a part of the limbic system that plays a central role in human memory; has been called a 'cognitive map'.

Holistic approach: The promotion of the concept of the mind–body connection, which ensures that the needs of an individual's mind, body and spirit are all met.

Homeostasis: Cannon's term (derived from the Greek *homos* = 'same' and *stasis* = 'stoppage') for the process by which an organism maintains a fairly constant internal (bodily) environment (i.e., physiological processes, such as body temperature and salt concentration levels in the blood, are kept in a state of relative balance/equilibrium).

Human Genome Project (HGP): Has successfully identified all the genes in the human *genome*; it has determined the sequences of chemical base pairs that comprise human *DNA*.

Hypothesis: A testable statement about the relationship between two or more variables, usually derived from a model or theory.

Hypothetical construct: A term that does not refer to anything that can be directly observed but to something which can only be *inferred* from observable behaviour and which helps explain the observed behaviour (such as intelligence and personality).

Ideal self: The kind of person we would like to be. Also known as *ego-ideal* or *idealised self-image*.

Ideological dogmatism: According to Rokeach, a closed mind, lack of flexibility, and authoritarianism, regardless of particular sociopolitical ideology (i.e., right- or left-wing).

Illusion of outgroup homogeneity: The tendency to see members of outgroups as 'all the same', rather than unique individuals.

Implementation intentions: The development of specific plans about what to do in a given set of environmental conditions (the 'what' and 'when' of a particular behaviour). Aims to overcome the *intention-behaviour gap*.

Implicit personality theory (IPT): Ready-made beliefs about how individuals' characteristics belong together. *Stereotypes* represent a special kind of IPT.

Individualism: One pole of one major cultural syndrome (individualism-collectivism), in which one's identity is defined by personal choices and achievements – the autonomous individual. Prevalent in Western and capitalist politico-economic societies.

Informational social influence (ISI): Conforming through a need to have an accurate perception of reality. Involves a social comparison with other group members and is related to *internalisation*.

Intention-behaviour gap: A serious limitation shared by all models of health behaviour, whereby they are unable to predict actual behaviour.

Internal desynchronisation: A very stressful bodily state, associated with changes in shift pattern, in which different physiological functions reverse at different times.

Internalisation: As a type of conformity, agreeing with others both privately and publicly. Also known as *true conformity*, it can be thought of as a conversion to others' views.

Internal validity: In the context of an experiment, the degree of control over relevant variables. In theory, complete control would exclude the influence of *experimenter bias* and *demand characteristics*.

Intimacy: According to Erikson, the ability to form close, meaningful relationships with others without fear of losing one's identity. The positive outcome of young adulthood.

Introspection: Observing and analysing the structure of our own conscious mental processes. Major method used by Wundt in his *structuralist* approach to psychology.

Jigsaw method: Aronson's technique for creating six-person, racially mixed, highly interdependent learning groups as a way of reducing race prejudice.

Korsakoff's syndrome: Damage to the *hippocampus* through excessive alcohol consumption, producing both *retrograde* and *anterograde amnesia*.

Learned helplessness: Seligman's term for the (acquired) belief that nothing the individual does will make any difference to what happens to him/her.

Likert scale: A method for measuring attitudes, which requires the participant to indicate how much s/he agrees or disagrees with a series of statements on a 5-point scale.

Locus of control: Rotter's term for the way that people perceive the influence they have over what happens to them. For example, *high external* locus denotes someone who believes they have little control; this is similar to *learned helplessness*.

Longitudinal study: A study of the *same* group of participants over a period (usually years). Also known as a *follow-up* study.

Marker events: A way of referring, collectively, to *age-graded* and *non-normative influences*. Also known as *critical life events*

Maternal deprivation hypothesis (MDH): Bowlby's claim that the mother–infant attachment could not be broken in the first 12 months (fo some children) or 3 years (for all children) without serious and permanent damage to social, emotional and intellectual development.

Milgram paradigm: An experimental method for testing obedience, in which a naive participant is required to deliver increasingly intense electric shocks to another participant (an actor) for making mistakes on a word-association task. Obedience rate is measured as how far up the shock scale the naive participant goes.

Minimal groups: Artificial groups created in the laboratory by randomly and arbitrarily dividing participants into two groups; according to Tajfel, knowledge of another group's existence is sufficient in itself to account for prejudice.

Minimally conscious state (MCS): The state to which some vegetative state (VS) patients progress in which they regain some (transient) level of awareness.

Mirror-image phenomenon: The tendency for enemies to attribute each other with the same negative characteristics and to see themselves as being in the right. Related to *autistic hostility*.

Model: A kind of *metaphor*, involving a single, fundamental idea or image; this makes it less complex than a theory (see later) (although sometimes the terms are used interchangeably).

Modern racism: Indirect, automatic, unconscious and ambiguous racism (as opposed to the crude, blatant traditional form); also known as *symbolic* racism.

Molecular genetic research (MGR): The search for *genes* that 'cause' specific behaviours or characteristics.

Monotropy: Bowlby's claim that infants display a strong, innate tendency to become attached to one particular adult female (not necessarily the biological mother).

Moratorium: According to Erikson, the status of adolescence is an authorised delay of adulthood in Western societies, aimed at making the transition to adulthood easier.

Mutations: Errors that sometimes occur during the *replication* of *genes*. Those that occur during division of the fertilised embryo (*mitosis* or *mitotic division*) are called *somatic mutations* and are not heritable. Those that occur during the production of sperm and egg cells (via *meiosis* or *meiotic division*) are called *germ-line mutations* and are heritable. Other kinds include *acquired mutations* (damage to DNA during a person's lifetime) and *point mutations* (involving a single base-pair).

Mutual pretence awareness: Everyone is pretending that they do not know that the patient is dying, including the patient him/herself.

Negative identity: Engaging in abnormal or delinquent behaviour in an attempt to resolve the adolescent's *identity crisis*. Represents one component of *role confusion*.

Neurogenetic determinism: The belief that a particular *genotype* inevitably produces a particular *phenotype*.

Non-declarative memory: The acquisition of skills displayed through behavioural change (knowing *how*), a form of memory shared by human and non-human animals.

Non-normative influences: Idiosyncratic transitions that can happen at varying times and which do not affect everyone (e.g., parental divorce, own divorce, illness, incest, emigration). Also known as *non-normative shifts*.

Non-shared environments: Within-family variations, such as how parents treat each child differently.

Normative age-graded influences: Biological (e.g., puberty, menopause) and social (e.g., adolescents' changed relationships with parents, marriage) that normally occur at fairly predictable ages. Also known as *normative, maturational shifts*.

Normative, history-graded influences: Historical events that affect entire *cohorts* at about the same time (e.g., wars, recessions).

Normative social influence (NSI): Conforming through a need to be approved of by other people, who have the power to accept or reject us. Related to *compliance*.

Normative, society-dependent shifts: Socially sanctioned changes that occur at the same/similar ages for entire *cohorts* (e.g., leaving school, acquiring legal rights re: alcohol, sex, driving, voting).

Nursing culture: The understanding of death and dying and associated practices and rituals that form part of the nurse's professional knowledge and experience.

Object permanence: Understanding that things continue to exist even when they cannot be perceived. A major development within Piaget's *sensorimotor stage*, usually complete at around 18 months.

Object relations school: A psychodynamic approach that emphasises the child's relationship with particular love objects (especially the mother), rather than instinctive drives. A major example is Bowlby's *attachment theory*.

Ontogenetic development: Development of the *individual* (as opposed to *phylogenetic or evolutionary development* – development of the *species*). Also called *ontogenesis*.

Open awareness: The acknowledgement, through actions and words, by the dying patient and all those around him/her, that death is inevitable.

Operant conditioning: A form of associative learning in which behaviour is shaped by its consequences (i.e., reinforcement or punishment). Also known as *Skinnerian* or *instrumental* conditioning.

Organisational culture: The practices and provision relating to death, dying and grief that form part of the hospital or other institution caring for the dying patient.

Palliative care: The management of physical symptoms and psychological, social and spiritual needs, reducing the suffering, and maintaining the dignity and quality of life, of people at the end of their lives. Often used interchangeably with, 'hospice care', 'terminal care' and 'end-of-life care'.

Paradigm: A common or global perspective shared by most of those working in a particular discipline. When this is achieved, the discipline has reached the stage of *normal science*.

Patient culture: The meaning of death, dying and grieving, including religious beliefs and practices, that are part of the culture that patients identify with.

Perceived behavioural control (PBC): Feeling confident that our current skills and resources will enable us to achieve the desired behaviour and overcome any external barriers. Crucial for understanding motivation and similar to *self-efficacy*, which Ajzen added to the *theory of planned behaviour* (TPB) (a modified form of the *theory of reasoned action* [TRA]).

Periaqueductal grey: A region of the midbrain that forms part of the circuit, which controls how much pain we experience. Electrical stimulation of this structure can bring significant – though temporary – relief to chronic pain patients.

Permanent vegetative state (PVS): In the United Kingdom, a diagnosis made of a vegetative state (VS) patient after at least 6 months for non-traumatic brain injury and 12 months for traumatic ones.

Perseverative cognition: The cognitive representation of (thinking about) stressors, before and after they occur.

Person-centred therapy (PCT): Originally called *client*-centred therapy, this is Rogers' application of his self-theory; the full complexity of the person is the focus of his/her therapy. It is central to most forms of counselling.

Perspective taking (PT): According to Flavell et al., the 2- to 3-year-old's understanding that another person experiences something differently (*level 1: perceptual PT*) and the 4- to 5-year-old's rules for working out what the other person experiences (*level 2: affective and cognitive PT*).

Phenomenal field: In Rogers' humanistic theory, each individual's unique perception of the world.

Phenomenology: A philosophical movement, associated with Husserl and the humanistic psychologists Rogers and Maslow, based on the belief that there is nothing more fundamental than people's *experience*, how something appears (i.e., the 'phenomenon').

Phenotype: The manifest behaviour or condition associated with a particular *genotype*.

Physiolological psychology: The scientific study of how the functions of the nervous system (especially the brain) and the endocrine (hormonal) system are related and influence behaviour and mental processes; also known as *bio-psychology*.

Placebo: An inactive/inert substance, designed to take account of the psychological (as opposed to pharmacological) influences (such as the expectation of improvement) on physiological change.

Placebo effect: The positive psychological or physiological changes associated with the administration of a *placebo*.

Plasticity: A key characteristic of the human brain, without which the developing nervous system would be unable to repair itself following damage or to tailor its responses to changing aspects of the external world. Demonstrated by the ability of undamaged areas to take over the functions usually performed by damaged areas. Complementary to plasticity is *specificity*.

Pre-frontal cortex (PFC): The front-most part of the brain (right behind the forehead), which links the sensory cortex with the emotional and survival-oriented sub-cortical structures; found only in humans.

Prejudice: An extreme attitude, comprising a *stereotyped* belief about entire groups, a strong feeling of hostility towards those groups, and discriminatory behaviour towards them.

Prescience: According to Kuhn, a stage in which a majority of those working in a particular discipline do not yet share a *paradigm*; there are several theoretical orientations.

Primary appraisal: Our judgement as to whether an environmental event or situation poses a potential threat (is a stressor).

Primary degeneration: A disease process, such as Alzheimer's disease (AD), that is more likely to affect us as we get older.

Principle of compatibility: According to Ajzen, the claim that measures of attitudes and behaviour are compatible to the extent that the target, action, context and time elements are assessed at identical levels of generality or specificity.

Privation: The absence of any opportunity to form an attachment with an attachment figure (as opposed to *deprivation*, in which the child is *separated* from the attachment figure – sometimes permanently).

Problem-focused coping (PFC): According to Lazarus and Folkman, taking direct action to solve a problem or seeking information that is relevant to a solution. Contrasted with *emotion-focused coping*.

Procedural memory (PM): Information from long-term memory (LTM) that cannot be inspected consciously (such as the difficulty of describing how to ride a bicycle), in contrast with declarative memory (DM). Knowing *how*.

Projective tests: Designed to reveal unconscious attitudes by presenting participants with ambiguous stimuli, these include the Rorschach ink-blot test and the Thematic Apperception Test (TAT).

Psychoactive drugs: Chemical substances that alter conscious awareness through their effect on the brain.

Psychoanalysis: The form of psychotherapy, based on Freud's *psychoanalytic theory*, which attempts to resolve unconscious conflicts through dream interpretation, free association and transference.

Psychoanalytic theory: Freud's original *psychodynamic* account of human behaviour, from which all others are derived (including those of Adler, Jung and Erikson, which challenge his emphasis on sexuality).

Psychodynamic approach: A general theoretical framework that focuses on active forces within the individual, which motivate behaviour, in particular the unconscious conflict between different personality structures.

Psychogenic emesis: Anticipatory nausea and vomiting (ANV), acquired when anything that becomes associated with chemotherapy-induced emesis becomes a conditioned stimulus.

Psychological pain: A multifaceted experience that includes feelings of hopelessness, guilt, unresolved anger and fear of the unknown. Often expressed through body language and physical symptoms.

Psychological safety: Feeling sufficiently secure to be able to disclose important emotional concerns, based on the provision of understanding, support and encouragement. Can be enhanced by *therapeutic conversation*.

Psychological self: Our view of the self as a private, thinking self that is not visible to others, unlike our *bodily self*. Related to *theory of mind* (ToM).

Psychometric personality theories: Theories based on the use of personality scales that quantify how much of a particular trait an individual displays. Personality is seen as comprising a number of traits, all of which everyone displays to varying degrees.

Psychoneuroendocrinology (PNE): The study of links between psychological and hormonal processes.

Psychoneuroimmunology (PNI): The investigation of interactions between the brain and the immune system at a neural and biochemical level, together with the resulting implications for health. It reflects a *holistic* view of the person and helps explain the stress–illness relationship.

Psychophysiology (PP): The study of the relationship between psychological manipulations and physiological responses in relation to diverse behaviours (e.g. sleep, reactions to stress, and memory).

Psychosexual stages: Freud's account of personality development in terms of the *oral, anal, phallic, latency* and *genital* stages. Related to *infantile sexuality.*

Psychosocial stages: Erikson's account of personality development in terms of the 'Eight Ages of Man': *identity* versus *role confusion* (adolescence); *intimacy* vs. *isolation* (young adulthood); *generativity* vs. *stagnation* (middle age); and *ego integrity* vs. *despair* (old age).

Psychosocial transition: Parkes' term for critical life events or marker events (i.e. life-changing events).

Psychosomatic medicine: The study and treatment of physical disorders caused or aggravated by psychological factors, or mental disorders caused or aggravated by physical factors.

Radical behaviourism: Skinner's rejection of inner (mental) states as variables that can explain behaviour; they are not just inaccessible (as argued by *methodological behaviourism*), but are irrelevant and can be translated into the language of *reinforcement theory.*

Rapid eye movement (REM) sleep: Sleep, in which pulse and respiration rates, and blood pressure, increase and become less regular. EEGs (brain wave activity) begin to resemble those of the waking state, showing that the brain is active. Also involves muscular paralysis and resistance to being woken (hence, 'paradoxical sleep'). Also referred to as 'dream sleep'.

Reduced (or minimal) parenting: The collective term for a range of reproductive techniques, in particular *in vitro fertilisation* (IVF), *egg donation, donor insemination* (DI), *embryo donation* and *surrogacy.*

Reductionism: Any attempt to explain some complex whole in terms of its component or constituent parts.

Referent social influence (RSI): Turner's term for conformity that depends on categorising oneself and others as belonging to the same group.

Reification: Thinking of abstract concepts (or *hypothetical constructs:*) as 'things' or 'entities'.

Reinforcement schedules (or contingencies): How often and regularly/predictably reinforcements are given following some desired behaviour.

Reminiscence: The process of recalling past events and experiences. Related to *ego integrity*. Butler's *life review* (LR) involves a more focused consideration of one's past life as a whole.

Replication: In the context of genetics, the process by which a gene makes a copy of itself. DNA can replicate indefinitely, while still containing the same information.

Resistance: The second stage of the *general adaptation syndrome* (GAS), in which adrenocorticotrophic hormone (ACTH) stimulates the adrenal cortex to release corticosteroids (or adrenocorticoid hormones), one group of which are the glucocorticoid hormones. Resistance involves the anterior pituitary–adrenal cortex system (or hypothalamic–pituitary–adrenal [HPA] axis).

Retrograde amnesia: Failure to remember what happened *before* the surgery or accident that caused the amnesia.

Reverse tolerance: With cannabis, the *lowering* of the amount needed to produce the initial effect with repeated use.

Revolution: In science, the establishment of a new *paradigm*.

Salience: In the context of *addiction*, the all-consuming importance of the substance or activity.

Scaffolding: The guidance and support that adults provide children in the *zone of proximal development (ZPD)* by which they acquire their knowledge and skills.

Schema (or scheme): According to Piaget, mental structures that organise past experiences and provide a way of interpreting future experiences. The basic building block/unit of intelligent behaviour.

Schematic memory: The automatic ability to make sense of new experiences and to recognise and put new objects and experiences in the right categories. Related to the distinction between *automatic* and *effortful memory*. Represents part of the self we normally take for granted.

Schizophreniform disorder: A mental disorder involving at least two symptoms of psychosis (such as hallucinations, delusions, and catatonia), observed for at least 1 month but less than 6 months. Compared with schizophrenia, the patient has a much better chance of recovery.

Science: The constructing of theories regarding a definable subject matter, and hypothesis testing using empirical methods to collect data (evidence) relevant to the hypothesis being tested.

Scientific method: An account of how the scientific process takes place, including the sequence of events and the relationship between theory construction and hypothesis testing.

Secondary appraisal: Assessing our resources for coping with an environmental event or situation that we have already judged to be a stressor (*primary appraisal*).

Selective (or focused) attention: The ability to focus or concentrate on just one of the many things going on around us at any one time.

Self-consciousness (or self-awareness): An organism's capacity for representing its own mental states (thoughts about thoughts). Closely related to *theory of mind (ToM)*.

Self-efficacy: Bandura's term for our belief that we can act effectively and exercise control over events that influence our lives.

Self-esteem: How we evaluate ourselves, how much we like our self-image. Partly determined by the discrepancy between our *self-image* and *ideal self*. Also known as *self-regard*.

Self-fulfilling prophecy: Treating people, based on our expectations of their personalities or abilities, which, in turn, influences their behaviour in such a way that it confirms our expectations.

Self-image: How we describe ourselves, including our social roles, personality traits and physical characteristics (*body image* or *bodily self*).

Self-management: An approach to pain management that involves a range of treatments, such as learning coping skills, progressive muscle relaxation training, and providing rewards for displaying coping behaviour. Related to *cognitive behavioural therapy* (CBT).

Self-schema: Complex and clear information relating to various aspects of ourselves, including *possible selves* and *future-orientated selves*.

Seriation: The ability to arrange objects on the basis of a particular dimension (e.g., increasing height).

Shared environments: Between-family variations, such as socio-economic status (SES).

Social cognition models: According to Ogden, models such as *theory of reasoned action* (TRA) and *theory of planned behaviour* (TPB), which try to account for social behaviour in general and are much broader than *cognition models* (of health).

Social constructivist: A way of describing Vygotsky's theory of cognitive development (*child-as-apprentice*).

Social learning theory (SLT): An account of human learning that, while not rejecting the role of conditioning, emphasises the role of other people (models) and cognitive processes as influences on the learning process. Bandura renamed it *social cognitive theory*.

Social Readjustment Rating Scale (SRRS): Holmes and Rahe's method of measuring stress in terms of life changes. The amount of stress a person has experienced in a given period (usually one year) is measured by the total number of life change units (LCUs).

Spiritual pain: Feelings of unfairness following the realisation that life is approaching its end combined with a desolate sense of meaninglessness.

Stereotype: A special kind of *implicit personality theory* (IPT) that relates to an entire social group.

Stereotyping: Attributing characteristics to individuals based on the stereotype of their membership group.

Strange Situation: A controlled observational procedure for studying attachment behaviours in 12- to 18-month-olds, comprising eight 3-minute episodes involving the child, its mother, and a female stranger. According to Ainsworth, the critical indicator is how the child responds to the mother's return (*reunion behaviours*).

Stress management: A range of psychological techniques used by professionals to help people reduce their stress. These include *biofeedback*, progressive muscle relaxation, and cognitive restructuring (a major feature of *cognitive behaviour therapy* [CBT]).

Subjective age: How old the individual feels deep down inside.

Subjective norms: In the *theory of reasoned action* (TRA), a person's beliefs about the desirability of carrying out a certain health behaviour in the context of the social group, society and culture she/he belongs to.

Substance abuse: As defined by the *diagnostic and statistical manual of mental disorders* (DSM), a maladaptive pattern of substance use that does not meet the criteria for *substance dependence*.

Substance dependence: As defined by DSM-IV-R, a maladaptive pattern of substance use involving *tolerance, withdrawal* (*physiological dependence*) and other behaviours indicating *psychological dependence*. These all constitute part of the *dependence syndrome*.

Suspected awareness: The dying patient's suspicion that she/he may be dying and attempts to find out the prognosis.

Systematic desensitisation (SD): A form of *behaviour therapy* in which the person relaxes while exposed to a series of stimuli that are increasingly likely to produce the problem behaviour.

Theory: A complex set of inter-related statements that attempt to explain certain observed phenomena. In practice, when we refer to a particular theory (for example, Freud's or Piaget's), we often include *description* as well. Thomas (1985) defines a theory as 'an explanation of how the facts fit together' and he likens a theory to a lens through which to view the subject matter, filtering out certain facts and giving a particular pattern to those it lets in.

Theory of mind (ToM): The ability to infer the existence of mental states (e.g., beliefs and intentions) in others (*mind-reading*).

Therapeutic conversation: According to Burnard, dialogue that focuses on the here-and-now and the patient's feelings, involves empathic understanding, a non-prescriptive approach, and active listening.

Thresholder: Apter's term for 18- to 24-year-olds who are only on the brink of achieving self-sufficiency and autonomy (two key adult qualities).

Tolerance: In relation to addiction, the increasing amount of the substance or activity needed to achieve the same effect.

Transactional model (of stress): A view of stress as arising from an imbalance between the individual's perception of the demands being made by the situation and his/her ability to meet those demands.

Transductive reasoning: Drawing an inference about the relationship between two things based on a single shared attribute.

Translation: In the context of genetics, the process by which a gene 'reads' itself. It begins with the text of a gene being transcribed into a copy by replication, but the copy is made of *ribonucleic acid* (RNA), very similar to *deoxyribonucleic acid* (DNA). RNA uses the same base letters as DNA, except that it uses uracil (U) instead of thymine (T).

Unilateral visual neglect: Completely ignoring stimuli presented to the opposite side of the parietal lobe that has been affected by a stroke – including the body on that side.

Variable: Anything that can have different values (i.e., that can 'vary'). Variables are of two main types: (1) **participant** (for example, personality, gender, age, cultural background, diet); and (2) **situational** (for example, the type and difficulty of a task, task instructions, time of day). Most participant variables cannot be manipulated (an exception, among the examples given here, being diet). Instead, participants are *selected* because they already possess these characteristics or already engage in certain activities. Such studies are called 'quasi' ('almost') experiments (as opposed to *true* experiments).

Vegetative state (VS): A state in which the patient appears to be awake (conscious) but where there the patient lacks awareness of anything around him/her.

Withdrawal: In the context of *addiction*, the unpleasant feelings and physical effects produced when the addictive behaviour is suddenly reduced or stopped.

Zeitgeber: An environmental (exogenous) factor (such as light-dark cycles and clocks) that provides clues to bodily rhythms (*zeitgeber* = German for 'time-giver').

Zone of proximal development (ZPD): Vygotsky's term for those functions that have not yet matured but which are in the process of maturing; it characterises mental development *prospectively*.

References

Abrams, D., Wetherell, M., Cochrane, S., Hogg, M.A. and Turner, J.C. (1990) Knowing what to think by knowing who you are: self-categorisation and the nature of norm formation. *British Journal of Social Psychology, 29*, 97–119.

Addington-Hall, J. (2002) Research sensitivities to palliative care patients. *European Journal of Cancer Care, 11*(3), 220–224.

Adler, A. (1927) *The Practice and Theory of Individual Psychology.* New York: Harcourt Brace Jovanovich.

Adler, R. (2000) Pigeonholed. *New Scientist, 167*(2258), 389–391.

Adorno, T.W., Frenkel-Brunswick, E., Levinson, J.D. and Sanford, R.N. (1950) *The Authoritarian Personality.* New York: Harper & Row.

Ainsworth, M.D.S., Bell, S.M.V. and Stayton, D.J. (1971) Individual differences in Strange Situation behaviour of one-year-olds. In H.R. Schaffer (ed.) *The Origins of Human Social Relations.* New York: Academic Press.

Ainsworth, M.D.S., Blehar, M.C., Waters, E. and Wall, S. (1978) *Patters of Attachment: A Psychological Study of the Strange Situation.* Hillsdale, NJ: Lawrence Erlbaum Associates Inc.

Ajzen, I. (1988) *Attitudes, Personality and Behaviour.* Milton Keynes, UK: Open University Press.

Ajzen, I. (1991) The theory of planned behaviour. *Organisational Behaviour & Human Decision Processes, 50*, 179–211.

Ajzen, I. and Fishbein, M. (1970) The prediction of behaviour from attitudinal and normative beliefs. *Journal of Personality & Social Psychology, 6*, 466–487.

Ajzen, I. and Fishbein, M. (1977) Attitude–behaviour relations: a theoretical analysis and review of empirical research. *Psychological Bulletin, 24*, 888–918.

Alexander, M.F., Fawcett, J.N. and Runciman, P.J. (eds.) (2006) *Nursing Practice Hospital and Home* (3rd edn.). London, UK: Churchill Livingstone.

Allen, V. and Levine, J.M. (1968) Social support, dissent and conformity. *Sociometry, 31*, 138–149.

Allen, V. and Levine, J.M. (1971) Social support and conformity: the role of independent assessment of reality. *Journal of Experimental Social Psychology, 7*, 48–58.

Allport, G.W. (1935) Attitudes. In C.M. Murchison (ed.) *Handbook of Social Psychology.* Worchester, MA: Clark University Press.

Allport, G.W. (1947) *The Use of Personal Documents in Psychological Science.* London: Holt, Rinehart & Winston.

Allport, G.W. (1954) *The Nature of Prejudice.* Reading, MA: Addison-Wesley.

Allport, G.W. (1968) The historical background of modern psychology. In G. Lindzey and E. Aronson (eds.) *Handbook of Social Psychology* (2nd edn., Vol. 1). Reading, MA: Addison-Wesley.

Alsaker, F.D. (1992) Pubertal timing, overweight, and psychological adjustment. *Journal of Early Adolescence, 12*, 396–419.

Alsaker, F.D. (1996) The impact of puberty. *Journal of Child Psychology & Psychiatry, 37*(3), 249–258.

American Academy of Paediatrics. (2006) Prevention and management of pain in the neonate: an update. *Paediatrics, 118*, 2231–2241.

American Psychiatric Association. (2000) *Diagnostic and Statistical Manual of Mental Disorders* (4th edn., revised). Washington: American Psychiatric Association.

Amir, Y. (1969) Contact hypothesis in ethnic relations. *Psychological Bulletin, 71*, 319–342.

Amir, Y. (1994) The contact hypothesis in intergroup relations. In W.J. Lonner and R.S. Malpass (eds.) *Psychology and Culture*. Boston, MA: Allyn & Bacon.

Anand, K.J. and Craig, K.D. (1996) New perspectives on the definition of pain. *Pain, 67*, 3–6.

Anthony, S. (1971) *The Discovery of Death in Childhood and After*. Harmondsworth, UK: Penguin.

Applegate, K.L., Keefe, F.J., Siegler, I.C., Bradley, L.A., McKee, D.C., Cooper, K.S. and Riordan, P. (2005) Does personality at college entry predict number of reported pain conditions at mid-life? A longitudinal study. *The Journal of Pain, 6*, 92–97.

Apter, T. (2001) *The Myth of Maturity*. New York: Norton.

Apter, T. (2010) Pathways to adulthood. In R. Gross (ed.) *Psychology: The Science of Mind and Behaviour* (6th edn.). London, UK: Hodder Education.

Archer, J. (1999) *The Nature of Grief: The Evolution and Psychology of Reactions to Loss*. London: Routledge.

Arendt, H. (1965) *Eichmann in Jerusalem: A Report on the Banality of Evil*. New York: Viking.

Armitage, C.J. (2004) Evidence that implementation intentions reduce dietary fat intake: a randomised trial. *Health Psychology, 23*, 319–323.

Arnsten, A., Mazure, C.M. and Sinha, R. (2012) The is your brain meltdown. *Scientific American, 306*(40), 38–43.

Aronson, E. (1980) *The Social Animal* (3rd edn.). San Francisco, CA: W.H. Freeman.

Aronson, E. (1988) *The Social Animal* (5th edn.). New York: W.H. Freeman.

Aronson, E. (1992) *The Social Animal* (6th edn.). New York: W.H. Freeman.

Aronson, E. (2000) The jigsaw strategy: reducing prejudice in the classroom. *Psychology Review, 7*(2), 2–5.

Aronson, E. and Carlsmith, J.M. (1963) Effect of the severity of threat on the devaluation of forbidden behaviour. *Journal of Abnormal & Social Psychology, 6*, 584–588.

Aronson, E., Bridgeman, D.L. and Geffner, R.F. (1978) The effects of a cooperative classroom structure on student behaviour and attitudes. In D. Bar-Tal and L. Saxe (eds.) *Social Psychology of Education*. New York: Wiley.

Arthur, H.M., Daniels, C., McKelvie, R., Hirsch, J. and Rush, B. (2000) Effect of a preoperative intervention on preoperative and postoperative outcomes in low-risk patients awaiting elective coronary artery bypass graft surgery: a randomised, controlled trial. *Annals of Internal Medicine, 133*(4), 253–262.

Asch, S.E. (1951) Effect on group pressure upon the modification and distortion of judgements. In H. Guetzkow (ed.) *Groups, Leadership and Men*. Pittsburgh, PA: Carnegie Press.

Asch, S.E. (1952) *Social Psychology*. Englewood Cliffs, NJ: Prentice Hall.

Asch, S.E. (1955) Opinions and social pressure. *Scientific American, 193*, 31–35.

Asch, S.E. (1956) Studies of independence and submission to group pressure: 1: a minority of one against a unanimous majority. *Psychological Monographs, 70*, (whole No. 416).

Aschoff, J. (1979) Circadian rhythms: general features and endocrinological aspects. In D.T. Krieger (ed.) *Endocrine Rhythms*. New York: Raven Press.

Ashworth, P. (1980) *Care to Communicate*. London: Royal College of Nursing.

Ashworth, P. (1990) High technology and humanity for intensive care. *Intensive Care Nursing, 6*(3), 150–160.

Asmundson, G.J.G., Vlaeyen, J.W.S. and Crombez, G. (eds.) (2004) *Understanding and Treating Fear of Pain*. Oxford: Oxford University Press.

Atkinson, R.L., Atkinson, R.C., Smith, E.E. and Bem, D.J. (1990) *Introduction to Psychology* (10th edn.). New York: Harcourt Brace Jovanovich.

Axelson, M.L., Brindberg, D. and Durand, J.H. (1983) Eating at a fast-food restaurant: a social-psychological analysis. *Journal of Nutrition Education, 15*, 94–98.

Badenhorst, J.C.C. (1990) Psychotherapeutic approach to management of the severely injured patient. *Psychotherapy and Psychosomatics, 53*(1–4), 156–160.

Bainbridge, D. (2012) Marvellous middle age. *New Scientist, 213*(2855), 48–51.

Baker, A. (2000) 'Even as I bought it I knew it wouldn't work'. In A. Baker (ed.) *Serious Shopping: Essays in Psychotherapy and Consumerism*. London: Free Association Books.

Baker Miller, J. (1976) *Towards a New Psychology of Women*. Harmondsworth, UK: Penguin.

Baltes, M.M. and Baltes, P.B. (1986) *The Psychology of Control and Ageing*. Hillsdale, NJ: Erlbaum.

Balluffi, A., Kassam-Adams, N., Kazak, A., Tucker, M., Dominguez, T. and Helfaer, M. (2004) Traumatic stress in parents of children admitted to the paediatric intensive care unit. *Paediatric Critical Care Medicine, 5*, 547–553.

Baltes, P.B. (1983) Life-span developmental psychology: observations on history and theory revisited. In R.M. Lerner (ed.) *Developmental Psychology: Historical and Philosophical Perspectives*. Hillsdale, NJ: Erlbaum.

Baltes, P.B. and Lindenberger, U. (1997) Emergence of a powerful connection between sensory and cognitive functions across the adult life span: a new window to the study of ageing? *Psychology and Ageing, 12*, 12–21.

Bandura, A. (1971) *Social Learning Theory*. Englewood Cliffs, NJ: Prentice Hall.

Bandura, A. (1977) Self-efficacy: toward a unifying theory of behaviour change. *Psychological Review, 84*, 191–215.

Bandura, A. (1986) *Social Foundations of Thought and Action*. Englewood Cliffs, NJ: Prentice Hall.

Bandura, A. (1989) Social cognitive theory. In R. Vasta (ed.) *Six Theories of Child Development*. Greenwich, CT: JAI Press.

Bandura, A. (1997) *Self-Efficacy: The Exercise of Control*. New York: W.H. Freeman.

Banks, C. (1991) Alleviating anticipatory vomiting. *Nursing Times, 87*(16), 42–43.

Barber, B.K. and Buehler, C. (1996) Family cohesion and enmeshment: different constructs, different effects. *Journal of Marriage & the Family, 58*(2), 433–515.

Bargh, J.A., Chen, M. and Burrows, L. (1996) The automaticity of social behaviour: direct effects of trait concept and stereotype activation on action. *Journal of Personality & Social Psychology, 71*, 230–244.

Baron, R.A. and Byrne, D. (1991) *Social Psychology* (6th edn.). Boston, MA: Allyn & Bacon.

Barrett, R. and Robinson, B. (1994) Gay dads. In A.E. Gottfried and A.W. Gottfried (eds.) *Redefining Families*. New York: Plenum Press.

Bartlett, D. (1998) *Stress: Perspectives and Processes*. Buckingham: Open University Press.

Basovich, S.N. (2010) The role of hypoxia in mental development and in the treatment of mental disorders: a review. *Bioscience Trends, 4*(6), 288–296.

Bassett, C. (2002) Nurses' and students' perceptions of care: a phenomenological study. *Nursing Times, 94*(34), 32–34.

Baum, A. and Posluszny, M.M. (1999) Health psychology: mapping biobehavioural contributions to health and illness. *Annual Review of Psychology, 50*, 137–163.

Baumeister, R.F. (1997) The self and society: changes, problems and opportunities. In R.D. Ashmore and L. Jussim (eds.) *Self and Identity: Fundamental Issues*. New York: Oxford University Press.

Baumeister, R.F. (1998) The self. In D.T. Gilbert, S.T. Fiske and G. Lindzey (eds.) *Handbook of Social Psychology* (4th edn.). New York: McGraw-Hill.

Becker, M.H. (ed.) (1974) The health belief model and personal health behaviour. *Health Education Monographs, 2*, 324–508.

Becker, M.H. and Rosenstock, I.M. (1984) Compliance and medical advice. In A. Steptoe and A. Mathews (eds.) *Health Care and Human Behaviour*. London: Academic Press.

Becker, M.H. and Rosenstock, I.M. (1987) Comparing social learning theory and the health belief model. In W.B. Ward (ed.) *Advances in Health Education and Promotion*. Greenwich, CT: JAI Press.

Becker, M.H., Maiman, L.A., Kirscht, J.P., Haefner, D.P. and Drachman, R.H. (1977) The health belief model and prediction of dietary compliance: a field experiment. *Journal of Health & Social Behaviour, 18*, 348–366.

Bee, H. (1994) *Lifespan Development*. New York: HarperCollins.

Bee, H. (2000) *The Developing Child* (9th edn.). Boston, MA: Allyn & Bacon.

Beecher, H.K. (1956) Relationship of significance of wound to the pain experienced. *Journal of the American Medical Association, 161*, 1609–1613.

Bell, S.M. and Ainsworth, M.D.S. (1972) Infant crying and maternal responsiveness. *Child Development, 43*, 1171–1190.

Bem, D.J. (1965) An experimental analysis of self-persuasion. *Journal of Experimental & Social Psychology, 1*, 199–218.

Bem, D.J. (1967) Self-perception: an alternative interpretation of cognitive dissonance phenomena. *Psychological Review, 74*, 183–200.

Benjamin, B. and Burns, A. (2010) Old-age psychiatry. In B.K. Puri and I. Treasaden (eds.) *Psychiatry: An Evidence-Based Text*. London: Hodder Arnold.

Bennett, L., Michie, P. and Kippax, S. (1991) Qualitative analysis of burnout and its associated factors in AIDS nursing. *AIDS Care, 3*, 181–192.

Bergevin, T., Bukowski, W.M. and Miners, R. (2003) Social development. In A. Slater and G. Bremner (eds.) *An Introduction to Developmental Psychology*. Oxford, UK: Blackwell Publishing.

Berry, J.W. (1994) *Cross-Cultural Health Psychology*. Keynote address presented to the International Conference of Applied Psychology. Madrid (July).

Berry, J.W. (1998) Acculturation and health: theory and research. In S.S. Kazarian and D.R. Evans (eds.) *Cultural Clinical Psychology: Theory, Research and Practice*. New York: Oxford University Press.

Bhakta, P., Donnelly, P. and Mayberry, J. (1995) Management of breast disease in Asian women. *Professional Nursing, 11*, 187–189.

Bildner, J. and Krechel, S.W. (1996) Increasing awareness of postoperative pain management in the NICU. *Neonatal Network, 15*, 11–16.

Billig, M. (1976) *Social Psychology and Intergroup Relations*. London: Academic Press.

Bird, C.E., Conrad, P. and Fremont, A.M. (2000) *Handbook of Medical Sociology* (5th edn.). Upper Saddle River, NJ: Prentice Hall.

Black, J. (1991) Death and bereavement: the customs of Hindus, Sikhs and Moslems. *Bereavement Care, 10*, 6–8.

Black, S.E., Blessed, G., Edwardson, J.A. and Kay, D.W.K. (1990) Prevalence rates of dementia in an ageing population: are low rates due to the use of insensitive instruments? *Age and Ageing, 19*, 84–90.

Blackmore, C. (1989) Altered images. *Nursing Times, 85*(12), 36–39.

Blakemore, S.-J. (2007) The social brain of a teenager. *The Psychologist, 20*(10), 600–602.

Blane, H.T. (1976) Issues in preventing alcohol problems. *Preventive Medicine, 5*(1), 176–186.

Blount, R.L., Piira, T., Cohen, L.L. and Cheng, P.S. (2006) Paediatric procedural pain. *Behaviour Modification, 30*(1), 24–49.

Bluebond-Langner, M. (1978) *The Private Worlds of Dying Children*. Princeton, NJ: Princeton University Press.

Boden, M. (1980) Artificial intelligence and intellectual imperialism. In A.J. Chapman and D.M. Jones (eds.) *Models of Man*. Leicester, UK: British Psychological Society.

Bond, J. and Bond, S. (1986) *Sociology and health care.* Edinburgh: Churchill Livingstone.

Bond, J., Coleman, P. and Peace, S. (eds.) (1993) *Ageing in Society: An Introduction to Social Gerontology.* London: Sage.

Bond, R.A. and Smith, P.B. (1996) Culture and conformity: a meta-analysis of studies using Asch's (1952b, 1956) line judgement task. *Psychological Bulletin, 119*, 111–137.

Boore, J. (1978) *Precription for Recovery.* London: RCN.

Borke, H. (1975) Piaget's mountains revisited: changes in the egocentric landscape. *Developmental Psychology, 11*, 240–243.

Borrill, C., Wall, T., West, M., Hardy, GE., Shapiro, D.A., Carter, A., Golya, D.A. and Haynes, C.E. (1996) *Mental Health of the Workforce in NHS Trusts: Phase 1, Final Report.* Sheffield: Institute of Work Psychology.

Bowlby, J. (1951) *Maternal Care and Mental Health.* Geneva: World Health Organization.

Bowlby, J. (1969) *Attachment and Loss. Vol. 1: Attachment.* Harmondsworth, UK: Penguin.

Bowlby, J. (1973) *Attachment and Loss. Vol. 2: Separation.* Harmondsworth, UK: Penguin.

Bowlby, J. (1980) *Attachment and Loss, Vol. 3: Loss, Sadness and Depression.* London: Hogarth Press.

Bowlby, J., Ainsworth, M., Boston, M. and Rosenbluth, D. (1956) The effects of mother–child separation: a follow-up study. *British Journal of Medical Psychology, 24*(3/4), 211–247.

Bowler, I.M.W. (1993) Stereotypes of women of Asian descent in midwifery: some evidence? *Midwifery, 9*, 7–16.

Bradley, L.A. (1995) Chronic benign pain. In D. Wedding (ed.) *Behaviour and Medicine* (2nd edn.). St Louis, MO: Mosby-Year Book.

Brady, M.J., Peterman, A.H., Fitchett, G., Mo, M. and Cella, Dl. (1999) A case for including spirituality in quality of life measurement in oncology. *Psycho-Oncology, 8*, 417–428.

Brewer, M.B. (1999) The psychology of prejudice: ingroup love or outgroup hate? *Journal of Social Issues, 55*, 429–444.

Brewer, M.B. and Brown, R.J. (1998) Intergroup relations. In D.T. Gilbert, S.T. Fiske and G. Lindzey (eds.) *Handbook of Social Psychology* (4th edn., Vol. 2). New York: McGraw-Hill.

Brewer, N.T., Chapman, G.B., Brownlee, S. and Leventhal, E.A. (2002) Cholesterol control, medication adherence and illness cogntion. *British Journal of Health Psychology, 7*, 433–447.

Brislin, R. (1981) *Cross-Cultural Encounters: Face-to-Face Interaction.* Elmsford, NY: Pergamon.

Brislin, R. (1993) *Understanding Culture's Influence on Behaviour.* Orlando, FL: Harcourt Brace Jovanovich.

British Medical Association & Royal Pharmaceutical Society of Great Britain. (2005) *British National Formulary.* London: British Medical Association & The Royal Pharmaceutical Society of Great Britain.

Bromley, D.B. (1977, 21 April) Speculations in social and environmental gerontology. *Nursing Times (Occasional Papers 21 April)*, 53–56.

Bromley, D.B. (1988) *Human Ageing: An Introduction to Gerontology* (3rd edn.). Harmondsworth, UK: Penguin.

Bronfenbrenner, U. (1960) Freudian theories of identification and their derivatives. *Child Development, 31*, 15–40.

Bronner, M.B., Peek, N., Knoester, H., Bos, A.P., Last, B.F. and Grootenhuis, M.A. (2010) Course and predictors of posttraumatic stress in disorder n parents after paediatric intensive care treatment of their child. *Journal of Paediatric Psychology, 35*(9), 966–974.

Brook. C. (1986) *All About Adolescence* (2nd edn.). Chichester, UK: John Wiley.

Brooking, J. (1991) Doctors and nurses: a personal view. *Nursing Standard, 6*(12), 24–28.

Brooks-Gunn, J. and Warren, M.P. (1985) The effects of delayed menarche in different contexts. Dance and non-dance students. *Journal of Youth & Adolescence, 14*, 285–300.

Brooks-Gunn, J., Attie, I., Burrow, C., Rosso, J.T. and Warren, M.P. (1989) The impact of puberty on body and eating concerns in athletic and non-athletic contexts. *Journal of Early Adolescence, 9*, 269–290.

Brosschot, J.F., Gerin, W. and Thayer, J.F. (2006) Worry and health: the perseverative cognition hypothesis. *Journal of Psychosomatic Research, 60*, 113–124.

Brown, G. (2007) The bitter end. *New Scientist, 196*(2625), 42–43.

Brown, H. (1985) *People, Groups and Society.* Milton Keynes, UK: Open University Press.

Brown, H. (1996) Themes in experimental research on groups from the 1930s to the 1990s. In M. Wetherell (ed.) *Identities, Groups and Social Issues.* London: Sage, in association with the Open University.

Brown, P. (1988) Punching the body clock. *Nursing Times, 84*(44), 26–28.

Brown, R. (1965) *Social Psychology.* New York: Free Press.

Brown, R. (1986) *Social Psychology* (2nd edn.). New York: Free Press.

Brown, R.J. (1988) Intergroup relations. In M. Haewstone, W. Stroebe, J.P. Codol and G.M. Stephenson (eds.) *Introduction to Social Psychology.* Oxford: Blackwell Publishing.

Brown, R. and Kulik, J. (1982) Flashbulb memories. In U. Neisser (ed.) *Memory Observed.* San Francisco, CA: Freeman.

Brown, R., Marsas, P., Masser, B., Vivian, J. and Hewstone, M. (2001) Life on the ocean wave: testing some intergroup hypotheses in a naturalistic setting. *Group Processes & Intergroup Relations, 4*, 81–98.

Brown, V. (1991) The family as victim in trauma. *Hawaii Medical Journal, 50*(4), 153–154.

Brubaker, C. and Wickersham, D. (1990) Encouraging the practice of testicular self-examination: a field application of the theory of reasoned action. *Health Psychology, 9*, 154–163.

Bruner, J.S. (1966) *Towards a Theory of Instruction.* Cambridge, MA: Harvard University Press.

Buggins, E. (1995) Mind your language. *Nursing Standard, 10*(1), 21–22.

BullyOnLine. www.bullyonline.com (25 march, 2006).

Bulman, C. and Schutz, S. (eds.) (2008) *Reflective Practice in Nursing* (4th edn.). Oxford: Wiley-Blackwell.

Burnard, P. (1987) Meaningful dialogue. *Nursing Times, 83*(20), 43–45.

Burnard, P., Edwards, D., Fothergill, A., Hannigan, B. and Coyle, D. (2000) When the pressure's too much. *Nursing Times, 96*(19), 28–30.

Burns, R.B. (1980) *Essential Psychology.* Lancaster, UK: MTP Press.

Burt, K. (1995) The effect of cancer on body image and sexuality. *Nursing Times, 91*(7), 36–37.

Buss, A.H. (1992) Personality: primate heritage and human distinctiveness. In R.A. Zucker, A.I. Rabin, J. Aronoff and S.J. Frank (eds.) *Personality Structure in the Life Course: Essays on Personality in the Murray Tradition.* New York: Springer.

Butler, R.N. (1963) The life review: an interpretation of reminiscence in the aged. *Psychiatry, 26*, 65–76.

Butler, L.D., Symons, B.K., Henderson, S.L., Shortliffe, L.D. and Spiegel, D. (2005) Hypnosis reduces distress and duration of an invasive medical procedure for children. *Paediatrics, 115*(1), e77–e85.

Cahill, C.D., Stuart, G.W., Laraia, M.T. and Arana, G.W. (1991) Inpatient management of violent behaviour: nursing prevention and intervention. *Issues in Mental Health Nursing, 12*, 239–252.

Calne, S. (1994) Dehumanisation in intensive care. *Nursing Times, 27*(90), 31–33.

Campbell, C.M., France, C.R., Robinson, M.E., Logan, H.L., Geffken, G.R. and Fillingim, R.B. (2008) Ethnic differences in diffuse noxious inhibitory controls. *The Journal of Pain, 8*, 759–766.

Cannon, W.B. (1929) *Bodily Changes in Pain, Hunger, Fear and Rage.* New York: Appleton.

Carlisle, D. (2012) Would you like help to quit? *Nursing Standard, 26*(25), 20.

Carlson, N.R. and Buskist, W. (1997) *Psychology: The Science of Behaviour* (5th edn.). Needham Heights, MA: Allyn & Bacon.

Carper, B.A. (1978) Fundamental patterns of knowing. *Advances in Nursing Science, 1*, 13–23. Also reprinted in J.F. Kicuchiand and H. Simmons (eds.) (1992) *Philosophical inquiry into nursing.* Newbury Park, CA: Sage.

Carroll, J.K., Cullinan, E., Clarke, L. and David, N.F. (2012) The role of anxiolytic premedication in reducing preoperative anxiety. *British Journal of Nursing, 21*(8), 479–483.

Carson, J., Fagin, L., Brown, D., Leary, J. and Bartlett, H. (1997) Self-esteem and stress in mental health nurses. *Nursing Times, 93*(44), 55–58.

Carstensen, L.L. (1991) Selectivity theory: social activity in life-span context. *Annual Review of Gerontology & Geriatrics, 11*, 195–217.

Carstensen, L.L (1992) Social and emotional patterns in adulthood: support for socioemotional selectivity theory. *Psychology & Ageing, 7*, 331–338.

Carstensen, L.L. (1993) Motivation for social contact across the life span: a theory of socioemotional selectivity. In J. Jacobs (ed.) *Nebraska Symposium on Motivation, 1992, Developmental Perspectives on Motivation,* Vol. 40. Lincoln: University of Nebraska Press.

Carstensen, L.L. (1995) Evidence for a life-span theory of sociemotional selectivity. *Current Directions in Psychological Science, 4*, 151–156.

Carstensen, L.L. (1996) Socioemotional selectivity: a life span developmental account of social behaviour. In M.R. Merrens and G.C. Brannigan (eds.) *The Developmental Psychologists: Research Adventures Across the Life Span.* New York: McGraw-Hill.

Carstensen, L.L. and Turk-Charles, S. (1994) The salience of emotion across the adult life course. *Psychology & Ageing, 9*, 259–264.

Carter, N.M. (2004) Implications for medicine in the 'post-genome era'. *Current Anaestheia and Critical Care, 15*, 37–43.

Catan, L. (2004) *Becoming Adult: Changing Youth Transitions in the 21st Century.* Brighton: Trust for the Study of Adolescence.

Catania, J.A., Kegeles, S.M. and Coates, D.J. (1990) Towards an understanding of risk behaviour: an AIDS risk reduction model (ARRM). *Health Education Quarterly, 17*, 53–72.

Chapman, G.E. (1983) Ritual and rational action in hospitals. *Journal of Advanced Nursing, 8*, 13–20.

Cheesman, S. (2006) Promoting concordance: the implications for prescribers. *Nurse Prescribing, 4*(5), 205–208.

Chesterfield, P. (1992) Communicating with dying children. *Nursing Standard, 6*(20), 30–32.

Chisolm, K., Carter, M.C., Ames, E.W. and Morison, S.J. (1995) Attachment security and indiscriminately friendly behaviour in children adopted from Romanian orphanages. *Development & Psychopathology, 7*, 283–294.

Chochinov, H.M. (2006) Dying, dignity and new horizons in palliative end-of-life care. *CA: A Cancer Journal for Clinicians, 56*, 84–103.

Chochinov, H.M., Hack, T., Hassard, T., Kristjanson, L.J., McClement, S. and Harlos, M. (2005) Dignity therapy: a novel psychotherapeutic intervention for patients near the end of life. *Journal of Clinical Oncology, 23*, 5520–5525.

Chochinov, H.M., Hack, T., McClement, S., Kristjanson, L. and Harlos, M. (2002) Dignity in the terminally ill: a developing empirical model. *Social Science & Medicine, 54*, 433–443.

Christensen, M. and Hewitt-Taylor, J. (2006) Empowerment in nursing: paternalism or maternalism? *British Journal of Nursing, 15*(1), 695–699.

Christensen, M. and Hewitt-Taylor J. (2006) Empowerment in nursing: paternalism or maternalism? *British Journal of Nursing, 15*(13), 696–699. www.ncbi.nlm.nih.gov/pubmed/16926716.

Christie, D. and Khatun, H. (2012) Adjusting to life with chronic illness. *The Psychologist, 25*(3), 194–197.

Christie, D. and Khatun, H. (2012) Adjusting life to chronic illness. *The Psychologist, 25*(3), 194–197.

Christie, D. and Viner, R. (2009) Chronic illness and transition. *Adolescent Medicine, 20*(3), 981–987.

Clark, K.E. and Miller, G.A. (eds.) (1970) *Psychology: Behavioural and Social Sciences Survey Committee.* Englewood Cliffs, NJ: Prentice Hall.

Clarke, A. and Clarke, A. (2000) *Early Experience and the Life Path.* London: Jessica Kingsley.

Clinical Standards Advisory Group. (2000) *Services for Patients with Pain.* London: National Pain Audit.

Cloninger, C.R. (1987) Neurogenetic adaptive mechanisms in alcoholism. *Science, 236,* 410–416.

Clow, A. (2001) The physiology of stress. In F. Jones and J. Bright (eds.) *Stress: Myth, Theory and Research.* Harlow, UK: Pearson.

Cochrane, R. (1983) *The Social Creation of Mental Illness.* London: Longman.

Coffey, L., Skipper, K. and Jung, F. (1988) Nurses and shift work: effects on job performance and job related stress. *Journal of Advanced Nursing, 13,* 245–254.

Cohen, F. and Lazarus, R.S. (1979) Coping with the stress of illness. In G.C. Stone, N.E. Adler and F. Cohen (eds.) *Health Psychology: A Handbook.* Washington, DC: Jossey-Bass.

Cohen, J. (1958) *Humanistic Psychology.* London: Allen & Unwin.

Cole, M. (1990) Cultural psychology: a once and future discipline? In J.J. Berman (ed.) *Nebrasksa Symposium on Motivation: Cross-Cultural Perspectives.* Lincoln, NA: University of Nebraska Press.

Coleman, J.C. (1980) *The Nature of Adolescence.* London: Methuen.

Coleman, J.C. (1995) Adolescence. In P.E. Bryant and A.M. Colman (eds.) *Developmental Psychology.* London: Longman.

Coleman, J.C. and Hendry, L.B. (1990) *The Nature of Adolescence* (2nd edn.). London: Routledge.

Coleman, J.C. and Roker, D. (1998) Adolescence. *The Psychologist, 11*(12), 593–596.

Coleman, P.G. and O'Hanlon, A. (2004) *Ageing and Development.* London: Arnold.

Collins, J. (1994) What is pain? In J. Robbins (ed.) *Caring for the Dying Patient and the Family* (2nd edn.). London: Chapman & Hall.

Colville, G. (2008) The psychologic impact on children of admission to intensive care. *Paediatric Clinics of North America, 55,* 605–616.

Colville, G. (2012) Paediatric intensive care. *The Psychologist, 25*(3), 206–209.

Colville, G., Darkins, J., Hesketh, J., Bennett, V., Alcock, J. and Noyes, J. (2009) The impact of a child's admission to intensive care: integration of qualitative findings from a cross-sectional study. *Intensive and Critical Care Nursing, 25,* 72–79.

Colville, G., Kerry, S. and Pierce, C. (2008) Children's factual and delusional stories of intensive care. *American Journal of Respiratory and Critical Care Medicine, 177,* 976–982.

Compas, B.E., Hinden, B.R. and Gerhardt, C.A. (1995) Adolescent development: pathways and processes of risk and resilience. *Annual Review of Psychology, 46,* 265–293.

Conrad, R., Schilling, G., Bausch, C., Nadstawek, J., Wartenberg, H.C., Wegener, I., Geiser, F., Imbierowicz, K. and Liedtke, R. (2007) Temprerament and character personality profiles and personality disorders in chronic pain patients. *Pain, 133,* 197–209.

Cooke, M.W., Cooke, H.M. and Glucksman E.E. (1992) Management of sudden bereavement in the accident and emergency department. *British Medical Journal, 304,* 1207–1209.

Coolican, H. (2004) *Research Methods and Statistics in Psychology* (4th edn.). London: Hodder & Stoughton.

Coolican, H., Cassidy, T., Chercher, A., Harrower, J., Penny, G., Sharp, R., Walley, M. and Westbury, T. (1996) *Applied Psychology.* London: Hodder & Stoughton.

Coolican, H., Cassidy, T., Dunn, O., Sharp, R., Tudway, J., Simmonds, K., Westbury, T. and Harrower, J. (2007) *Applied Psychology* (2nd edn.). London: Hodder and Stoughton.

Cooper, A. M. and Palmer, A. (2003) *Mentoring, Preceptorship and Clinical Supervision: A Guide to Professional Roles in Clinical Practice* (2nd edn.). New York: Wiley-Blackwell.

Cooper, C. and Faragher, B. (1993) Psychological stress and breast cancer: the interrelationship between stress events, coping strategies and personality. *Psychological Medicine, 23*, 653–662.

Cooper, D. (1995) NT guide to working with people who misuse drugs. *Nursing Times Guides*.

Cooper, J., Kelly, K.A. and Weaver, K. (2004) Attitudes, norms and social groups. In M.B. Brewer and M. Hewstone (eds.) *Social Cognition*. Oxford: Blackwell Publishing.

Coopersmith, S. (1967) *The Antecedents of Self-Esteem*. San Francisco: Freeman.

Costa, P.T. and McCrae, R.R. (1992) *Revised NEO Personality Inventory (NEO-PI-R)*. Odessa, FL: Psychological Assessment Resources.

Costa, P.T., Yang, J. and McCrae, R.R. (2008) Ageing and personality traits: Generalisations and clinical implications. In I.H. Nordhus, G.R. VandenBos, S. Ber and P. Fromholt (eds.) *Clinical Geropsychology*. Washington, DC: American Psychological Association.

Costello, J. (2000) Truth telling and the dying patient: a conspiracy of silence? *International Journal of Palliative Care, 6*(8), 398–405.

Cox, T. (1978) *Stress*. London: Macmillan Education.

Craig, G.J. (1992) *Human Development* (6th edn.). Englewood Cliffs, NJ: Prentice Hall.

Craig, K.D., Prkachin, K.M. and Grunau, R.E. (2001) The facial expression of pain. In D.C. Turk and R. Melzack (eds.) *Handbook of Pain Assessment* (2nd edn.). New York: Guilford Press.

Cramer, D. (1995) Special issue on personal relationships. *The Psychologist, 8*, 58–59.

Crawford, M. and Unger, R.K. (1995) Gender issues in psychology. In A.M. Colman (ed.) *Controversies in Psychology*. London: Longman.

Crawford, R. (1984) A cultural account of health: self-control, release and the social body. In J. McKinlay (ed.) *Issues in the Political Economy of Health Care*. London: Tavistock.

Crombez, G., Eccleston, C., Van Hamme, G. and De Vlieger, P. (2008) Attempting to solve the problem of pain: a questionnaire study in acute and chronic pain patients. *Pain, 137*, 556–563.

Crouch, D. (2003) Tackling substance abuse. *Nursing Times, 99*(33), 20–23.

Crutchfield, R.S. (1954) A new technique for measuring individual differences in conformity to group judgement. *Proceedings of the Invitational Conference on Testing Problems*, 69–74.

Cumming, E. (1975) Engagement with an old theory. *International Journal of Ageing & Human Development, 6*, 187–191.

Cumming, E. and Henry, W.E (1961) *Growing Old: The Process of Disengagement*. New York: Basic Books.

Curry, C. (1998) Adolescence. In K. Trew and J. Kremer (eds.) *Gender and Psychology*. London: Arnold.

Curtiss, A. (1999) The psychology of pain. *Psychology Review, 5*(4), 15–18.

Cuthbertson, B.H., Rattray, J., Campbell, M.K., Gager, M., Roughton, S., Smith, A., Hull, A. et al. (2009) The practical study of nurse led, intensive care follow-up programmes for improving long term outcomes from critical illness. *British Medical Journal, 339*, b3723.

Dacey, J.S. (1982) *Adolescents Today* (2nd edn.). Glenview, IL: Scott, Foresman & Co.

Damasio, A.R., Van Hoesen, G.W. and Hyman, B.T. (1990) Reflections on the selectivity of neuropathological changes in Alzheimer's disease. In M.F. Schwartz (ed.) *Modular Deficits in Alzheimer's Dementia*. Cambridge, MA: MIT Press.

Damon, W. and Hart, D. (1988) *Self-Understanding in Childhood and Adolescence*. Cambridge: Cambridge University Press.

Damrosch, S. (1995) Facilitating adherence to preventive and treatment regimes. In D. Wedding (ed.) *Behaviour and Medicine* (2nd edn.). St Louis, MO: Mosby-Year Book.

Daniel, H.C. and de C Williams, A.C. (2010) Pain. In D. French, K. Vedhara, A.A. Kaptein and J. Weinman (eds.) *Health Psychology* (2nd edn.). Oxford: BPS Blackwell.

Darbyshire, P. (1986a, 2 April) 'Can Tiger come, too?' *Nursing Times*, 40–42.

Darwin, C. (1859) *The Origin of Species by Means of Natural Selection*. London: John Murray.

Dasen, P.R. (1994) Culture and cognitive development from a Piagetian perspective. In W.J. Lonner and R.S. Malpass (eds.) *Psychology and Culture*. Boston, MA: Allyn & Bacon.

Dasen, P.R. (1999) Rapid social change and the turmoil of adolescence: a cross-cultural perspective. *International Journal of Group Tensions, 29*(1–2), 17–49.

Davey, G. (2008) *Psychopathology: Research, Assessment and Treatment in Clinical Psychology*. Chichester, UK: BPS Backwell.

David, D.J. and Barrit, J.A. (1977) Psychological aspects of head and neck cancer surgery. *Australia and New Zealand Journal of Surgery, 47*, 584–589.

David, D.J. and Barrit, J.A. (1982) Psychological implications of surgery for head and neck cancer. *Clinical Plactic Surgery, 9*, 327–336.

Davidson, A.R. and Jaccard, J. (1979) Variables that moderate the attitude–behaviour relation: results of a longitudinal survey. *Journal of Personality & Social Psychology, 37*, 1364–1376.

Davies, E. and Furnham, A. (1986) Body satisfaction in adolescent girls. *British Journal of Medical Psychology, 59*, 279–288.

Davies, N.J. (2012) Alcohol misuse in adolescents. *Nursing Standard, 26*(42), 43–48.

Davison, G.C. and Neale, J.M. (1994) *Abnormal Psychology* (6th edn.). New York: John Wiley.

Davison, G.C., Neale, J.M. and Kring, A.M. (2004) *Abnormal Psychology* (9th edn.). New York: John Wiley.

Davitz, L.L., Davitz, J.R. and Higuchi, Y. (1977) Cross-cultural inferences of physical pain and psychological distress, 2. *Nursing Times*, 556–558 (21 April).

Davydow, D.S., Richardson, L.P., Zatzick, D.F. and Katon, W.J. (2010) Psychiatric morbidity in paediatric critical illness survivors. *Archives of Paediatrics and Adolescent Medicine, 64*(4), 377–383.

Dean, A. (2002) Talking to dying patients of their hopes and needs. *Nursing Times, 98*(43), 34–35.

Deese, J. (1972) *Psychology as Science and Art*. New York: Harcourt Brace Jovanovich.

Denholm, C. (1987) The adolescent patient at discharge and in the post-hospitalisation environment: a review. *Maternal Child Nursing Journal, 16*(2), 95–101.

Department of Health (2008) *End of Life Care Strategy: Promoting High Quality Care for All Adults at the End of Life*. London: DOH.

DeSantis, L. (1994) Making anthropology clinically relevant to nursing care. *Journal of Advanced Nursing, 20*(4), 707–715.

Deutsch, M. and Gerard, H.B. (1955) A study of normative and informational social influence upon individual judgement. *Journal of Abnormal & Social Psychology, 51*, 629–636.

Devine, P.G. and Zuwerink, J.R. (1994) Prejudice and guilt: the internal struggle to control prejudice. In W.J. Lonner and R.S. Malpass (eds.) *Psychology and Culture*. Boston, MA: Allyn & Bacon.

Devlin, R. (1989) Robertson's revolution. *Nursing Times, 85*(5), 18.

DeWolff, M.S. and van Ijzendoorn, M.H. (1997) Sensitivity and attachment: a meta-analysis on parental antecedents of infant attachment. *Child Development, 68*, 571–591.

Dex, S. and Phillipson, C. (1986) Social policy and the older worker. In C. Phillipson and A. Walker (eds.) *Ageing and Social Policy: A Critical Assessment*. Aldershot: Gower.

Digman, J.M. (1990) Personality structure: emergence of the five-factor model. *Annual Review of Psychology, 41*, 417–440.

Dignity in Dying. (2010) *DPP's Policy on Assisted Suicide*. http://tiny.cc/DPP_assisted_dying.

Dimatteo, M.R. (2004) Variations in patients' adherence to medical recommendations: a quantitative review of 50 years of research. *Medical Care, 42*, 200–209.

Dimatteo, M.R., Giordani, P.J., Lepper, H.S. and Croghan, T.W. (2002) Patient adherence and medical treatment outcomes: a meta-analysis. *Medical Care, 40*, 794–811.

Dimatteo, M.R., Sherbourne, C., Hays, R., Ordway, L., Kravitz, R., McGlynn, E., Kaplan, S. and Rogers, W.H. (1993) Physicians' characteristics influence patients' adherence to medical treatment: results from the medical outcomes study. *Health Psychology, 12*, 245–286.

Dimond, B. (2008) *Legal Aspects of Nursing* (5th edn.). London: Longman Publishing Group.

Dollard, J., Doob, L.W., Mowrer, O.H. and Sears, R.R. (1939) *Frustration and Aggression.* New Haven, CT: Harvard University Press.

Donaldson, M. (1978) *Children's Minds.* London: Fontana.

Donnelly, C. (1991) Ending the torment. *Nursing Times, 87*(11), 36–38.

Dovidio, J.F., Brigham, J.C., Johnson, B.T. and Gaertner, S.L. (1996) Stereotyping, prejudice, and discrimination: another look. In C.N. Macrae, C. Stangor and M. Hewstone (eds.) *Stereotypes and Stereotyping.* New York: McGraw-Hill.

Downie, C.M. and Basford, P.R (eds.) (2003) *Mentoring in Practice: A Reader.* London: Greenwich University Press.

Dropkin, M.J. (1981) Changes in body image associated with head and neck cancer. *Cancer Nursing, 4*, 560–581.

Duchene, P. (1990) Using biofeedback for childbirth pain. *Nursing Times, 86*(25), 56.

Duck, S. (1991) *Friends for Life* (2nd edn.). Hemel Hempstead, UK: Harvester Wheatsheaf.

Dunn, V. (1988) Life after mastectomy. *Nursing Times* (Community Outlook), August, 34.

Durie, M.H. (1994) Maori perspectives of health and illness. In J. Spicer, A. Trlin and J.A. Walton (eds.) *Social Dimensions of Health and Disease: New Zealand Perspectives.* Palmerston North, NZ: Dunmore Press.

Durkin, K. (1995) *Developmental Social Psychology: From Infancy to Old Age.* Oxford: Blackwell.

Dyer, C. (2009) House of Lords votes against immunity from prosecution for relatives who help in assisted suicide abroad. *British Medical Journal, 339*, b2797.

Earp, J.A., Eng, E., O'Malley, M.S., Altpeter, M., Rauscher, G., Mayne, L., Mathews, H.F. et al. (2002) Increasing use of mammography among older, rural African American women: results from a community trial. *American Journal of Public Health, 92*, 646–654.

Eccleston, C. (2011) A normal psychology of chronic pain. *The Psychologist, 24*(6), 422–425.

Eccleston, C. and Crombez, G. (2007) Worry and chronic pain. *Pain, 132*, 233–236.

Eccleston, C., Malleson, P.M., Clinch, J., Connell, H. and Sourbut, C. (2003) Chronic pain in adolescents. *Archives of Disease in Childhood, 88*, 881–885.

Edwards, G. (1986) The alcohol dependence syndrome: a concept as stimulus to enquiry. *British Journal of Addiction, 81*, 71–84.

Egan, G. (1977) *You and Me.* California: Brooks/Cole.

Ekerling, L. and Kohrs, M.B. (1984) Research on compliance with diabetic regimens: application to practice. *Journal of the American Dietetic Association, 84*, 805–809.

Elkind, D. (1970) Erik Erikson's eight ages of man. *New York Times Magazine,* 5 April, 25–27, 84–92, 110–119.

Embriaco, N., Azoulay, E., Barrau, K., Kentish, N., Pochard, F., Loundou, A. and Papazian, L. (2007) High level of burnout in intensivists. *American Journal of Respiratory and Critical Care Medicine, 175*(7), 686–692.

Engel, G.L. (1977) The need for a new medical model: a challenge for bio-medicine. *Science, 196*, 129–135.

Engel, G.L. (1980) The clinical application of the biopsychosocial model. *American Journal of Psychiatry, 137*, 535–544.

Erikson, E.H. (1950) *Childhood and Society.* New York: Norton.

Erikson, E.H. (1963) *Childhood and Society* (2nd edn.). New York: Norton.

Evans, D. and Allen, H. (2002) Emotional intelligence: its role in training. *Nursing Times, 98*(27), 41–42.

Ewins, D. and Bryant, J. (1992) Relative comfort. *Nursing Times, 88*(52), 61–63.

Eysenck, H.J. (1985) *Decline and Fall of the Freudian Empire.* Harmondsworth, UK: Penguin.

Facione, N.C., Giancarlo, C. and Chan, L. (2000) Perceived risk and help-seeking behaviour for breast cancer: a Chinese-American perspective. *Cancer Nursing, 23*, 258–267.

Fairbairn, R. (1952) *Psychoanalytical Studies of the Personality.* London: Tavistock.

Fancher, R.E. (1979) *Pioneers of Psychology.* New York: Norton.

Fancher, R.E. (1996) *Pioneers of Psychology* (3rd edn.). New York: Norton.

Fawcett, J. and Fry, S. (1980) An exploratory study of body image dimensionality. *Nursing Research, 29*(5), 324–327.

Fazio, R.H. (1986) How do attitudes guide behaviour? In R.M. Sorrentino and E.T. Higgins (eds.) *Handbook of Motivation and Cognition: Foundations of Social Behaviour.* New York: Guilford.

Fazio, R.H. (1990) Multiple processes by which attitudes guide behaviour: the MODE model as an integrative framework. In M.P. Zanna (ed.) *Advances in Experimental Social Psychology, Vol. 23.* San Diego, CA: Academic Press.

Fazio, R.H. and Zanna, M.P. (1978) Attitudinal qualities relating to the strength of the attitude–behaviour relation. *Journal of Experimental Social Psychology, 14*, 398–408.

Fennell, G., Phillipson, C. and Evers, H. (1988) *The Sociology of Old Age.* Milton Keynes, UK: Open University Press.

Fergusson, D.M., Horwood, L.J. and Ridder, E.M. (2006) Abortion in young women and subsequent mental health. *Journal of Child Psychology & Psychiatry, 47*(1), 16–24.

Fernando, S. (1991) *Mental Health, Race and Culture.* London: Macmillan, in conjunction with MIND.

Festinger, L. (1950) Informal social communication. *Psychological Review, 57*, 271–282.

Festinger, L. (1954) A theory of social comparison processes. *Human Relations, 7*, 117–140.

Festinger, L. (1957) *A Theory of Cognitive Dissonance.* New York: Harper & Row.

Festinger, L. and Carlsmith, J.M. (1959) Cognitive consequences of forced compliance. *Journal of Abnormal & Social Psychology, 58*, 203–210.

Field, D. and Copp, G. (1999) Communication and awareness about dying in the 1990s. *Palliative Medicine, 13*(6), 459–468.

Fields, H.L. (2009) The psychology of pain. *Scientific American Mind, 20*(5), 42–49.

Fife, B.L., Huster, G.A., Cornetta, K.G., Kennedy, V.N., Akard, L.P. and Broun, E.R. (2000) Longitudinal study of adaptation to the stress of bone marrow transplantation. *Journal of Clinical Oncology, 18*(7), 1539–1549.

Firn, S. and Norman, I.J. (1995) Psychological and emotional impact of an HIV diagnosis. *Nursing Times, 91*(8), 37–39.

Fishbein, M. (1967) Attitudes and the prediction of behaviour. In M. Fishbein (ed.) *Readings in Attitude Theory and Measurement.* New York: John Wiley.

Fishbein, M. and Ajzen, I. (1974) Attitudes towards objects as predictors of single and multiple behavioural criteria. *Psychological Review, 81*, 59–74.

Fishbein, M. and Ajzen, I. (1975) *Belief, Attitude, Intention and Behaviour: An Introduction to Theory and Research.* Reading, MA: Addison-Wesley.

Fiske, A.P., Kitayama, S., Markus, H.R. and Nisbett, R.E. (1998) The cultural matrix of social psychology. In D.T. Gilbert, S.T. Fiske and G. Lindzey (ed.) *Handbook of Social Psychology* (4th edn., Vol. 2). New York: McGraw-Hill.

Fiske, S.T. (2004) *Social Beings: A Core Motives Approach to Social Psychology.* New York: John Wiley.

Fiske, S.T. and Taylor, S.E. (1991) *Social Cognition* (2nd edn.). New York: McGraw-Hill.

Flavell, J.H. (1982) Structures, stages and sequences in cognitive development. In W.A. Collins (ed.) *The Concept of Development: The Minnesota Symposia on Child Development, Vol. 15.* Hillsdale, NJ: Erlbaum.

Flavell, J.H. (1986) The development of children's knowledge about the appearance–reality distinction. *American Psychologist, 41,* 418–425.

Flavell, J.H., Green, F.L. and Flavell, E.R. (1990) Developmental changes in young children's knowledge about the mind. *Cognitive Development, 5,* 1–27.

Flavell, J.H., Shipstead, S.G. and Croft, K. (1978) *What Young Children Think You See When Their Eyes Are Closed.* Unpublished report, Stanford University.

Fletcher, B.C. (1995) The consequences of stress. In D. Messer and C. Meldrum (eds.) *Psychology for Nurses and Health Care Professionals.* Hemel Hempstead, UK: Prentice Hall/Harvester Wheatsheaf.

Folkman, S. and Lazarus, R.S. (1988) *Manual for the Ways of Coping Questionnaire.* Palo Alto, CA: Consulting Psychologists Press.

Forshaw, M. (2002) *Essential Health Psychology.* London: Arnold.

Foxcroft, D.R., Ireland, D., Lister-Sharp, D.J., Lowe, G. and Breen, R. (2008) Primary prevention for alcohol misuse in young people. *Cochrane Database Systems* (3rd edn.), CD003024.

Franklin, L.L., Ternestedt, B.M. and Nordenfelt, L. (2006) Views on dignity of elderly nursing home residents. *Nursing Ethics, 13,* 130–146.

Freedman, J.L. (1963) Attitudinal effects of inadequate justification. *Journal of Personality, 31,* 371–385.

Freedman, J.L. (1965) Long-term behavioural effects of cognitive dissonance. *Journal of Experimental & Social Psychology, 1,* 145–155.

French, D., Vedhara, K., Kaptein, A.A. and Weinman, J. (eds.) (2010) *Health Psychology* (2nd edn.). Oxford: BPS Blackwell.

French, D.P. and Cooke, R. (2012) Using the theory of planned behaviour to understand binge drinking: the importance of beliefs for developing interventions. *British Journal of Health Psychology, 17*(1), 1–17.

Freud, A. and Dann, S. (1951) An experiment in group upbringing. *Psychoanalytic Study of the Child, 6,* 127–168.

Freud, S. (1914) *Remembering, Repeating and Working Through. The Standard Edition of Complete Psychological Works of Sigmund Freud, Volume XII.* London: Hogarth Press.

Freud, S. (1926) Inhibitions, symptoms and anxiety. In *Standard Edition of the Complete Psychological Works of Sigmund Freud,* Vol. XX. London: Hogarth Press.

Freud, S. (1949) *An Outline of Psychoanalysis.* London: Hogarth Press.

Friedman, M. and Rosenman, R.H. (1974) *Type A Behaviour and Your Heart.* New York: Harper Row.

Frith, M. (2006) Warning: campaigns to promote health are a waste of money. *Independent,* 18 April, 7.

Froggatt, A. (1988) Self-awareness in early dementia. In B. Gearing, M. Johnson and T. Heller (eds.) *Mental Health Problems in Old Age: A Reader.* Chichester, UK: John Wiley.

Fromant, S. (1988) Helping each other. *Nursing Times, 84*(36), 30–32.

Funnell, E. (1996) The single case study and Alzheimer-type dementia. In R.G. Morris (ed.) *The Cognitive Neuropsychology of Alzheimer-Type Dementia.* Oxford: Oxford University Press.

Fursland, E. (1998) Finding ways to cope. *Nursing Times, 94*(33), 30–31.

Galaal, K.A., Deane, K., Sangal, S. and Lopes, A.D. (2007) Interventions for reducing anxiety in women undergoing colopscopy. *Cochrane Database Systems* (3rd edn.), CD006013.

Gallagher, M., Millar, R., Hargie, O. and Ellis, R. (1992) The personal and social worries of adolescents in Northern Ireland: results of a survey. *British Journal of Guidance & Counselling, 30*(3), 274–290.

Gallup, C.G. (1970) Chimpanzees: self-recognition. *Science, 167,* 86–87.

Garrard, P. (2010) Neurology for psychiatrists. In B.K. Puri and I. Treasaden (eds.) *Psychiatry: An Evidence-Based Text.* London: Hodder Arnold.

Garrett, R. (1996) Skinner's case for radical behaviourism. In W. O'Donohue and R.F. Kitchener (eds.) *The Philosophy of Psychology.* London: Sage.

Gauntlett-Gilbert, J. and Connell, H. (2011) Coping and acceptance in chronic childhood conditions. *The Psycholgist, 25*(3), 198–201.

Gaze, H. (1988) Stressed to the limit. *Nursing Times, 84*(36), 16–17.

Gelder, M., Mayou, R. and Geddes, J. (1999) *Psychiatry* (2nd edn.). Oxford: Oxford University Press.

Gelman, R. (1979) Preschool thought. *American Psychologist, 34,* 900–905.

Gentleman, J.F. and Lee, J. (1997) Who doesn't get a mammography? *Health Reports* (Statistic Canada, Catalogue 82-003-XPB), *9,* 20–28.

George, M. (1995) Crisis of silence. *Nursing Standard, 10*(10), 20–21.

Gibbs, G. (1988) *Learning by Doing: A Guide to Teaching and Learning Methods.* Oxford: Oxford Polytechnic Further Education Unit.

Gidron, Y., Russ, K., Tissarchondou, H. and Warner, J. (2006) The relation between psychololgical factors and DNA damage: a critical review. *Biological Psychology, 72,* 291–304.

Gilbert, S.J. (1981) Another look at the Milgram obedience studies: the role of the graduated series of shocks. *Personality & Social Psychology Bulletin, 7,* 690–695.

Gill, M. and McGrath, J. (2010) Genetics. In B.K. Puri and I. Treasaden (eds.) *Psychiatry: An Evidence-Based Text.* London: Hodder Arnold.

Gillies, M. (1992) Teenage traumas. *Nursing Times, 88*(27), 26–29.

Gilligan, C. (1982) *In a Different Voice: Psychological Theory and Women's Development.* Cambridge, MA: Harvard University Press.

Glaser, B.G. and Strauss, A.L. (1968) *Time for Dying.* Chicago, IL: Aldine.

Glassman, W.E. (1995) *Approaches to Psychology* (2nd edn.). Buckingham, PA: Open University Press.

Glide, S. (1994) Maintaining sensory balance. *Nursing Times, 27*(90), 33–34.

Goetsch, V.L. and Fuller, M.G. (1995) Stress and stress management. In D. Wedding (ed.) *Behaviour and Medicine* (2nd edn.). St Louis, MO: Mosby-Year Book.

Gogtay, N., Giedd, J.N., Lusk, L., Hayashi, K.M., Greenstein, D., Vaituzis, A.C., Nugent, T.F. et al. (2009) Dynamic mapping of human cortical development during childhood through early adulthood. *Proceedings of the National Academy of Sciences, 101*(21), 8174–8179.

Goldberg, L.R. (1993) The structure of phenotypic personality traits. *American Psychologist, 48,* 26–34.

Goldberg, S. (2000) *Attachment and Development.* London: Arnold.

Goldfarb, W. (1943) The effects of early institutional care on adult personality. *Journal of Experimental Education, 12,* 106–129.

Gollwitzer, P.M. (1993) Goal achievement: the role of intentions. In W. Stroebe and M. Hewstone (eds.) *European Review of Social Psychology, Vol. 4.* Chichester, UK: John Wiley.

Golombok, S. (2010) Children in new family forms. In R. Gross (ed.) *Psychology: The Science of Mind and Behaviour* (6th edn.). London: Hodder Education.

Golombok, S., Brewaeys, A., Cook, R., Giavazzi, M.T., Guerra, D., Mantovani, A., van Hall, E., Crosignani, P.G. and Dexeus, S. (1996) The European Study of Assisted Reproduction Families. *Human Reproduction, 11*(10), 2324–2331.

Golombok, S., Brewaeys, A., Giavazzi, M.T., Guerra, D., MacCallum, F. and Rust, J. (2002a) The European Study of Assisted Reproduction Families: the transition to adolescence. *Human Reproduction, 17*(3), 830–840.

Golombok, S., Cook, R., Bish, A. and Murray, C. (1995) Families created by the new reproductive technologies: quality of parenting and social and emotional development of the children. *Child Development, 66*, 285–289.

Golombok, S., MacCallum, F. and Goodman, E. (2001) The 'test tube' generation: parent–child relationships and the psychological well-being of in vitro fertilisation children at adolescence. *Child Development, 72*, 599–608.

Golombok, S., MacCallum, F., Goodman, E. and Rutter, M. (2002b) Families with children conceived by donor insemination: a follow-up at age 12. *Child Development, 73*(3), 952–968.

Golombok, S., Owen, L., Blake, L., Murray, C. and Jadva, V. (2009) Parent-child relationships and the psychological well-being of 18-year-old adolescents conceived by in vitro fertilisation. *Human Fertility, 12*(2), 63–72.

Golombok, S., Perry, B., Burston, A., Murray, C., Mooney-Somers, J., Stevens, M. and Golding, J. (2003) Children with lesbian parents: a community study. *Developmental Psychology, 39*(1), 20–33.

Golombok, S. and Tasker, F. (1996) Do parents influence the sexual orientation of their children? Findings from a longitudinal study of lesbian families. *Developmental Psychology, 32*(1), 3–11.

Golombok, S., Tasker, F. and Murray, C. (1997) Children raised in fatherless families from infancy: family relationships and the socioemotional development of children of lesbian and single heterosexual mothers. *Journal of Child Psychology & Psychiatry, 38*(7), 83–92.

Goodman, N. (1978) *Ways of World Making.* Indianapolis, IN: Hackett Publishing.

Gopnik, A. and Astington, J.W. (1988) Children's understanding of representational change and its relation to the understanding of false belief and the appearance–reality distinction. *Child Development, 59*, 26–37.

Gopnik, A. and Wellman, H.M. (1994) The theory theory. In L.A. Hirschfield and S.A. Gelman (eds.) *Mapping the Mind.* Cambridge: Cambridge University Press.

Gosline, A. (2009) Five ages of the brain: 3. Adolescence. *New Scientist, 202*(2702), 29–30.

Granja, C., Gomes, E., Amarao, A., Ribeiro, O., Jones, C., Carneiro, A., Costa-Pereira, A. and JMIP Study Group. (2008) Understanding posttraumatic stress disorder-related symptoms after critical care: the early illness amnesia hypothesis. *Critical Care Medicine, 36*(10), 2801–2809.

Granja, C., Lopes, A., Moreira, S., Dias, C., Costa-Pereira, A. and Carneiro, A. (2005) Patients' recollections of experiences in the intensive care unit may affect their quality of life. *Critical Care, 9*(2), R96–R109.

Greer, S. (1991) Psychological response to cancer and survival. *Psychological Medicine, 21*, 43–49.

Greer, S. and Morris, T. (1975) Psychological attributes of women who develop breast cancer: a controlled study. *Journal of Psychosomatic Research, 19*, 147–153.

Greer, S., Morris, T. and Pettingale, K.W. (1979) Psychological response to breast cancer: effect on outcome. *The Lancet, 13*, 785–787.

Greer, S., Morris, T., Pettingale, K.W. and Haybittle, J.L. (1990) Psychological responses to breast cancer and fifteen year outcome. *Lancet, 335*, 49–50.

Greisinger, A.J., Lorimor, R.J., Aday, L.A., Winn, R.J. and Baile, W.F. (1997) Terminally ill cancer patients: their most important concerns. *Cancer Practitioners, 5*, 147–154.

Griffiths, E. (1989) More than skin deep. *Nursing Times, 85*(40), 34–36.

Griffiths, M.D. (1995) Technological addictions. *Clinical Psychology Forum, 76*, 14–19.

Griffiths, M.D. (2010) Addictions. In R. Gross *Psychology: The Science of Mind and Behaviour* (6th edn.). London: Hodder Education.

Griffiths, R.D. and Jones, C. (2001) Filling the intensive care memory gap? *Intensive Care Medicine, 27*, 344–346.

Groskop, V. (2004) Minding the parent gap. *Observer*, 25 April, 4.

Gross, R. (2009) *Themes, Issues and Debates in Psychology* (3rd edn.). London: Hodder Education.

Gross, R. (2010) *Psychology: The Science of Mind & Behaviour* (6th edn.). London: Hodder Arnold.

Gross, R. (2012a) *Being Human: Psychological and Philosophical Perspectives*. London: Hodder Education.

Gross, R. (2012b) *Key Studies in Psychology* (6th edn.). London: Hodder Education.

Grunau, R.V. and Craig, K.D. (1987) Pain expression in neonates: facial action and cry. *Pain, 28*, 395–410.

Grunau, R.V., Johnston, C.C. and Kenneth, D. (1990) Neonatal facial and cry responses to invasive and non-invasive procedures. *Pain, 42*, 295–205.

Grunau, R.V., Oberlander, T., Holsti, L. and Whitfield, M.F. (1998) Bedside application of the neonatal facial coding system in pain assessment of premature neonates. *Pain, 76*, 277–286.

Hadjistavropoulos, T., vonBaeyer, C. and Craig, K.D. (2001) Pain assessment in persons with limited ability to communicate. In D.C. Turk and R. Melzack (eds.) *Handbook of Pain Assessment* (2nd edn.). New York: Guilford Press.

Haigh, C. (2012) Exploring the case for assisted dying in the UK. *Nursing Standard, 26*(18), 33–39.

Hall, G.S. (1904) *Adolescence*. New York: Appleton & Co.

Hall, S. and Payne, S. (2010) Palliative and end-of-life care. In D. French, K. Vedhara, A.A. Kaptein and J. Weinman (eds.) *Health Psychology* (2nd edn.). Oxford: BPS Blackwell.

Hall, S., Chochinov, H., Maurray, S., Harding, R., Richardson, A. and Higginson, I.J. (2009) Assessing the feasibility, acceptability and potential effectiveness of dignity therapy for older people in care homes: Study Protocol. *BMC Geriatrics, 9*.

Hamilton, L. and Timmons, C.R. (1995) Psychopharmacology. In D. Kimble and A.M. Colman (eds.) *Biological Aspects of Behaviour*. London: Longman.

Hamilton, V.L. (1978) Obedience and responsibility: a jury simulation. *Journal of Personality & Social Psychology, 36*, 126–146.

Hamilton-West, K. (2011) *Psychobiological Processes in Health and Illness*. London: Sage.

Hammersley, R. (1999) Substance use, abuse and dependence. In D. Messer and F. Jones (eds.) *Psychology and Social Care*. London: Jessica Kingsley Publishers.

Harcourt, D. and Rumsey, N. (2008) Psychology and visible difference. *The Psychologist, 21*(6), 486–489.

Hare, J. and Pratt, C. (1989) Nurses' fear of death and comfort level with dying patients. *Death Studies, 13*, 349–360.

Harlow, H.F. (1959) Love in infant monkeys. *Scientific American, 200*, 68–74.

Harlow, H.F. and Zimmerman, R.R. (1959) Affectional responses in the infant monkey. *Science, 130*, 421–432.

Harris, P. and Middleton, W. (1995) Social cognition and health behaviour. In D. Messer and C. Meldrum (eds.) *Psychology for Nurses and Health Care Professionals*. Hemel Hempstead, UK: Prentice Hall/Harvester Wheatsheaf.

Hartley, J. and Branthwaite, A. (1997) Earning a crust. *Psychology Review, 3*(3), 24–26.

Hartley, J. and Branthwaite, A. (2000) Prologue: the roles and skills of applied psychologists. In J. Hartley and A. Branthwaite (eds.) *The Applied Psychologist* (2nd edn.). Buckingham: Open University Press.

Hasher, L. and Zacks, T.T. (1979) Automatic and effortful processes in memory. *Journal of Experimental Psychology: General, 108*, 356–388.

Havighurst, R.J. (1964) Stages of vocational development. In H. Borrow (ed.) *Man in a World at Work*. Boston, MA: Houghton Mifflin.

Havighurst, R.J., Neugarten, B.L. and Tobin, S.S. (1968) Disengagement and patterns of ageing. In B.L. Neugarten (ed.) *Middle Age and Ageing*. Chicago, IL: University of Chicago Press.

Hawkins, L.H. and Armstrong-Esther, C.A. (1978) Circadian rhythms and night shift working in nurses. *Nursing Times*, 49–52, May 4.

Hayes, S.C., Strosahl, K. and Wilson, K.G. (1999) *Acceptance and Commitment Therapy: An Experiential Approach to Behaviour Change.* New York: Guilford.

Hayslip, B. and Panek, P.E. (1989) *Adult Development and Ageing.* New York: Harper & Row.

Heather, N. (1976) *Radical Perspectives in Psychology.* London: Methuen.

Hedge, B. (1995) Psychological implications of HIV infection. In D. Messer and C. Meldrum (eds.) *Psychology for Nurses and Health Care Professionals.* Hemel Hempstead, UK: Prentice Hall/Harvester Wheatsheaf.

Heenan, A. (1990) Playing patients. *Nursing Times, 86*(46), 46–48.

Hegarty, J. (2000) Psychologists, doctors and cancer patients. In J. Hartley and A. Branthwaite (eds.) *The Applied Psychologist* (2nd edn.). Buckingham: Open University Press.

Heinonen, H., Volin, L., Zevon, M.A., Uutela, A., Barrick, C. and Ruutu, T. (2005) Stress among allogenic bone marrow transplantation patients. *Patient Education and Counselling, 56*(1), 62–71.

Helman, C. (1994) *Culture, health and illness.* London: Butterworth-Heinemann.

Hemingway, H. and Marmot, M. (1999) Psychosocial factors in the aetiology and prognosis of coronary heart disease: systematic review of prospective cohort studies. *British Medical Journal, 318,* 160–167.

Hendry, L.B. (1999) Adolescents and society. In D. Messer and F. Jones (eds.) *Psychology and Social Care.* London: Jessica Kingsley.

Hendry, L.B. and Kloep, M. (1999) Adolescence in Europe – an important life phase? In D. Messer and S. Millar (eds.) *Exploring Developmental Psychology: From Infancy to Adolescence.* London: Arnold.

Hendry, L.B., Shucksmith, J., Love, J.G. and Glendinning, A. (1993) *Young People's Leisure and Lifestyles.* London: Routledge.

Hennessy, J. and West, M.A. (1999) Intergroup behaviour in organisations: a field test of social identity theory. *Small Group Research, 30,* 361–382.

Hetherington, E.M. and Baltes, P.B. (1988) Child psychology and life-span development. In E.M. Hetherington, R. Lerner and M. Perlmutter (eds.) *Child Development in Life-Span Perspective.* Hillsdale, NJ: Erlbaum.

Hewitt, J. (2002) Psycho-affective disorder in Intensive Care Units: a review. *Journal of Clinical Nursing, 11*(5), 695–699.

Hewstone, M. (2003) Intergroup contact: panacea for prejudice? *The Psychologist, 16*(7), 352–355.

Hewstone, M., Rubin, M. and Willis, H. (2002) Intergroup bias. *Annual Review of Psychology, 53,* 575–604.

Hill, A. (2007) Cancer warning for stressed-out men. *Observer,* 2 September, 24.

Hill, P. (1993) Recent advances in selected aspects of adolescent development. *Journal of Child Psychology & Psychiatry, 34*(1), 69–99.

Hillan, E. (1991) Caesarean section: psychosocial effects. *Nursing Standard, 5*(50), 30–33.

Hinton, J. (1975) *Dying.* Harmondsworth, UK: Penguin.

Hochschild, A.R. (1983) *The Managed Heart: Commercialisation of Human Feeling.* Berkeley, CA: University of California Press.

Hodges, C. (1998) Easing children's pain. *Nursing Times, 94*(10), 55–58.

Hodges, J. and Tizard, B. (1989) Social and family relationships of ex-institutional adolescents. *Journal of Child Psychology & Psychiatry, 30,* 77–97.

Hofling, K.C., Brotzman, E., Dalrymple, S., Graves, N. and Pierce, C.M. (1966) An experimental study in the nurse–physician relationship. *Journal of Nervous & Mental Disorders, 143,* 171–180.

Hofstede, G. (1980) *Culture's consequences.* Beverly Hills, CA: Sage.

Hogg, M.A. and Abrams, D. (1988) *Social Identifications: A Social Psychology of Intergroup Relations and Group Processes.* London: Routledge.

Hogg, M.A. and Abrams, D. (2000) Social psychology. In N.R. Carlson, W. Buskist and G.N. Martin (eds.) *Psychology: The Science of Behaviour* (European Adaptation). Harlow, UK: Pearson Education Limited.

Hogg, M.A. and Vaughan, G.M. (1995) *Social Psychology: An Introduction*. Hemel Hempstead, UK: Prentice Hall/Harvester Wheatsheaf.

Holahan, C.K. and Sears, R.R. (1995) *The Gifted Group in Later Maturity*. Stanford, CA: Stanford University Press.

Hole, L. (1998) More than skin deep. *Nursing Times, 94*(33), 28–30.

Holland, K. and Hogg, C. (2001) *Cultural Awareness in Nursing and Health Care: An Introductory Text*. London: Arnold.

Holm, S. (1993) What is wrong with compliance? *Journal of Medical Ethics, 19*(2), 108–110.

Holmes, T.H. and Rahe, R.H. (1967) The social readjustment rating scale. *Journal of Psychosomatic Research, 11*, 213–218.

Holyoake, D.-D. (1998) Disentangling caring from love in a nurse–patient relationship. *Nursing Times, 94*(49), 56–58.

Horn, J.L (1982) The ageing of human abilities. In B. Wolman (ed.) *Handbook of Developmental Psychology*. Englewood Cliffs, NJ: Prentice Hall.

Horne, R. (2001) Compliance, adherence, and concordance. In K. Taylor and G. Harding (eds.) *Pharmacy Practice*. London: Taylor and Francis.

Horne, R. and Clatworthy, J. (2010) In D. French, K. Vedhara, A.A. Kaptein and J. Weinman (eds.) *Health Psychology* (2nd edn.). Oxford: BPS Blackwell.

Horne, R., Weinman, J., Barber, N., Elliott, R.A. and Morgan, M. (2006) *Concordance, Adherence and Compliance in Medicine Taking: A Conceptual Map and Research Priorities*. London: National Coordinating Centre for NHS Service Delivery and Organisation (NCCSDO).

Horton, M. (1999) Prejudice and discrimination: group approaches. In D. Messer and F. Jones (eds.) *Psychology and Social Care*. London: Jessica Kingsley Publishers.

Hortsman, W. and McKusick, L. (1986) The impact of AIDS on the physician. In L. McKusick (ed.) *What to Do about AIDS*. Berkeley, CA: University of California Press.

Hovland, C.I. and Sears, R.R. (1940) Minor studies in aggression, VI: correlation of lynching with economic indices. *Journal of Psychology, 2*, 301–310.

Hovland, C.I. and Janis, I.L. (1959) *Personality and Persuasibility*. New Haven, CT: Yale University Press.

Howarth, A. (2002) Management of chronic pain. *Nursing Times, 98*(32), 52–53.

Hudcova, J., McNichol, E., Quah, C., Lau, J. and Carr, D.B. (2006) Patient controlled opioid analgesia versus conventional opioid analgesia for postoperative pain. *Cochrane Database Systems* (4th edn.), CD003348.

Hunt, M. and Meerabeau, L. (1993) Purging the emotions: the lack of emotional expression in sub-fertility and in care of the dying. *International Journal of Palliative Care, 30*(2), 115–123.

IASP (International Association for the Study of Pain) (1986) Classification of chronic pain syndrome and definition of pain terms. *Pain, 3*(Supp.): S1–S226.

Jackson, S., Cicogani, E. and Charman, L. (1996) The measurement of conflict in parent–adolescent relationships. In L. Verhofstadt-Deneve, I. Kienhorst and C. Braet (eds.) *Conflict and Development in Adolescence*. Leiden, UK: DSWO Press.

Jacobs, M. (1992) *Freud*. London: Sage Publications.

James, T., Harding, I. and Corbett, K. (1994) Biased care? *Nursing Times, 90*(51), 28–30.

James, W. (1890) *The Principles of Psychology*. New York: Henry Holt & Company.

Jamieson, S. (1996) Altered body image. *Nursing Standard, 10*(16), 51–53.

Janis, I. and Feshbach, S. (1953) Effects of fear-arousing communication. *Journal of Abnormal & Social Psychology, 48*, 78–92.

Janis, I. and Terwillinger, R.T. (1962) An experimental study of psychological resistance to fear-arousing communication. *Journal of Abnormal & Social Psychology, 65*, 403–410.

Janis, I.L., Kaye, D. and Kirschner, P. (1965) Facilitating effects of 'eating-while-reading' on responsiveness to persuasive communications. J*ournal of Personality & Social Psychology, 1*, 181–186.

Janz, N.K. and Becker, M.H. (1984) The health belief model: a decade later. *Health Education Quarterly, 11*, 1–47.

Jarrett, C. (2011) Ouch! The different ways people experience pain. *The Psychologist, 24*(6), 416–420.

Jasper, M. (2003) *Beginning Reflective Practice*. Cheltenham: Nelson Thornes.

Jefferis, B.J., Power, C. and Manor, O. (2005) Adolescent drinking level and adult binge drinking in a national birth cohort. *Addiction, 100*(4), 543–549.

Jellinek, E.M. (1946) Phases in the drinking history of alcoholics. *Quarterly Journal of Studies on Alcohol, 7*, 1–88.

Jellinek, E.M. (1952) The phases of alcohol addiction. *Quarterly Journal of Studies on Alcohol, 13*, 673–684.

Jenness, A. (1932) The role of discussion in changing opinion regarding matter of fact. *Journal of Abnormal & Social Psychology, 27*, 279–296.

Jensen, M.P. and Karoly, P. (2001) Self-report scales and procedures for assessing pain in adults. In D.C. Turk and R. Melzack (eds.) *Handbook of Pain Assessment* (2nd edn.). New York: Guilford Press.

Johnson, J.H. and Sarason, I.G. (1978) Life stress, depression and anxiety: internal/external control as a moderator variable. *Journal of Psychosomatic Research, 22*, 205–208.

Jonas, K., Eagly, A.H. and Stroebe, W. (1995) Attitudes and persuasion. In M. Argyle and A.M. Colman (eds.) *Social Psychology*. London: Longman.

Jones, C., Backman, C., Capuzzo, M., Egerod, I., Flaatten, H., Granja, C., Rylander, C., Griffiths, R.D. and RACHEL group. (2010) Intensive care diaries reduce new onset post traumatic stress disorder following critical illness. *Critical Care, 14*(5), R168.

Jones, F. (1995) Managing stress in health care: issues for staff and patient care. In D. Messer and C. Meldrum (eds.) *Psychology for Nurses and Health Care Professionals*. Hemel Hempstead, UK: Prentice Hall/Harvester Wheatsheaf.

Joseph, J. (2003) *The Gene Illusion: Genetic Research in Psychiatry and Psychology under the Microscope*. Herefordshire, UK: PCCS Books.

Joynson, R.B. (1980) Models of man: 1879–1979. In A.J. Chapman and D.M. Jones (eds.) *Models of Man*. Leicester, UK: British Psychological Society.

Judd, D. (1989) *Give Sorrow Words: Working with a Dying Child*. London: Free Association Books.

Judd, D. (1993) Communicating with dying children. In D. Dickinson and M. Johnson (eds.) *Death, Dying & Bereavement*. London: Sage, in association with the Open University.

Jung, C.G. (ed.) (1964) *Man and His Symbols*. London: Aldus-Jupiter Books.

Jurrett, C. (2006) Physical therapists providing psychological support. *The Psychologist, 19*(3), 134.

Kabat-Zinn, J. (1990) Full catastrophe living: *Using the Wisdom of Your Body and Mind to Face Stress, Pain and Illness;* the program of the Stress Reduction Clinic at the University of Massachusetts Medical Centre. New York: Dell.

Kagan, J., Kearsley, R.B. and Zelago, P.R. (1978) *Infancy: Its Place in Human Development*. Cambridge, MA: Harvard University Press.

Kalish, R.A. (1982) *Late Adulthood: Perspectives on Human Development* (2nd edn.). Monterey, CA: Brooks-Cole.

Kastenbaum, R. (1979) *Growing Old – Years of Fulfilment*. London: Harper & Row.

Katz, D. (1960) The functional approach to the study of attitudes. *Public Opinion Quarterly, 24*, 163–204.

Katz, D. and Braly, K. (1933) Racial stereotypes of one hundred college students. *Journal of Abnormal & Social Psychology, 28*, 280–290.

Kauhanen, M.L., Korpelainen, J.T., Hiltunen, P.A., Brusin, E., Mononen, H., Määttä, R., Nieminen, P., Sotaniemi, K.A. and Myllylä, V.V. (1999) Poststroke depression correlates with cognitive impairment and neurological deficits. *Stroke, 30*(9), 1875–1880.

Kearney, M. and Mount, B. (2000) Spiritual care of the dying patient. In H.M. Cochinov and W. Reitbart (eds.) *Handbook of Psychiatry in Palliative Care*. New York: Oxford University Press.

Keefe, F.J., Williams, D.A. and Smith, S.J. (2001) In D.C. Turk and R. Melzack (eds.) *Handbook of Pain Assessment* (2nd edn.). New York: Guilford Press.

Kenrick, D.T. (1994) Evolutionary social psychology: from sexual selection to social cognition. *Advances in Experimental Social Psychology, 26*, 75–121.

Kerns, R.D., Haythornthwaite, J., Rosenberg, R., Southwick, S., Gller, E.L. and Jacob, M.C. (1991) The pain behaviour check list (PBCL): factor structure and psychometric properties. *Journal of Behavioural Medicine, 14*, 55–167.

Kessler, T. and Mummendey, A. (2008) Prejudice and intergroup relations. In M. Hewstone, W. Stroebe and K. Jonas (eds.) *Introduction to Social Psychology: A European Perspective* (4th edn.). Oxford: BPS Blackwell.

Khan, M.A., Sehgal, A., Mitra, B., Agarwal, P.N., Lal, P. and Malik, V.K. (2000) Psychobehavioural impact of mastectomy. *Journal of the Indian Academy of Applied Psychology, 26*(1–2), 65–71.

Khan, S. (2003) New wave of heroin sucks in pre-teens. *Observer*, 6 July, 6.

Kiecolt-Glaser, J.K., Garner, W., Speicher, C.E., Penn, G.M., Holliday, J. and Glaser, R. (1984) Psychosocial modifiers of immunocompetence in medical students. *Psychosomatic Medicine, 46*, 7–14.

Kiecolt-Glaser, J.K., Marucha, P.T., Malarkey, W.B., Mercado, A.M. and Glaser, R. (1995) Slowing of wound healing by psychological stress. *Lancet, 346*, 1194–1196.

Kiecolt-Glaser, J.K., Page, G.G., Marucha, P.T., MacCallum, R.C. and Glaser, R. (1998) Psychological influences on surgical recovery: perspectives from psychoneuroimmunology. *American Psychologist, 53*(11), 1209–1218.

Kiger, A.M. (1994) Student nurses' involvement with death: the image and the experience. *Journal of Advanced Nursing, 20*, 679–686.

King, T.L. and McCool, W.F. (2004) The definition and assessment of pain. *Journal of Midwifery and Women's Health 49*, 71–472.

Kitzinger, C. and Coyle, A. (1995) Lesbian and gay couples: speaking of difference. *The Psychologist, 8*, 64–69.

Kitzinger, C., Coyle, A., Wilkinson, S. and Milton, M. (1998) Towards lesbian and gay psychology. *The Psychologist, 11*(11), 529–533.

Klein, M. (1932) *The Psycho-Analysis of Children*. London: Hogarth.

Kleinman, A. (1980) *Patients and Healers in the Context of Culture: An Explanation of the Borderland between Anthropology, Medicine and Psychiatry*. Berekeley, CA: University of California Press.

Kline, P. (1984) *Personality and Freudian Theory*. London: Methuen.

Kline, P. (1988) *Psychology Exposed*. London: Routledge.

Kline, P. (1989) Objective tests of Freud's theories. In A.M. Colman and J.G. Beaumont (eds.) *Psychology Survey No. 7*. Leicester, UK: British Psychological Society.

Kloep, M. and Hendry, L.B. (1999) Challenges, risks, and coping in adolescence. In D. Messer and S. Millar (eds.) *Exploring Developmental Psychology: From Infancy to Adolescence*. London: Arnold.

Kloep, M. and Tarifa, F. (1993) Albanian children in the wind of change. In L.E. Wolven (ed.) *Human Resource Development*. Hogskolan: Ostersund.

Knotkova, H., Clark, W.C., Mokrejs, P., Padour, F. and Kuhl, J. (2004) What do ratings on unidimensional pain and emotion scales really mean? A multidimensional affect and pain survey (MAPS) analysis of cancer patient responses. *Journal of Pain and Symptom Management, 28*, 19–27.

Knowles, R.E. and Tarrier, N. (2009) Evaluation of the effect of prospective patient diaries on emotional well-being in intensive care unit survivors. *Critical Care Medicine, 37*(1), 184–191.

Kobasa, S.C. (1979) Stressful life events, personality and health: an inquiry into hardiness. *Journal of Personality & Social Psychology, 37*, 1–11.

Kobasa, S.C., Maddi, S.R. and Kahn, S. (1982) Hardiness and health: a prospective study. *Journal of Personality & Social Psychology, 42*, 168–177.

Kohli, N. and Dalal, A.K. (1988) Culture as a factor in causal understanding of illness: A study of cancer patients. *Psychology & Developing Societies, 10*, 115–129.

Koluchova, J. (1972) Severe deprivation in twins: a case study. *Journal of Child Psychology & Psychiatry, 13*, 107–114.

Koluchova, J. (1991) Severely deprived twins after 22 years' observation. *Studia Psychologica, 33*, 23–28.

Koster, M.E.T.A. and Bergsma, J. (1990) Problems in coping behaviour official cancer patients. *Social Science Medicine, 30*(5), 569–578.

Krackow, A. and Blass, T. (1995) When nurses obey or defy inappropriate physician orders: attributional differences. *Journal of Social Behaviour and Personality, 10*(3), 585–594.

Krantz, D.S., Arabian, J.M., Davia, J.E. and Parker, J.S. (1982) Type A behaviour and coronary bypass surgery: intraoperative blood pressure and perioperative complications. *Psychosomatic Medicine, 44*(3), 273–284.

Krebs, D. and Blackman, R. (1988) *Psychology: A First Encounter*. New York: Harcourt Brace Jovanovich.

Krieger, D. (2002) *Therapeutic Touch as Transpersonal Healing*. Englewood Cliffs, NJ: Lantern Books.

Kripalani, S., Yao, X. and Haynes, R.B. (2007) Interventions to enhance medication adherence in chronic medical conditions: a systematic review. *Archives of Internal Medicine, 167*, 540–550.

Kroger, J. (2007) *Identity Development: Adolescence through Adulthood* (2nd edn.). Thousand Oaks, CA: Sage.

Kroll, D. (1990) Equal access to care? *Nursing Times, 86*(23), 72–73.

Krupat, E. and Garonzik, R. (1994) Subjects' expectations and the search for alternatives to deception in social psychology. *British Journal of Social Psychology, 33*, 211–222.

Kübler-Ross, E. (1969) *On Death and Dying*. London: Tavistock/Routledge.

Kuhn, H.H. and McPartland, T.S. (1954) An empirical investigation of self attitudes. *American Sociological Review, 47*, 647–652.

Kuhn, T.S. (1962) *The Structure of Scientific Revolutions*. Chicago, IL: University of Chicago Press.

Kuhse, H. (1997) *Caring: Nurses, Women and Ethics*. New York: Wiley-Blackwell.

Kulik, J.A. and Mahler, H.I.M. (1989) Stress and affiliation in a hospital setting: pre-operative room-mate preference. *Personality & Social Psychology Bulletin, 15*, 183–193.

Kuppens, M., de Wit, J. and Stroebe, W. (1996) Angstaanjagenheid in gezondheids-voorlichting: Een dual process analyse. *Gedrag en Gezondheid, 24*, 241–248.

Kuykendall, J. (1989) Teenage trauma. *Nursing Times, 85*(27), 26–28.

Labouvie-Vief, G. (2005) The psychology of emotions and ageing. In M. Johnson, V.L. Bengston, P.G. Coleman and T. Kirkwood (eds.) *The Cambridge Handbook of Age and Ageing*. Cambridge: Cambridge University Press.

Lang, A.R. and Marlatt, G.A. (1982) Problem drinking: a social learning perspective. In R.J. Gatchel, A. Baum and J.E. Singer (eds.) *Handbook of Psychology and Health, Vol. 1. Clinical Pychology and Behavioural Medicine: Overlapping Disciplines.* Hillsdale, NJ: Erlbaum.

Lang, E.V., Benotsch, E.G., Fick, L.J., Lutgendorf, S., Berbaum, M.L., Bernbaum, K.S., Logan, H. et al. (2000) Adjunctive non-pharmacological analgesia for invasive medical procedures: a randomised trial. *Lancet, 355*(9214), 1486–1490.

Lang, F.R. and Carstensen, L.L. (1998) Social relationships and adapation in late life. In A.S. Bellack and M. Herson (eds.) *Comprehensive Clinical Psychology, Vol. 7.* Oxford: Pergamon.

Lang, F.R. and Carstensen, L.L. (2002) Time counts: future time perspective, goals, and social relationships. *Psychology and Ageing, 17*, 125–139.

Lansdown, R. and Benjamin, G. (1985) The development of the concept of death in children aged 5–9 years. *Child Care, Health and Development, 11*(1), 13–20.

Laswell, H.D. (1948) The structure and function of communication in society. In L. Bryson (ed.) *Communication of Ideas.* New York: Harper.

Lau, R.R. (1995) Cognitive representations of health and illness. In D. Gochman (ed.) *Handbook of Health Behaviour Research Vol. 1.* New York: Plenum.

Laurance, J. (2000) Young cocaine users run higher risk of strokes. *Independent,* 13 May, 5.

Laurance, J. (2005) Stress can reduce breast cancer risk researchers find. *Independent,* 9 September, 18.

Laureys, S. (2005) The neural correlate of (un) awareness: lessons from the vegetative state. *Trends in Cognitive Science, 9*(12), 556–559.

Lawler, J. (1991) *Behind the Screens: Nursing, Somology and the Problem of the Body.* Melbourne, VIC: Churchill Livingstone.

Lazarus, R.S. and Averill, J. (1978) Emotion and cognition. In C.D. Spielberger (ed.) *Anxiety: Current Trends in Theory and Research.* New York: New York Academy Press.

Lazarus, R.S. (1966) *Psychological Stress and the Coping Process.* New York: McGraw-Hill.

Lazarus, R.S. (1999) *Stress and Emotion: A New Synthesis.* London: Free Association Books.

Lazarus, R.S. and Folkman, S. (1984) *Stress, Appraisal and Coping.* New York: Springer.

Leekam, S. (1993) Children's understanding of mind. In M. Bennett (ed.) *The Child as Psychologist: An Introduction to the Development of Social Cognition.* Hemel Hempstead, UK: Harvester Wheatsheaf.

LeFrancois, G.R. (1983) *Psychology.* Belmont, CA: Wadsworth Publishing Co.

Legge, D. (1975) *An Introduction to Psychological Science.* London: Methuen.

Leidy, N.K., Margolis, M.K., Marcin. J.P., Flynn, J.A., Frankel, L.R., Johnson, S., Langkamp, D. and Simoes, E.A. (2005) The impact of severe respiratory syncytial virus on the child, caregiver and family during hospitalisation and recovery. *Paediatrics, 115*(6), 1536–1546.

Le Page, M. (2010) 'RNA rules, OK'. *New Scientist, 206*(2765), 34–35.

Leslie, J.C. (2002) *Essential Behaviour Analysis.* London: Arnold.

Leventhal, H., Benyamini, Y., Brownlee, S., Deifenbach, M., Leventhal, E.A., Patrick-Miller, L. and Robitaille, C. (1997) Illness representations: theoretical foundations. In K.J. Petrie and J.A. Weinman (eds.) *Perceptions of Health and Illness.* Amsterdam, the Netherlands: Harwood.

Leventhal, H., Meyer, D. and Nerenz, D. (1980) The common sense representation of illness danger. *Medical Psychology, 2*, 7–30.

Levinson, D.J. (1986) A conception of adult development. *American Psychologist, 41*, 3–13.

Levinson, D.J., Darrow, D.N., Klein, E.B., Levinson, M.H. and McKee, B. (1978) *The Seasons of a Man's Life.* New York: A.A. Knopf.

Levinson, D.J. and Levinson, J.D. (1997) *The Seasons of a Woman's Life.* New York: Ballantine Books.

Lewis, M. (1990) Social knowledge and social development. *Merrill–Palmer Quarterly, 36*, 93–116.

Lewis, M. and Brooks-Gunn, J. (1979) *Social Cognition and the Acquisition of Self.* New York: Plenum.

Ley, P. (1981) Professional non-compliance: a neglected problem. *British Journal of Clinical Psychology, 20*, 151–154.

Ley, P. (1989) Improving patients' understanding, recall, satisfaction and compliance. In A. Broome (ed.) *Health Psychology.* London: Chapman & Hall.

Likert, R. (1932) A technique for the measurement of attitudes. *Archives of Psychology, 22*, 140.

Lilienfeld, S.O. (1995) *Seeing Both Sides: Classic Controversies in Abnormal Psychology.* Pacific Grove, CA: Brooks/Cole Publishing Co.

Lipowski, Z.J. (1984) What does the word 'psychosomatic' really mean? A historical and semantic inquiry. *Psychosomatic Medicine, 46*, 53–171.

Lippmann, W. (1922) *Public Opinion.* New York: Harcourt.

Lipsedge, M. (1997) Addictions. In L. Rees, M. Lipsedge and C. Ball (eds.) *Textbook of Psychiatry.* London: Arnold.

Littlewood, R. and Lipsedge, M. (1989) *Aliens and Alienists: Ethnic Minorities and Psychiatry.* London: Unwin Hyman.

Lock, M. (1986) Ambiguities of ageing: Japanese experience and perceptions of menopause. *Culture, Medicine and Psychiatry, 10*, 23–46.

Lock, M. (1999) The politics of health, identity and culture. In R. Contrada and R. Ashmore (eds.) *Self, Social Identity and Physical Health.* New York: Oxford University Press.

Lombardo, V.S. and Lombardo, E.F. (1986) *Kids Grieve Too.* Chicago, IL: Charles C. Thomas.

Lorentz, M.M. (2006) Stress and psychoneuroimmunology revisted: using mind-body interventions to reduce stress. *Alternative Journal of Nursing, 11*, 1–11.

Lorenz, K. (1935) The companion in the bird's world. *Auk, 54*, 245–273.

Lowe, G. (1995) Alcohol and drug addiction. In A.A. Lazarus and A.M. Colman (eds.) *Abnormal Psychology.* London: Longman.

Lowes, L., Gregory, J.W. and Lyne, P. (2005) Newly diagnosed childhood diabetes: a psychosocial transition for parents? *Journal of Advanced Nursing, 50*(3), 253–261.

Maccoby, E.E. (1980) *Social Development: Psychological Growth and the Parent–Child Relationship.* New York: Harcourt Brace Jovanovich.

MacCallum, F. and Golombok, S. (2004) Children raised in fatherless families from infancy: a follow-up of children of lesbian and single heterosexual mothers at early adolescence. *Journal of Child Psychology & Psychiatry, 45*(7), 1407–1419.

MacKenzie, H. (1988) Teenagers in hospital. *Nursing Times, 84*(32), 58–61.

Maddox, G.L. (1964) Disengagement theory: a critical evaluation. *The Gerontologist, 4*, 80–83.

Maes, S. and van Elderen, T. (1998) Health psychology and stress. In M.W. Eysenck (ed.) *Psychology: An Integrated Approach.* London: Longman.

Maitland, J. and Goodliffe, H. (1989) The Alexander technique. *Nursing Times, 85*(42), 55–57.

Mann, L. (1969) *Social Psychology.* New York: Wiley.

Manthorpe, J. (1994) Life changes. *Nursing Times, 90*(18), 66–67.

March, P. (1995) Dying and bereavement. In D. Messer and C. Meldrum (eds.) *Psychology for Nurses and Health Care Professionals.* Hemel Hempstead, UK: Prentice Hall/Harvester Wheatsheaf.

March, P. and Doherty, C. (1999) Dying and bereavement. In D. Messer and F. Jones (eds.) *Psychology and Social Care.* London: Jessica Kingsley Publishers.

Marcia, J.E. (1998) Peer Gynt's life cycle. In E. Skoe and A. von der Lippe (eds.) *Personality Development in Adolescence: A Cross National and Lifespan Perspective.* London: Routledge.

Marcus, H.R. and Kitayama, S. (1991) Culture and the self: implications for cognition, emotion and motivation. *Psychological Review, 98*, 224–253.

Markus, H. and Nurius, P. (1986) Possible selves. *American Psychologist, 41*, 954–969.

Marland, G. (1998) Partnership encourages patients to comply with treatment. *Nursing Times, 94*(27), 58–59.

Marlatt, G.A., Baer, J.S., Kivlahan, D.R., Dimeff, L.A., Larimer, M.E., Quigley, L.A., Somers, J.M. and Williams, E. (1998) Screening and brief intervention for high-risk college student drinkers: results from a 2-year follow-up assessment. *Journal of Consulting & Clinical Psychology, 66*(4), 604–615.

Marrone, M. (1998) *Attachment and Interaction.* London: Jessica Kingsley Publishers.

Marsland, D. (1987) *Education and Youth.* London: Falmer.

Martin, R. and Hewstone, M. (2001) Conformity and independence in groups: majorities and minorities, In M.A. Hogg and R.S. Tindale (eds.) *Blackwell Handbook of Social Psychology: Group Processes.* Malden, MA: Blackwell Publishing.

Maslach, C. and Jackson, S.E. (1986) *Maslach Burn-Out Inventory.* San Francisco, CA: Consulting Psychologists Press.

Maslach, C. and Jackson, S.E. (1981) The measurement of experienced burnout. *Journal of Occupational Behaviour, 2*, 99–113.

Maslow, A. (1954) *Motivation and Personality.* New York: Harper & Row.

Maslow, A. (1968) *Towards a Psychology of Being* (2nd edn.). New York: Van Nostrand Reinhold.

Mason, P. (1991) Jobs for the boys. *Nursing Times, 87*(7), 26–28.

Matarazzo, J.D. (1982) Behavioural health's challenge to academic, scientific, and professional psychology. *American Psychologist, 37*, 1–14.

Mazhindu, D. (1998) Emotional healing. *Nursing Times, 94*(6), 26–28.

McCaffrey, M. and Beebe, A. (1994) *Pain: Clinical Manual for Nursing Practice.* London: Mosby.

McCann, M.E. and Kain, Z.N. (2001) The management of preoperative anxiety in children. *Anaesthesia and Analgesia, 93*(1), 98–105.

McCauley, C. and Stitt, C.L. (1978) An individual and quantitative measure of stereotypes. *Journal of Personality & Social Psychology, 36*, 929–940.

McClain, C.S., Rosenfeld, B. and Breitbart, W. (2003) Effect of spiritual well-being on end-of-life despair in terminally-ill cancer patients. *Lancet, 361*, 1603–1607.

McCraken, L.M. and Eccleston, C. (2003) Coping or acceptance? What to do about chronic pain. *Pain, 105*, 197–204.

McCracken, L.M. and Gauntlett-Gilbert, J. (2011) The role of psychological flexibility in parents of adolescents with chronic pain: development of a measure and preliminary correlation analyses. *Pain, 152*, 780–785.

McCrae, R.R. and Costa, P.T. (1989) More reasons to adopt the five-factor model. *American Psychologist, 44*, 451–452.

McDonald, D.D. (1994) Gender and ethnic stereotyping and narcotic analgesic administration. *Research in Nursing and Health, 17*(1), 45–49.

McDonald, S., Hetrick, S. and Green, S. (2004) Pre-operative education for hip or knee replacement. *Cochrane Database Systems* (1st edn.). CD003526.

McDowell, I. and Newell, C. (1996) *Measuring health: A guide to rating scales and questionnaires* (2nd edn.). New York: Oxford University Press.

McEleney, M. (1992) Facing facts. *Nursing Times, 88*(25), 56–58.

McEwen, B.S. and Seeman, T. (1999) Protective and damaging effects of mediators of stress: elaborating and testing the concepts of allostasis and allostatic load. *Annals of the New York Academy of Sciences, 896*, 30–47.

McGlone, F., Park, A. and Roberts, C. (1996) *Relative Values*. Family Policy Centre: BSA.

McGuire, W.J. (1968) Personality and susceptibility to social influence. In E.F. Borgatta and W.W. Lambert (eds.) *Handbook of Personality: Theory and Research*. Chicago, IL: Rand-McNally.

McGuire, W.J. (1969) The nature of attitudes and attitude change. In G. Lindzey and E. Aronson (eds.) *Handbook of Social Psychology* (2nd edn., Vol. 3). Reading, MA: Addison-Wesley.

McHaffie, H. (1994) Breaking down prejudices. *Nursing Times*, *90*(14), 34–35.

McIlfatrick, S., Sullivan, K., McKenna, H. and Parahoo, K. (2007) Patients' experiences of having chemotherapy in a day hospital setting. *Journal of Advanced Nursing, 59*(3), 254–273.

McVeigh, T. (2009) How Britain is coming to terms with growing old. *Observer*, 17 May.

Meadows, S. (1993) *The Child as Thinker: The Acquisition and Development of Cognition in Childhood*. London: Routledge.

Meadows, S. (1995) Cognitive development. In P.E. Bryant and A.M. Colman (eds.) *Developmental Psychology*. London: Longman.

Medawar, P.B. (1963) *The Art of the Soluble*. Harmondsworth, UK: Penguin.

Meier, D.E., Emmons, C.A., Wallenstein, S., Quill, T., Morrison, R.S. and Cassel, C.K. (1998) A national survey of physician-assisted suicide and euthanasia in the United States. *New England Journal of Medicine, 338*, 1193–1201.

Meins, E. (2003) Emotional development and early attachment relationships. In A. Slater and G. Bremner (eds.) *An Introduction to Developmental Psychology*. Oxford: Blackwell Publishing.

Meltzoff, A. and Moore, M. (1983) Newborn infants imitate adult facial gestures. *Child Development, 54*, 702–709.

Melzack, R. (1975) McGill pain questionnaire: major properties and scoring methods. *Pain, 1*, 277–299.

Melzack, R. (1987) The short form McGill pain questionnaire. *Pain, 30*, 191–197.

Melzack, R. and Wall, P.D. (1988) *The Challenge of Pain* (2nd edn.). Harmondsworth, UK: Penguin.

Melzack, R. and Wall, P.D. (1991) *The Challenge of Pain* (3rd edn.). Harmondsworth, UK: Penguin.

Mencap. (2007) *Death by indifference*. London: Mencap. www.mencap.org.uk/document.asp?id = 284.

Meyer, V. and Chesser, E.S. (1970) *Behaviour Therapy in Clinical Psychiatry*. Harmondsworth, UK: Penguin.

Middleton, W., Moylan, A., Raphael, B., Burnett, P. and Martinek, N. (1993) An international perspective on bereavement-related concepts. *Australian & New Zealand Journal of Psychiatry, 27*, 457–463.

Milgram, S. (1963) Behavioural study of obedience. *Journal of Abnormal & Social Psychology, 67*, 391–398.

Milgram, S. (1965) Liberating effects of group pressure. *Journal of Personality & Social Psychology, 1*, 127–134.

Milgram, S. (1974) *Obedience to Authority*. New York: Harper & Row.

Miller, C. and Newton, S.E. (2006) Pain perception and expression: the influence of gender, personal self-efficacy and lifespan socialisation. *Pain Management Nursing, 7*, 148–152.

Miller, E. and Morris, R. (1993) *The Psychology of Dementia*. Chichester, UK: John Wiley.

Miller, W.R. and Rollnick, S. (2002) *Motivational Interviewing: Preparing People for Change* (2nd edn.). New York: Guilford Press.

Milne, S., Sheeran, P. and Orbell, S. (2000) Prediction and intervention in health-related behaviour: a meta-analytic review of protection motivation theory. *Journal of Applied Social Psychology, 30*, 106–143.

Minardi, H.A. and Riley, M. (1988) Providing psychological safety through skilled communication. *Nursing, 27*, 990–992.

Mo, B. (1992) Modesty, sexuality and breast health in Chinese-American women. *Western Journal of Medicine, 157*, 260–264.

Moghaddam, F.M., Taylor, D.M. and Wright, S.C. (1993) *Social Psychology in Cross-Cultural Perspective*. New York: W.H. Freeman.

Monti, M.M. and Owen, A.M. (2010) The aware mind in the motionless body. *The Psychologist, 23*(6), 478–481.

Moos, R.H. and Schaefer, J.A. (1984) The crisis of physical illness: an overview and conceptual approach. In R.H. Moos (ed.) *Coping with Physical Illness: New Perspectives, 2.* New York: Plenum.

Morris, P.L.P., Robinson, R.G., Andrezejewski, P., Samuels, J. and Price, T.R. (1993) Association of depression with 10-year poststroke mortality. *American Journal of Psychiatry, 150*(1), 124–129.

Morris, R.G. (1996a) Neurobiological correlates of cognitive dysfunction. In R.G. Morris (ed.) *The Cognitive Neuropsychology of Alzheimer-Type dementia.* Oxford: Oxford University Press.

Morris, R.G. (1996b) A cognitive neuropsychology of Alzheimer-type dementia. In R.G. Morris (ed.) *The Cognitive Neuropsychology of Alzheimer-Type dementia.* Oxford: Oxford University Press.

Morrison, R. (1992) Diagnosing spiritual pain in patients. *Nursing Standard, 6*(25), 36–38.

Moscovici, S. (1976) *Social Influence and Social Change.* London: Academic Press.

Moscovici, S. (1980) Towards a theory of conversion behaviour. In L. Berkowitz (ed.) *Advances in Experimental Social Psychology 13,* 209–239. New York: Academic press.

Moscovici, S. and Faucheux, C. (1972) Social influence, conforming bias and the study of active minorities. In L. Berkowitz (ed.) *Advances in Experimental Social Psychology, Vol. 6.* New York: Academic Press.

Motluck, A. (1999) Jane behaving badly. *New Scientist, 164*(2214), 28–33.

Muller, D., Harris, J. and Whattley, L. (1988) *Nursing Children: Psychology, Research and Practice.* London: Harper and Row.

Munro, R. (2000) In serious pain or just bellyaching? *Nursing Times, 96*(28), 13.

Murphy, G. (1947) *Personality: A Bio-Social Approach to Origins and Structure.* New York: Harper & Row.

Murray, S.A., Kendall, M., Boyd, K., Worth, A. and Benton, T.F. (2004) Exploring the spiritual needs of people dying of lung cancer or heart failure: a prospective qualitative interview study of patients and their carers. *Palliative Medicine, 18,* 39–45.

Muslim Law (Shariah) Council (1996) The Muslim Law (Shariah) Council and organ transplant. *Accident and Emergency Nursing, 4,* 73–75.

Nagayama Hall, G.C. and Barongan, C. (2002) *Multicultural Psychology.* Upper Saddle River, NJ: Prentice Hall.

Nagera, H. (1969) The imaginary companion: its significance for ego development and conflict solution. *The Psychoanalytic Study of the Child, 24,* 165–196.

Naryanasamy, A. (1991) *Spiritual Care: A Resource Guide for Nurses.* Lancaster: Quay Publishing.

Neugarten, B.L. and Neugarten, D.A. (1987) The changing meanings of age. *Psychology Today, 21,* 29–33.

New Scientist. (1999) Desperate remedies. *New Scientist, 164*(2214), 34–36.

NICE. (2009a) *Clinical Guideline 76: Medicines Adherence: Involving Patients in Decisions about Prescribed Medicines and Supporting Adherence.* London: National Institute for Health and Clinical Excellence.

NICE. (2009b) *Costing Statement: Medicines Adherence: Involving Patients in Decisions about Prescribed Medicines and Supporting Adherence.* London: National Institute for Health and Clinical Excellence.

Nichols, K. (2003) *Psychological Care for Ill and Injured People – A Clinical Guide.* Maidenhead: Open University Press.

Nichols, K. (2005) Why is psychology still failing the average patient? *The Psychologist, 18*(1), 26–27.

North, N. (1988) Psychosocial aspects of coronary artery bypass surgery. *Nursing Times, 84*(1), 26–29.

Norton, C. (2000) Brains can fight breast cancer. *Independent on Sunday,* 16 April, 12.

Nursing. (1974) Probe. *Nursing, 4*(9), 35–44, September.

Nursing Times. (1990) Questionnaire: are you a racist? *Nursing Times, 86*(14), 30–32.

Nydegger, R. (2008) Psychologists and hospice: where we are and where we can be. *Professional Psychology: Research and Practice, 39,* 459–463.

Nye, R.D. (2000) *Three Psychologies: Perspectives from Freud, Skinner and Rogers* (6th edn.). Belmont, CA: Wadsworth/Thompson Learning.

Oakes, P.J., Haslam, S.A. and Turner, J.C. (1994) *Stereotyping and Social Reality*. Oxford: Blackwell Publishing.

Oakley, A. (1980) *A Woman Confined*. Oxford: Martin Robertson.

Oakley, A. (1983) Social consequences of obstetric technology: the importance of measuring 'soft' outcomes. *Birth, 10*, 99–108.

O'Connell, S. (2000) Pain? Don't give it another thought. *Independent Review*, 16 June, 8.

O'Donnell, E. (1996) Stressing the point. *Nursing Standard, 10*(16), 22–23.

O'Donohue, W. and Ferguson, K.E. (2001) *The Psychology of B.F. Skinner*. Thousand Oaks, CA: Sage Publications.

O'Dowd, A. (1998) Handmaidens and battleaxes. *Nursing Times, 94*(36), 12–13.

Ogden, J. (2000) *Health Psychology: A Textbook* (2nd edn.). Buckingham: Open University Press.

Ogden, J. (2004) *Health Psychology: A Textbook* (3rd edn.). Maidenhead, UK: Open University Press/ McGraw-Hill Education.

Ogden, J. (2010a) Eating behaviour. In D. French, K. Vedhara, A.A. Kaptein and J. Weinman (eds.) *Health Psychology* (2nd edn.). Oxford: BPS Blackwell.

Ogden, J. (2010b) Issues of control in applied settings. In R. Gross (ed.) *Psychology: The Science of Mind and Behaviour* (6th edn.). London: Hodder Education.

Ogden, J., Boden, J., Caird, R., Chor, C., Flynn, M., Hunt, M., Khan, K., MacLurg, K., Swade, S. and Thapar, V. (1999) You're depressed; no, I'm not: GPs' and patients' different models of depression. *British Journal of General Practice, 49*, 123–124.

Ogden, J., Clementi, C. and Aylwin, S. (2006) Having obesity surgery: a qualitative study and the paradox of control. *Psychology & Health, 21*, 273–293.

O'Halloran, C.M. and Altmaier, E.M. (1995) The efficacy of preparation for surgery and invasive medical procedures. *Patient Education and Counselling, 25*(1), 9–16.

Operario, D. and Fiske, S.T. (2004) Stereotypes: content, structures, processes and context. In M.B. Brewer and M. Hewstone (eds.) *Social Cognition*. Oxford: Blackwell Publishing.

Orne, M.T. (1962) On the social psychology of the psychological experiment: with particular reference to demand characteristics and their implications. *American Psychologist, 17*, 776–783.

Orne, M.T. and Holland, C.C. (1968) On the ecological validity of laboratory deceptions. *International Journal of Psychiatry, 6*, 282–293.

Ott, A., Breteler, M.M.B., van Hasrkamp, F., Clasu, J.J., van der Cammen, T.J.M., Grobbe, D.E. and Hofman, A. (1995) Prevalence of Alzheimer's disease and vascular dementia: association with education. The Rotterdam study. *British Medical Journal, 310*, 970–973.

Owen, W. (1990) After Hillsborough. *Nursing Times, 86*(25), 16–17.

Ozegovic, D., Carroll, L.J. and Cassidy, J.D. (2009) Does expecting mean achieving? The association between expecting to return to work and recovery in whiplash associated disorders: a population-based prospective cohort study. *European Spine Journal, 18*(6), 893–899.

Palermo, D.S. (1971) Is a scientific revolution taking place in psychology? *Psychological Review, 76*, 241–263.

Palmer, B., Macfarlane, G., Afzal, C., Esmail, A., Silman, A. and Lunt, M. (2007) Acculturation and the prevalence of pain amongst South Asian minority ethnic groups in the UK. *Rheumatology, 46*, 1009–1014.

Panda, N., Bajaj, A., Pershad, D., Yaddanapudi, L.N. and Chari, P. (1996) Preoperative anxiety. *Anaesthesia, 51*, 344–346.

Pandey, M., Sarita, G.P., Devi, N., Thomas, B.C., Hussain, B.M. and Krishnan, R. (2006) Distress, anxiety and depression in cancer patients undergoing chemotherapy. *World Journal of Surgical Oncology, 4*, 68.

Parke, R.D. (2002) Fathers and families. In M.H. Bornstein (ed.) *Handbook of Parenting* (2nd edn., Vol. 3). Mahwah, NJ: Erlbaum.

Parkes, C.M. (1972) *Bereavement: Studies of Grief in Adult Life.* Harmondsworth, UK: Penguin.

Parkes, C.M. (1986) *Bereavement: Studies of Grief in Adult Life* (2nd edn.). London: Tavistock.

Parkes, C.M. (1993) Bereavement as a psychosocial transition: processes of adaptation to change. In M.S. Stroebe, W. Stroebe and R.O. Hansson (eds.) *Handbook of Bereavement: Theory, Research and Intervention.* New York: Cambridge University Press.

Parkes, C.M. (1995) Attachment and bereavement. In T. Lundin (ed.) *Grief and Bereavement: Proceedings from the Fourth International Conference on Grief and Bereavement in Contemporary Society,* Stockholm, 1994. Stockholm, Sweden: Swedish Association for Mental Health.

Parkes, C.M. and Weiss, R.S. (1983) *Recovery from Bereavement.* New York: Basic Books.

Parkinson, P. (1992) Coping with dying and bereavement. *Nursing Standard, 6*(17), 36–38.

Partridge, J. and Pearson, A. (2008) 'Don't worry…it's the inside that counts'. *The Psychologist, 21*(6), 490–491.

Paulson, P.E., Minoshima, S., Morrow, T.J. and Casey, K.L. (1998) Gender differences in pain perception and patterns of cerebral activation during noxious heat stimulation in humans. *Pain, 76,* 223–229.

Payne, D. (2000) Shock study triggers call to ban ageist slur. *Nursing Times, 96*(18), 13.

Pearlin, L. and Lieberman, M. (1979) Social sources of emotional distress. In R. Simmons (ed.) *Research in Community Mental Health.* Greenwich, CT: JAI Press.

Pediani, R. (1992) Preparing to heal. *Nursing Times, 88*(27), 68–70.

Penedo, F., Hernandez, M. and Dahn, J. (2010) Ageing, health and illness. In D. French, K. Vedhara, A.A. Kaptein and J. Weinman (eds.) *Health Psychology* (2nd edn.). Oxford: BPS Blackwell.

Penny, G. (1996) Health psychology. In H. Coolican (ed.) *Applied Psychology.* London: Hodder & Stoughton.

Perry, R.J. and Hodges, J.R. (1999) Attention and executive deficits in Alzheimer's disease. *Brain, 122,* 383–404.

Peters, M., Vlaeyen, J.W.S. and Weber, W.E.J. (2005) The joint contribution of physical pathology, pain-related fear and catastrophising to chronic back pain disability. *Pain, 113,* 45–50.

Petersen, A.C. and Crockett, L. (1985) Pubertal timing and grade effects on adjustment. *Journal of Youth & Adolescence, 14,* 191–206.

Petersen, A.C., Sarigiani, P.A. and Kennedy, R.E. (1991) Adolescent depression: why more girls? *Journal of Youth & Adolescence, 20,* 247–271.

Petit-Zeman, S. (2000) Mmm, guilt-free chocolate. *The Times,* 18 July, 10.

Pettigrew, T.F. (1959) Regional differences in antinegro prejudice. *Journal of Abnormal & Social Psychology, 59,* 28–56.

Pettigrew, T.F. (1971) *Racially Separate or Together?* New York: McGraw-Hill.

Pettigrew, T.F. (1998) Intergroup contact theory. In J.T. Spence, J.M. Darley and D.J. Foss (eds.) *Annual Review of Psychology, Vol. 49.* Palo Alto, CA: Annual Reviews.

Pettigrew, T.F. and Meertens, R.W. (1995) Subtle and blatant prejudice in Western Europe. *European Journal of Social Psychology, 25,* 57–75.

Pettigrew, T.F. and Tropp, L.R. (2006) A meta-analytic test of intergroup contact theory. *Journal of Personality & Social Psychology, 90,* 751–783.

Phillips, J.L. (1969) *The Origins of Intellect: Piaget's Theory.* San Francisco, CA: W.H. Freeman.

Piaget, J. (1952) *The Child's Conception of Number.* London: Routledge & Kegan Paul.

Piaget, J. and Inhelder, B. (1956) *The Psychology of the Child.* London: Routledge & Kegan Paul.

Piaget, J. and Szeminska, A. (1952) *The Child's Conception of Number.* New York: Humanities Press.

PICANET (Paediatric Intensive Care Audit Network). (2010) *Annual Report 2007–2009.* Universities of Leeds, Leicester and Sheffield.

Pike, A. and Plomin, R. (1999) Genetics and development. In D.J. Messer and S. Millar (eds.) *Exploring Developmental Psychology: From Infancy to Adolescence.* London: Arnold.

Pinel, J.P.J. (1993) *Biopsychology* (2nd edn.). Boston, MA: Allyn & Bacon.

Piot-Ziegler, C., Sassi, M.-L, Raffoul, W. and Delaloye, J.-F. (2010) Mastectomy, body deconstruction, and impact on identity: a qualitative study. *British Journal of Health Psychology, 15,* 479–510.

Plant, S. (1999) *Writing on Drugs.* London: Faber & Faber.

Playfor, S., Thomas, D. and Choonara, I. (2000) Recollection of children following intensive care. *Archives of Disease in Childhood, 83,* 445–448.

Plomin, R., DeFries, J.C., McClearn, G.E. and McGuffin, P. (2000) *Behavioural Genetics* (4th edn.). New York: W.H. Freeman.

Poliakoff, M. (1993) Cancer and cultural attitudes. In R. Masi, L. Mensah and K.A. McLeod (eds.) *Health and Cultures: Policies, Professional Practice and Education.* New York: Mosaic Press.

Popper, K. (1959) *The Logic of Scientific Discovery.* London: Hutchinson.

Popper, K. (1972) *Objective Knowledge: An Evolutionary Approach.* Oxford: Oxford University Press.

Porter, S. (1995) *Nursing's Relationship with Medicine: A Critical Realist Ethnography.* Aldershot, UK: Avebury.

Povey, R., Conner, M., Sparks, P., James, R. and Shepherd, R. (2000) The theory of planned behaviour and healthy eating: examining additive and moderating effects of social influence variables. *Psychology & Health, 14,* 991–1006.

Powell, J. (2000) Drug and alcohol dependence. In L. Champion and M. Power (eds.) *Adult Psychological Problems: An Introduction* (2nd edn.). Hove, UK: Psychology Press.

Premack, D. and Woodruff, G. (1978) Does the chimpanzee have a theory of mind? *Behavioural & Brain Sciences, 4,* 515–526.

Price, B. (1986) Keeping up appearances. *Nursing Times,* 58–61, 1 October.

Price, B. (1988) What are nurses like? *Nursing Times, 84*(1), 42–43.

Price, B. (1990) *Body Image: Nursing Concepts and Care.* Hemel Hempstead, UK: Prentice Hall.

Price, W.F. and Crapo, R.H. (1999) *Cross-Cultural Perspectives in Introductory Psychology* (3rd edn.). Belmont, CA: Wadsworth Publishing Co.

Prochaska, J.A. and DiClemente, D.D. (1984) *The Transtheoretical Approach: Crossing Traditional Boundaries of Therapy.* Homewood, IL: Dow Jones Irwin.

Professional Practice Board of the BPS (2008) *The Role of Psychology in End of Life Care.* Leicester: BPS.

Pud, D., Yarnitsky, D., Sprecher, E., Rogowski, Z., Adler, R. and Eisenberg, E. (2006) Can personality traits and gender predict the response to morphine. An experimental cold pain study. *European Journal of Pain, 10,* 103–112.

Pullen, M. (1998) Support role. *Nursing Times, 94*(47), 57.

Quinton, D. and Rutter, M. (1988) *Parental Breakdown: The Making and Breaking of Intergenerational Links.* London: Gower.

Rabbitt, P.M.A. (1993) Does it all go together when it goes? *Quarterly Journal of Experimental Psychology, 46A,* 385–434.

Rainey, N. (1998) Old age. In K. Trew and J. Kremer (eds.) *Gender & Psychology.* London: Arnold.

Ramachandran, V.S. and Blakeslee, S. (1998) *Phantoms in the Brain.* London: Fourth Estate.

Ramsay, M. (1997) How well are the emotional support needs of carers of demented elderly supported by hospital nurses? *Scottish Nurse,* 8 March, 34–35.

Ramsay, R. and de Groot, W. (1977) A further look at bereavement. Paper presented at EATI conference, Uppsala. Cited in P.E. Hodgkinson (1980) Treating abnormal grief in the bereaved. *Nursing Times*, 17 January, 126–128.

Randle, J., Coffey, F. and Bradbury, M. (2009) *Clinical Skills in Adult Nursing.* Oxford: Oxford University Press.

Rank, S.G. and Jacobson, C.K. (1977) Hospital nurses' compliance with medication overdose orders: a failure to replicate. *Journal of Health & Social Behaviour, 18*, 188–193.

Raphael, B. (1984) *The Anatomy of Bereavement*. London: Hutchinson.

Raven, B.H. and Haley, R.W. (1980) Social influence in a medical context. In L. Bickman (ed.) *Applied Social Psychology Annual, Volume 1*. Beverly Hills, CA: Sage. RCNONLINE www.rcn.org.uk/direct. (Published 2003-04-14.)

Reason, J. (2000) The Freudian slip revisited. *The Psychologist, 13*(12), 610–611.

Redfearn, D.J. (1982) *Predictors of Nurses' Compliance with Physicians' Inappropriate Orders*. Ann Arbor, MI: UMI Research Press.

Rees, M. (1993) He, she or it? *Nursing Times, 89*(10), 48–49.

Reich, B. and Adcock, C. (1976) *Values, Attitudes and Behaviour Change*. London: Methuen.

Richards, G. (1996) *Putting Psychology in Its Place*. London: Routledge.

Richardson, K. (1991) *Understanding Intelligence*. Milton Keynes, UK: Open University Press.

Ridley, M. (1999) *Genome: The Autobiography of a Species in 23 Chapters*. London: Fourth Estate.

Rifkin, A. (2001) Is it denial or wisdom to accept life threatening illness? *British Medical Journal, 323* (7320), 1071.

Robertson, J. and Robertson, J. (1967–73) *Film Series, Young Children in Brief Separation: No.3 (1969): John, 17 months, 9 days, in a Residential Nursery*. London: Tavistock.

Robinson, R.G., Lipsey, J.R., Rao, K. and Price, T.R. (1986) Two-year longitudinal study of poststroke mood disorders: comparison of acute-onset with delayed-onset depression. *American Journal of Psychiatry, 143*(10), 1238–1244.

Robinson, R.G., Schultz, S.K., Castillo, C., Kopel, T., Kosier, J.T., Newman, R.M., Curdue, K., Petracca, G. and Starkstein, S.E. (2000) Nortriptyline versus fluoxetine in the treatment of depression and in short-term recovery after stroke: a placebo-controlled double-blind study. *American Journal of Psychiatry, 157*(3), 351–359.

Robinson, V. and Scott, H. (2012) Why assisted suicide must remain illegal in the UK. *Nursing Standard, 26*(18), 40–48.

Robotham, M. (1999) What you think of doctors. *Nursing Times, 95*(2), 24–27.

Rochlin, G. (1967) How younger children view death and themselves. In E. Grollman (ed.) *Explaining Death to Children*. Boston, MA: Beacon.

Roger, D. and Nash, P. (1995) Coping. *Nursing Times, 91*(29), 42–43.

Rogers, C.R. (1951) *Client-Centred Therapy: Its Current Practices, Implications and Theory*. Boston, MA: Houghton Mifflin.

Rogers, C.R. (1959) A theory of therapy, personality and interpersonal relationships as developed in the client-centred framework. In S. Koch (ed.) *Psychology: A Study of Science, Volume III, Formulations of the Person and the Social Context*. New York: McGraw-Hill.

Rogers, J., Meyer, J. and Mortel, K. (1990) After reaching retirement age physical activity sustains cerebral perfusion and cognition. *Journal of the American Geriatric Society, 38*, 123–128.

Rogers, R.W. (1975) A protection motivation theory of fear appeals and attitude change. *Journal of Psychology, 91*, 93–114.

Rogers, R.W. (1985) Attitude change and information integration in fear appeals. *Psychological Reports, 56*, 179–182.

Rogers, R.W. and Prentice-Dunn, S. (1997) Protection motivation theory. In D.S. Gochman (ed.) *Handbook of Health Behaviour Research 1: Personal and Social Determinants*. New York: Plenum.

Rogoff, B. (1990) *Apprenticeship in Thinking: Cognitive Development in Social Context*. New York: Oxford University Press.

Rokeach, M. (1960) *The Open and Closed Mind*. New York: Basic Books.

Roper, N., Logan, W. and Tierney, A. (1996) *The Elements of Nursing* (4th edn.). Edinburgh: Churchill Livingstone.

Rose, N. (1996) Identity, geneology, history. In S. Hall and P. duGay (eds.) *Questions of Cultural Identity*. London: Sage.

Rose, P. (1993) Out in the open? *Nursing Times*, 89(30), 50–52.

Rose, P. and Platzer, H. (1993) Confronting prejudice. *Nursing Times*, 89(31), 52–54.

Rose, S. (1997) *Lifelines: Biology, Freedom, Determinism*. Harmondsworth, UK: Penguin.

Rose, S. (2003) *The Making of Memory: From Molecules to Mind* (revised edn.). London: Vintage.

Rose, S.A. and Blank, M. (1974) The potency of context in children's cognition: an illustration through conservation. *Child Development*, 45, 499–502.

Rosenberg, M.J. and Hovland, C.I. (1960) Cognitive, affective and behavioural components of attitude. In M.J. Rosenberg, C.I. Hovland, W.J. McGuire, R.P. Abelson and J.W. Brehm (eds.) *Attitude Organisation and Change: An Analysis of Consistency Among Attitude Components*. New Haven, CT: Yale University Press.

Rosenblatt, P.C. (1993) The social context of private feelings. In M.S. Stroebe, W. Stroebe and R.O. Hansson (eds.) *Handbook of Bereavement: Theory, Research and Intervention*. New York: Cambridge University Press.

Rosenthal, R. and Jacobson, L. (1968) *Pygmalion in the Classroom: Teacher Expectation and Pupils' Intellectual Development*. New York: Holt.

Rosnow, I. (1985) Status and role change through the life cycle. In R.H. Binstock and E. Shanas (eds.) *Handbook of Ageing and the Social Sciences* (2nd edn.). New York: Van Nostrand Reinhold.

Rotter, J. (1966) Generalised expectancies for internal versus external control of reinforcement. *Psychological Monographs*, 30(1), 1–26.

Rowe, A. (1999) Spectre at the feast. *Nursing Times*, 95(2), 28–29.

Rowe, J.W. and Kahn, R.L. (1998) *Successful Ageing*. New York: Plenum.

Royal College of Nursing. (2005) *Dealing with Bullying and Harassment at Work: A Guide for RCN Members*. London: RCN.

Royal College of Nursing. (2009) *RCN Moves to Neutral Position on Assisted Suicide*. London: RCN.

Royal College of Psychiatrists. (1987) *Drug Scenes: A Report on Drugs and Drug Dependence by the Royal College of Psychiatrists*. London: Gaskell.

Ruiter, R.A.C. and Kok, G. (2006) Response to Hammond et al. Showing leads to doing, but doing what? The need for experimental pilot-testing. *European Journal of Public Health, 16*, 225.

Ruiz, F.J. (2010) A review of acceptance and commitment therapy (ACT) empirical evidence: correlational, experimental, psychopathology, component and outcome studies. *International Journal of Psychology and Psychological Therapy*, 10, 125–162.

Rutter, M. (1981) *Maternal Deprivation Reassessed* (2nd edn.). Harmondsworth, UK: Penguin.

Rutter, M. (1989) Pathways from childhood to adult life. *Journal of Child & Psychology & Psychiatry*, 30, 23–25.

Rutter, M. (2006) The psychological effects of institutional rearing. In P. Marshall and N. Fox (eds.) *The Development of Social Engagement: Neurobiological Perspectives*. New York: Oxford University Press.

Rutter, M., Colvert, E., Kreppner, J., Beckett, C., Castle, J., Groothues, C., Hawkins, A. et al. (2007) Early adolescent outcomes for institutionally-deprived and non-deprived adoptees 1: disinhibited attachment. *Journal of Child & Psychology & Psychiatry, 48*(1), 17–30.

Rutter, M. and The English and Romanian Adoptees (ERA) study team. (1998) Developmental catch-up, and deficit following adoption after severe global early privation. *Journal of Child Psychology & Psychiatry, 39*(4), 465–476.

Rutter, M. and the English and Romanian Adoptees (ERA) study team. (2004) Are there biological programming effects for psychological development? Findings from a study of Romanian adoptees. *Developmental Psychology, 40*, 81–94.

Rutter, M., Graham, P., Chadwick, D.F.D. and Yule, W. (1976) Adolescent turmoil: fact or fiction? *Journal of Child Psychology & Psychiatry, 17*, 35–56.

Ryan, R.M. and Lynch, J.H. (1989) Emotional autonomy versus detachment: revisiting the vicissitudes of adolescence and young adulthood. *Child Development, 60*, 340–356.

Rydstrom, I., Dalheim-Englund, A.C., Segesten, K. and Rasmussen, B.H. (2004) Relations governed by uncertainty: part of life for families of a child with asthma. *Journal of Paediatric Nursing, 19*(2), 85–94.

Sabat, S.R. (2001) *The Experience of Alzheimer's Disease: Life through a Tangled Veil*. Malden, MA: Blackwell Publishing.

Sabat, S.R. and Harré, R. (1992) The construction and deconstruction of self in Alzheimer's disease. *Ageing and Society, 12*, 443–461.

Saffran, E.M., Fitzpatrick-DeSalme, E.J. and Coslett, H.B. (1990) Visual disturbances in dementia. In M.F. Schwartz (ed.) *Modular Deficits in Alzheimer-Type Dementia*. Cambridge, MS: MIT Press.

Salmon, P. (1993) The reduction of anxiety in surgical patients: an important nursing task or the medicalisation of preparatory worry? *International Journey of Nursing Studies, 30*(4), 323–330.

Salovey, J.D. and Mayer, P. (1990) Emotional Intelligence. *Imagination, Cognition and Personality, 9*(3), 185–211.

Samuel, J. and Bryant, P. (1984) Asking only one question in the conservation experiment. *Journal of Child Psychology & Psychiatry, 25*, 315–318.

Saradjian, A., Thompson, A.R. and Datta, D. (2007) The experience of men using an upper limb prosthesis following amputation: positive coping and minimising feeling different. *Disability and Rehabilitation, 30*(11), 871–873.

Saunders, C. (1988) Spiritual pain. *Journal of Palliative Care, 4*(3), 29–32.

Savage, R. and Armstrong, D. (1990) Effect of a general practitioner's consulting style on patients' satisfaction: a controlled study. *British Medical Journal, 301*, 968–970.

Sayette, M.A. (1993) An appraisal-disruption model of alcohol's effects on stress responses in social drinkers. *Psychological Bulletin, 114*, 459–476.

Schaffer, H.R. (1971) *The Growth of Sociability*. Harmondsworth, UK: Penguin.

Schaffer, H.R. (1996a) *Social Development*. Oxford: Blackwell Publishing.

Schaffer, H.R. (1996b) Is the child father to the man? *Psychology Review, 2*(3), 2–5.

Schaffer, H.R. (1998) Deprivation and its effects on children. *Psychology Review, 5*(2), 2–5.

Schaffer, H.R. (2004) *Introducing Child Psychology*. Oxford: Blackwell Publishing.

Schaffer, H.R. and Emerson, P.E. (1964) The development of social attachments in infancy. *Monographs of the Society for Research in Child Development, 29* (whole No. 3).

Schaie, K.W. and Hertzog, C. (1983) Fourteen-year cohort-sequential analysis of adult intellectual development. *Developmental Psychology, 19*, 531–543.

Scheer, S.D. and Unger, D.G. (1995) Parents' perceptions of their adolescents – implications for parent–youth conflict and family satisfaction. *Psychological Reports, 76*(1), 131–136.

Schiffman, R. and Wicklund, R.A. (1992) The minimal group paradigm and its minimal psychology. *Theory & Psychology, 2*, 29–50.

Schifter, D.E. and Ajzen, I. (1985) Intention, perceived control and weight loss: an application of the theory of planned behaviour. *Journal of Personality & Social Psychology, 49*, 843–851.

Schliefer, S.J., Keller, S.E., Camerino, M., Thornton, J.C. and Stein, M. (1983) Suppression of lymphocyte stimulation following bereavement. *Journal of the American Medical Association, 250*, 374–377.

Schlossberg, N.K. (1984) Exploring the adult years. In A.M. Rogers and C.J. Scheirer (eds.) *The G. Stanley Hall Lecture Series, Vol. 4*. Washington, DC: American Psychological Association.

Schlossberg, N.K., Troll, L.E. and Leibowitz, Z. (1978) *Perspectives on Counselling Adults: Issues and Skills*. Monterey, CA: Brooks/Cole.

Schott, G.D. (2004) Communicating the experience of pain: the role of analgy. *Pain, 108*, 209–212.

Schott, J. and Henley, A. (1999) *Culture, Religion & Childbearing in a Multi-Racial Society*. Oxford: Butterworth Heinemann.

Schuchter, S.R. and Zisook, S. (1993) The course of normal grief. In M.S. Stroebe, W. Stroebe and R.O. Hansson (eds.) *Handbook of Bereavement: Theory, Research and Intervention*. New York: Cambridge University Press.

Schwarzer, R. (1992) Self-efficacy in the adoption and maintenance of health behaviours: theoretical approaches and a new model. In R. Schwarzer (ed.) *Self Efficacy: Thought Control of Action*. Washington, DC: Hemisphere.

Schwartz, G.E. and Weiss, S.M. (1977) What is behavioural medicine? *Psychosomatic Medicine, 39*, 377–381.

Segall, M.H., Dasen, P.R., Berry, J.W. and Poortinga, Y.H. (1999) *Human Behaviour in Global Perspective: An Introduction to Cross-Cultural Psychology* (2nd edn.). Needham Heights, MA: Allyn & Bacon.

Seligman, M.E.P. (1975) *Helplessness: On Depression, Development and Death*. San Francisco, CA: W.H. Freeman.

Selye, H. (1956) *The Stress of Life*. New York: McGraw-Hill.

Shatz, M. (1994) *A Toddler's Life: Becoming a Person*. New York: Oxford University Press.

Sheahan, P. (1996) Psychological pain and care. *Nursing Times, 92*(17), 63–67.

Shepherd, R. (1988) Belief structure in relation to low-fat milk consumption. *Journal of Human Nutrition and Dietetics, 1*, 421–428.

Shepherd, R. and Farleigh, C.A. (1986) Attitudes and personality related to salt intake. *Appetite, 7*, 343–354.

Shepherd, R. and Stockley, L. (1985) Fat consumption and attitudes towards food with a high fat content. *Human Nutrition: Applied Nutrition, 39A*, 431–442.

Shepherd, R. and Stockley, L. (1987) Nutrition knowledge, attitudes and fat consumption. *Journal of the American Dietetic Association, 87*, 615–619.

Sherif, M. (1935) A study of social factors in perception. *Archives of Psychology, 27* (whole No. 187).

Sherif, M. (1966) *Group Conflict and Co-operation: Their Social Psychology*. London: RKP.

Sherr, L. (1989) Death of a baby. In L. Sherr (ed.) *Death, Dying and Bereavement*. Oxford: Blackwell Publishing.

Shontz, F.C. (1975) *The Psychological Aspects of Physical Illness and Disability*. New York: Macmillan Co.

Siegal, M. (2003) Cognitive development. In A. Slater and G. Bremner (eds.) *An Introduction to Developmental Psychology*. Oxford: Blackwell Publishing.

Siegel, K., Schrimshaw, E.W. and Dean, L. (1999) Symptom interpretation and medication adherence among late middle-aged and older HIV-affected adults. *Journal of Health Psychology, 4*, 247–257.

Simmons, R.G. and Blyth, D.A. (1987) *Moving into Adolescence: The Impact of Pubertal Change and School Context*. New York: Aldine de Gruyter.

Simpson, S.H., Eurich, D.T., Majumdar, S.R., Padwal, R.S., Tsuyuki, R.T., Varney, J. and Johnson, J.A. (2006) A meta-analysis of the association between adherence to drug therapy and mortality. *British Medical Journal, 333*, 15.

Sinha, D. (1997) Indigenising psychology. In J.W. Berry, Y.H. Poortinga and J. Pandey (eds.) *Handbook of Cross-Cultural Psychology* (2nd edn., Vol. 1). Boston, MA: Allyn & Bacon.

Sissons Joshi, M. (1995) Lay explanations of the causes of diabetes in India and the UK. In I. Markova and R.M. Farr (eds.) *Representations of Health, Illness and Handicap*. Philadelphia: Harwood.

Sjodahl, G., Gard, G. and Jarnlo, G.-B. (2004) Coping after trans-femoral amputation due to trauma or tumour: a phenomenological apparaoch. *Disability and Rehabilitation, 26*(14/15), 851–861.

Skinner, B.F. (1974) *About Behaviourism*. New York: Alfred Knopf.

Skinner, B.F. (1987) Skinner on behaviourism. In R.L. Gregory (ed.) *The Oxford Companion to the Mind*. Oxford: Oxford University Press.

Smith, A.D. (1998) Ageing of the brain: is mental decline inevitable? In S. Rose (ed.) *From Brain to Consciousness: Essays on the New Science of the Mind*. Harmondsworth, UK: Penguin.

Smith, J. and Baltes, P.B. (1997) Profiles of psychological functioning in the old and oldest old. *Psychology and Ageing, 12*, 458–472.

Smith, K. (2002) In M. Snyder and R. Lindquist (eds.) *Complementary/Alternative Theories in Nursing* (4th edn.). New York: Springer.

Smith, K.R. and Zick, C.D. (1996) Risk of mortality following widowhood: age and sex differences by mode of death. *Social Biology, 43*, 59–71.

Smith, P. (1992) *The Emotional Labour of Nursing: How Nurses Care*. London: Macmillan.

Smith, P.B. and Bond, M.H. (1998). *Social Psychology Across Cultures* (2nd edn.). Hemel Hempstead, UK: Prentice-Hall Europe.

Smith, P.K. and Cowie, H. (1988) *Understanding Children's Development*. Oxford: Basil Blackwell.

Smith, S. (1997) A time to die. *Nursing Times, 93*(44), 34–35.

Smolderen, K.G. and Vingerhoets, A. (2010) Hospitalisation and stressful medical procedures. In D. French, K. Vedhara, A.A. Kaptein and J. Weinman (eds.) *Health Psychology* (2nd edn.). Oxford: BPS Blackwell.

Smyth, J.M. and Filipkowski, K.B. (2010) Coping with Stress. In D. French, K. Vedhara, A.A. Kaptein and J. Weinman (eds.) *Health Psychology* (2nd edn.). Oxford: BPS Blackwell.

Snell, J. (1995) It's tough at the bottom. *Nursing Times, 91*(43), 55–58.

Snell, J. (1997) Joke over. *Nursing Times, 93*(11), 26–28.

Snyder, S. (1977) Opiate receptors and internal opiates. *Scientific American, 236*, 44–56.

Sparks, P., Conner, M., James, R., Shepherd, R. and Povey, R. (2001) Ambivalence about health-related behaviours: an exploration in the domain of food choice. *British Journal of Health Psychology, 6*, 53–68.

Spencer, C. and Perrin, S. (1998) Innovation and conformity. *Psychology Review, 5*(2), 23–26.

Sperling, H.G. (1946) An experimental study of some psychological factors in judgement, Master's thesis, New york: New School for Social Research.

Spinetta, J.J. (1975) Death anxiety in the outpatient leukaemic child. *Paediatrics, 56*(6), 1034–1037.

Spinetta, J.J., Rigler, D. and Karon, M. (1973) Anxiety in the dying child. *Paediatrics, 52*(6), 841–845.

Spitz, R.A. (1945) Hospitalism: an inquiry into the genesis of psychiatric conditions in early childhood. *Psychoanalytic Study of the Child, 1*, 53–74.

Spitz, R.A. (1946) Hospitalism: a follow-up report on investigation described in Vol. 1, 1945. *Psychoanalytic Study of the Child, 2*, 113–117.

Spitz, R.A. and Wolf, K.M. (1946) Anaclitic depression. *Psychoanalytic Study of the Child, 2*, 313–342.

Sroke Association. (2006) Retrieved from www.stroke.org.uk/information/index.html, November, 2006.

Stahlberg, D. and Frey, D. (1988) Attitudes 1: structure, measurement and functions. In M. Hewstone, W. Stroebe, J.P. Codol and G.M. Stephenson (eds.) *Introduction to Social Psychology*. Oxford: Blackwell Publishing.

Stainton Rogers, R., Stenner, P., Gleeson. K. and Stainton Rogers, W. (1995) *Social Psychology: A Critical Agenda*. Cambridge: Polity Press.

Stanley, J. (1998) Mixed messages. *Nursing Times, 94*(49), 58–59.

Starr, B.S. (1995) Approaches to pain control. In D. Messer and C. Meldrum (eds.) *Psychology for Nurses and Health Care Professionals*. Hemel Hempstead, UK: Prentice Hall/Harvester Wheatsheaf.

Starr, B.S. and Chandler, C.J. (1995) Common addictive behaviours. In D. Messer and C. Meldrum (eds.) *Psychology for Nurses and Health Care Professionals*. Hemel Hempstead, UK: Prentice Hall/Harvester Wheatsheaf.

Stattin, H. and Klackenberg, G. (1992) Family discord in adolescence in the light of family discord in childhood. Paper presented at Conference Youth–TM, Utrecht.

Stattin, H. and Magnusson, D. (1990) *Pubertal Maturation in Female Development*. Hillsdale, NJ: Erlbaum.

Stein, L. (1967) The doctor-nurse game. *Archives of General Psychiatry, 16*, 699–703.

Stein, L., Watts, D.T. and Howell, T. (1990) The doctor-nurse game revisited. *The New England Journal of Medicine, 322*, 546–549.

Stephan, W.G. and Stephan, C.W. (1985) Intergroup anxiety. *Journal of Social Issues, 41*, 157–175.

Steptoe, A., Gardner, B. and Wardle, J. (2010) The role of behaviour in health. In D. French, K. Vedhara, A.A. Kaptein and J. Weinman (eds.) *Health Psychology* (2nd edn.). Oxford: BPS Blackwell.

Sterling, P. and Eyer, J. (1988) Allostasis: a new paradigm to explain arousal pathology. In S. Fisher and J. Reason (eds.) *Handbook of Life Stress, Cognition and Health*. Oxford: John Wiley.

Sternberg, E. (2000) *The Balance Within: The Science Connecting Health and Emotions*. New York: W.H. Freeman.

Sternberg, E. and Gold, P.W. (1997) The mind-body interaction in disease. *Scientific American Mysteries of the Mind, 7*(1), 8–15.

Stevens, R. (1995) Freudian theories of personality. In S.E. Hampson and A.M. Colman (eds.) *Individual Differences and Personality*. London: Longman.

Stouffer, S.A., Suchman, E.A., DeVinney, L.C., Starr, S.A. and Williams, R.M. (1949) *The American Soldier: Adjustment During Army Life, Vol. 1*. Princeton, NJ: Princeton University Press.

Strawbridge, W.J., Shema, S., Balfour, J.L., Higby, H.R. and Kaplan, G.A. (1998) Antecedents of frailty over three decades in an older cohort. *Journal of Gerontology: Social Sciences, 53B*, S9-S16.

Stroebe, M.S. and Stroebe, M. (1993) The mortality of bereavement: a review. In M.S. Stroebe, W. Stroebe and R.O. Hansson (eds.) *Handbook of Bereavement: Theory, Research and Intervention*. New York: Cambridge University Press.

Stroebe, M.S., Stroebe, W. and Hansson, R.O. (1993) Contemporary themes and controversies in bereavement research. In M.S. Stroebe, W. Stroebe and R.O. Hansson (eds.) *Handbook of Bereavement: Theory, Research and Intervention*. New York: Cambridge University Press.

Stroebe, W. (2000) *Social Psychology and Health* (2nd edn.). Buckingham: Open University Press.

Stroke Association. (2009) *Dementia after stroke*. (Factsheet 29). London: Stroke Association.

Stroke Association. (2010) *Cognitive problems after stroke*. (Factsheet 7). London: Stroke Association.

Stroke Association. (2011a) *Communication problems after stroke*. (Factsheet 3). London: Stroke Association.

Stroke Association. (2011b) *Depression after stroke*. (Factsheet 10). London: Stroke Association.

Stroke Association. (2011c) *Emotional changes after stroke*. (Factsheet 36). London: Stroke Association.

Stroke Association. (2011d) *Stroke in younger adults.* (Factsheet 9). London: Stroke Association.

Stuart-Hamilton, I. (1994) *The Psychology of Ageing: An Introduction* (2nd edn.). London: Jessica Kingsley.

Stuart-Hamilton, I. (1997) Adjusting to later life. *Psychology Review, 4*(2), 20–23.

Stuart-Hamilton, I. (2000) Ageing and intelligence. *Psychology Review, 6*(4), 19–21.

Stuart-Hamilton, I. (2003) Intelligence and ageing: is decline inevitable? *Psychology Review, 9*(3), 14–16.

Sudnow, D. (1967) *Passing On: The Social Organisation of Dying.* Englewood Cliffs, NJ: Prentice-Hall.

Sullivan, P.J. (1993) Occupational stress in psychiatric nursing. *Journal of Advanced Nursing, 18,* 591–601.

Swendsen, M. (1934) Children's Imaginary Companions. *Archives of Neurological Psychiatry, 32,* 985–999.

Swensen, C.H. (1983) A respectable old age. *American Psychologist, 46,* 1208–1221.

Swift, C.R., Seidman, F. and Stein, H. (1967) Adjustment problems in juvenile diabetes. *Psychosomatic Medicine, 29*(6), 555–571.

Sykes, E.A. (1995) Psychopharmacology. In D. Messer and C. Meldrum (eds.) *Psychology for Nurses and Health Care Professionals.* Hemel Hempstead, UK: Prentice Hall/Harvester Wheatsheaf.

Taenzer, P.A., Melzack, R. and Jeans, M.E. (1986) Influence of psychological factors in postoperative pain, mood and analgesic requirements. *Pain, 24,* 331–342.

Taggart, P., Parkinson, P. and Carruthers, M. (1972) Cardiac responses to thermal, physical and emotional stress. *British Medical Journal, 3*(5818), 71–76.

Tait, A., Maguire, P., Faulkener, A., Brooke, M., Wilkinson, S., Thomson, L. and Sellwood, R. (1982) Improving communication skills. *Nursing Times, 78*(51), 2181–2184.

Tajfel, H. (1969) Social and cultural factors in perception. In G. Lindzey and E. Aronson (eds.) *Handbook of Social Psychology, Vol. 3.* Reading, MA: Addison-Wesley.

Tajfel, H. (1972) Experiments in a vacuum. In J. Israel and H. Tajfel (eds.) *The Context of Social Psychology: A Critical Assessment.* London: Academic Press.

Tajfel, H. (ed.) (1978) *Differentiation between Social Groups: Studies in the Social Psychology of Intergroup Relations.* London: Academic Press.

Tajfel, H., Billig, M.G. and Bundy, R.P. (1971) Social categorisation and intergroup behaviour. *European Journal of Social Psychology, 1,* 149–178.

Tajfel, H. and Turner, J.C. (1986) The social identity theory of intergroup behaviour. In S. Worchel and W. Austin (eds.) *Psychology of Intergroup Relations.* Monterey, CA: Brooks Cole.

Talaska, C., Fiske, S.T. and Chaiken, S. (2003) Biases hot and cold: emotional prejudices and cognitive stereotypes as predictors of discriminatory behaviour. Unpublished manuscript, Princeton University (cited in S.T. Fiske, 2004).

Tanner, J.M. (1978) *Foetus into Man; Physical Growth from Conception to Maturity.* Cambridge, MA: Harvard University Press.

Tanner, J.M. and Whitehouse, R.H. (1976) Clinical longitudinal standards for height, weight, velocity, weight velocity and stages of puberty. *Archives of Disease in Childhood, 51,* 170–179.

Tasker, F. and Golombok, S. (1995) Adults raised as children in lesbian families. *American Journal of Orthopsychiatry, 65*(2), 203–215.

Taylor, G. (1993) Challenges from the margins. In J. Clarke (ed.) *A Crisis in Care.* London: Sage.

Taylor, J., Miller, D., Wattley, L. and Harris, P. (1999) *Nursing Children. Psychology, Research and Practice* (3rd edn.). Cheltenham, UK: Stanley Thornes (Publishers) Ltd.

Taylor, P. (1994) Beating the taboo. *Nursing Times, 90*(13), 51–53.

Tedeschi, J.T. and Rosenfield, P. (1981) Impression management theory and the forced compliance situation. In J.T. Tedeschi (ed.) *Impression Management Theory and Social Psychological Research.* New York: Academic Press.

Tellis-Nyak, M. and Tellis-Nyak, V. (1984) Games that physicians play: the social psychology of physician-nurse interaction. *Social Science and Medicine, 18*(12), 1063–1069.

Temoshok, L. (1987) Personality, coping style, emotions and cancer: towards an integrative model. *Cancer Surveys, 6*(Supp.), 545–567.

Thayer, J.F. and Brosschott, J.F. (2010) Stress, health and illness. In D. French, K. Vedhara, A.A. Kaptein and J. Weinman (eds.) *Health Psychology* (2nd edn.). Oxford: BPS Blackwell.

Thekkumpurath, P., Venkateswaran, C., Kumar, M. and Bennett, M.I. (2008) Screening for psychological distress in palliative care: a systematic review. *Journal of Pain and Symptom Management, 36*, 520–528.

Thomas, B. (1993) Gender loving care. *Nursing Times, 89*(10), 50–51.

Thomas, R.M. (1985) *Comparing Theories of Child Development* (2nd edn.). Belmont, CA: Wadsworth Publishing Company.

Thorne, B. (1992) *Rogers*. London: Sage Publications.

Thurber, C.A. and Walton, E. (2007) Preventing and treating homesickness. *Paediatrics, 119*(1), 192–201.

Tizard, B. (1977) *Adoption: A Second Chance*. London: Open Books.

Tizard, B. and Hodges, J. (1978) The effects of early institutional rearing on the development of eight-year-old children. *Journal of Child Psychology & Psychiatry, 19*, 99–118.

Toates, F. (2001) *Biological Psychology: An Integrative Approach*. Harlow, UK: Pearson Education Ltd.

Tobin, S.S. (1999) *Preservation of the Self in the Oldest Years: With Implications for Practice*. New York: Springer.

Toogood, L. (1999) White-knuckle ride to theatre. *Nursing Times, 95*(14), 50–51.

Topping, A. (1990) Sexual activity and the stoma patient. *Nursing Standard, 4*(41), 24–26.

Tredre, R. (1996, May 12) Untitled article. *Observer Life*, 16–19.

Triandis, H. (1990) Theoretical concepts that are applicable to the analysis of ethnocentrism. In R.W. Brislin (ed.) *Applied Cross-Cultural Psychology*. Newbury Park, CA: Sage.

Triandis, H.C. (1994) *Culture and Social Behaviour*. New York: McGraw-Hill.

Triandis, H. (1995) *Individualism and Collectivism*. Boulder, CO: Westview Press.

Tschudin, V. (2003) *Ethics in Nursing* (3rd edn.). Oxford: Butterworth Heinemann.

Tucker, J.A., Vuchinich, R.E. and Downey, K.K. (1992) Substance abuse. In S.M. Turner, K.S. Calhoun and H.E. Adams (eds.) *Handbook of Clinical Behaviour Therapy*. New York: Wiley.

Turk, D.C. and Okifuji, A. (2003) Clinical assessment of the person with chronic pain. In T.S. Jensen, P.R. Wilson and A. Rice (eds.) *Clinical Pain Management: Chronic Pain*. London: Arnold.

Turnbull, S.K. (1995) The middle years. In D. Wedding (ed.) *Behaviour and Medicine* (2nd edn.). St Louis, MO: Mosby-Year Book.

Turner, J.C. (1991) *Social Influence*. Milton Keynes, UK: Open University Press.

Turner, J.S. and Helms, D.B. (1989) *Contemporary Adulthood* (4th edn.). Fort Worth, FL: Holt, Rinehart & Winston.

Turpin, G. and Slade, P. (1998) Clinical and health psychology. In P. Scott and C. Spencer, *Psychology: A Contemporary Introduction*. Oxford: Blackwell.

Tyrer, P. (2010) Personality disorders. In B.K. Puri and I. Treasaden (eds.) *Psychiatry: An Evidence-Based Text*. London: Hodder Arnold.

UKCC. (1992) *Code of Professional Conduct*. London: UKCC.

Uman, L.S., Chambers, C.T., McGrath, P.J. and Kisely, S. (2006) Psychological interventions for needle-related procedural pain and distress in children and adolescents. *Cochrane Database Systems* (4th edn.). CD005179.

Unruh, A.M., Versnel, J. and Kerr, N. (2002) Spirituality unplugged: a review of commonalities and contentions and a resolution. *Canadian Journal of Occupational Therapy, 69*, 5–19.

Uskul, A.K. (2010) Sociocultural aspects of health and illness. In D. French, K. Vedhara, A.A. Kaptein and J. Weinman (eds.) *Health Psychology* (2nd edn.). Oxford: BPS Blackwell.

Uskul, A.K. and Ahmad, F. (2003) Physician-patient interaction: a gynaecology clinic in Turkey. *Social Science & Medicine, 57,* 205–215.

Uskul, A.K. and Hynie, M. (2007) Self-construal and concerns elicited by imagined and real health problems. *Journal of Applied Social Psychology, 37,* 2156–2189.

Uskul, A.K. and Oyserman, D. (2010) When message-frame fits silent cultural-frame, messages feel more persuasive. *Psychology & Health, 25,* 321–337.

Valentine, E.R. (1992) *Conceptual Issues in Psychology.* London: Routledge.

Van Avermaet, E. (1996) Social influence in small groups. In M. Hewstone, W. Stroebe and G.M. Stephenson (eds.) *Introduction to Social Psychology* (2nd edn.). Oxford: Blackwell Publishing.

Van Broeck, N. (1993) Medical play. In *Treatment of Ill Children.* Houten, The Netherlands: Bohn Stafleu Van Loghum.

van de Leur, J.P., van der Schans, C.P., Loef, B.G., Deelman, B.G., Geertzen, J.H. and Zwaveling, J.H. (2004) Discomfort and factual recollection in intensive care unit patients. *Critical Care, 8*(6), R467–R473.

Van Ijzendoorn, M.H. and Schuengel, C. (1999) The development of attachment relationships: infancy and beyond. In D. Messer and S. Millar (eds.) *Exploring Developmental Psychology: From Infancy to Adolescence.* London: Arnold.

Veitia, M.C. and McGahee, C.L. (1995) Ordinary addictions: tobacco and alcohol. In D. Wedding (ed.) *Behaviour and Medicine* (2nd edn.). St Louis, MO: Mosby-Year Book.

Vetter, N.J., Clay, E.I. Philip, A.E. and Strange, R.C. (1977) Anxiety on admission to coronary care unit. *Journal of Psychosomatic Medicine, 21*(1), 73–78.

Vivian, J. and Brown, R. (1995) Prejudice and intergroup conflict. In M. Argyle and A.M. Colman (eds.) *Social Psychology.* London: Longman.

Voss, S. (2002) The winter years: understanding ageing. *Psychology Review, 8*(3), 26–28.

Vossen, H.G., van Os., J. and Lousberg, R. (2006) Evidence that trait-anxiety and trait-depression differentially moderate cortical processing of pain. *Clinical Journal of Pain, 22,* 725–729.

Vowles, K.E. and McCracken, L.M. (2009) Acceptance and values-based action in chronic pain: a study of treatment effectiveness and process. *Journal of Consulting and Clinical Psychology, 76,* 397–407.

Vygotsky, L.S. (1978) *Mind in Society.* Cambridge, MA: Harvard University Press.

Vygotsky, L.S. (1981) The genesis of higher mental functions. In J.V. Wretch (ed.) *The Concept of Activity in Soviet Psychology.* Armonk, NY: Sharpe.

Vygotsky, L.S. (1987) Thinking and speech. In R.W. Rieber and A.S. Carton (eds.) *The Collected Works of L.S. Vygotsky.* New York: Plenum.

Wade, C. and Tavris, C. (1999) *Invitation to Psychology.* New York: Longman.

Walker, J., Payne, S., Smith, P. and Jarrett, N. (2004) *Psychology for Nurses and the Caring Professions* (2nd edn.). Maidenhead, UK: Open University Press/McGraw-Hill Education.

Wallander, J.L., Varni, J.W., Babani, L., Banis, H.T. and Wilcox, K.T. (1989) Family resources as resistance factors for psychological maladjustment in chronically ill and handicapped children. *Journal of Psychology, 14,* 157–173.

Walsh, D., Caraceni, A.T., Fainsinger, R., Foley, K., Glare, P., Goh, C. Lloyd-Williams, M. et al. (2008) *Palliative Medicine.* Philadelphia, PA: Saunders.

Warr, P.B. (1987) Job characteristics and mental health. In P.B. Warr (ed.) *Psychology at Work.* Harmondsworth, UK: Penguin.

Warren, S. and Jahoda, M. (1973) *Attitudes* (2nd edn.). Harmondsworth, UK: Penguin.

Watkins, E.R. (2008) Constructive and unconstructive repetitive thought. *Psychological Bulletin, 134*(2), 163–206.

Watson, J.B. (1913) Psychology as the behaviourist views it. *Psychological Review, 20,* 158–177.

Watson, J.B. (1919) *Psychology from the Standpoint of a Behaviourist.* Philadelphia, PA: J.B. Lippincott.

Watts, F. (1986) Listening to the client. *Changes, 4*(1), 164–167.

Webster, M.E. (1981) Communicating with dying patients. *Nursing Times, 77*(23), 999–1002.

Weddington, W.W., Miller, N.J. and Sweet, D.L. (1984) Anticipatory nausea and vomiting associated with cancer chemotherapy. *Journal of Psychosomatic Research, 28*(1), 73–77.

Weinman, J. (1995) Health psychology. In A.M. Colman (ed.) *Controversies in Psychology.* London: Longman.

Weinstein, N. (1983) Reducing unrealistic optimism about illness susceptibility. *Health Psychology, 2,* 11–20.

Weinstein, N. (1984) Why it won't happen to me: perceptions of risk factors and susceptibility. *Health Psychology, 3,* 431–457.

Wellisch, D., Landsverk, J., Guidera, K., Pasnau, R.O. and Fawzy, F. (1983) Evaluation of psychological problems of the homebound cancer patient. *Psychosomatic Medicine, 45,* 11–21.

Wellman, H.M. (1990) *The Child's Theory of Mind.* Cambridge, MA: MIT Press.

Westedorp, R.G.J. and Kirkwood, T.B.L. (2007) The biology of ageing. In J. Bond, S. Peace, F. Dittmann-Kohli and G. Westerhof (eds.) *Ageing in Society* (3rd edn.). London: Sage Publications.

Wetherell, M. (1982) Cross-cultural studies of minimal groups: implications for the social identity theory of intergroup relations. In H. Tajfel (ed.) *Social Psychology and Intergroup Relations.* Cambridge: Cambridge University Press.

Wetherell, M. (1996) Group conflict and the social psychology of racism. In M. Wetherell (ed.) *Identities, Groups and Social Issues.* London: Sage, in association with the Open University.

Whyte, A. (1998) Weight on our minds. *Nursing Times, 94*(14), 29–31.

Wickelgren, I. (2009) I do not feel your pain. *Scientific American Mind, 20*(5), 51–57.

Wichstrom, L. (1998) Self-concept development during adolescence: do American truths hold for Norwegians? In E. Skoe and A. von der Lippe (eds.) *Personality Development in Adolescence: A Cross National and Life Span Perspective.* London: Routledge.

Wilkinson, S. (1991) Factors which influence how nurses communicate with cancer patients. *Journal of Advanced Nursing, 16*(6), 667–688.

Williams, A.C. deC. (2002) Facial expression of pain: an evolutionary account. *Behavioural and Brain Sciences, 25,* 439–488.

Williams, A.C. deC. (2007a) Chronic pain: investigation. In S. Lindsay and G. Powell (eds.) *The Handbook of Clinical Adult Psychology* (3rd edn.). Hove, UK: Routledge.

Williamson, H. and Wallace, M. (2012) When Treatment Affects Appearance. In N. Rumsey and D. Harcourt (eds.) *The Oxford Handbook of the Psychology of Appearance.* Oxford: Oxford University Press.

Willis, J. (1998) Inner strength. *Nursing Times, 94*(40), 36–37.

Wilson, G.T., O'Leary, K.D., Nathan, P.E. and Clark, L.A. (1996) *Abnormal Psychology: Integrating Perspectives.* Needham Heights, MA: Allyn & Bacon.

Wink, P. (1999) Life review and acceptance in older adulthood. Paper presented at the 3rd Reminiscence and Life Review Conference, New York.

Wink, P. and Schiff, B. (2002) To review or not to review? The role of personality and life events in life review and adaptation to older age. In J.D. Webster and B.K. Haight (eds.) *Critical Advances in Reminiscence Work: From Therapy to Applications.* New York: Springer.

Witte, K. and Allen, M. (2000) A meta-analysis of fear appeals: implications for effective public health campaigns. *Health Education & Behaviour, 27,* 591–615.

Wood, D. and Wood, H. (1996) Vygotsky, tutoring and learning. *Oxford Review of Education, 22,* 5–16.

Wood, D.J., Bruner, J.S. and Ross, G. (1976) The role of tutoring in problem-solving. *Journal of Child Psychology & Psychiatry, 17*, 89–100.

Wood, W. (2000) Attitude change: persuasion and social influence. In S.T. Fiske, D.L. Schachter and C. Zahn-Waxler (eds.) *Annual Review of Psychology, Vol. 51*. Palo Alto, CA: Annual Reviews.

Wood, W., Lundgren, S., Ouellette, J.A., Busceme, S. and Blackstone, T. (1994) Minority influence: a meta-analytic review of social influence processes. *Psychological Bulletin, 115*, 323–345.

Woods, N.F. (1975) Influences on sexual adaptation to mastectomy. *Journal of Obstetric Gynaecololgical and Neonatal Nursing, 4*, 33–37.

World Health Organisation. (1947) *Constitution of the World Health Organisation.* Geneva, Switzerland: WHO.

World Health Organisation. (1982) *Medium Term Programme.* Geneva, Switzerland: WHO.

World Health Organisation. (2003) *Adherence to long-term therapies: Evidence for action.* Geneva, Switzerland: WHO.

Wright, A.J. (2010) The impact of perceived risk on risk-reducing behaviours. In D. French, K. Vedhara, A.A. Kaptein and J. Weinman (eds.) *Health Psychology* (2nd edn.). Oxford: BPS Blackwell.

Wright, S. and Neuberger, J. (2012) Why spirituality is essential for nurses. *Nursing Standard, 26*(40), 19–21.

Yeo, M. and Sawyer, S. (2005) Chronic illness and disability. In R. Viner (ed.) *ABC of Adolescence.* Oxford: Blackwell Publishing.

Zborowski, M. (1952) Cultural components in response to pain. *Journal of Social Issues, 8*, 16–30.

Zeldow, P.B. (1995) Psychodynamic formulations of human behaviour. In D. Wedding (ed.) *Behaviour and Medicine* (2nd edn.). St Louis, MO: Mosby-Year Book.

Zeltzer, L., LeBaron, S. and Zeltzer, P.M. (1984) The effectiveness of behavioural intervention for reduction of nausea and vomiting in children and adolescents receiving chemotherapy. *Journal of Clinical Oncology, 2*(6), 683–690.

Zeman, A. and Torrens, L. (2010) Cognitive assessment. In B.K. Puri and I. Treasaden (eds.) *Psychiatry: An Evidence-Based Text.* London: Hodder Arnold.

Zimbardo, P.G. (1992) *Psychology and Life* (13th edn.). New York: HarperCollins.

Zimbardo, P.G. and Leippe, M. (1991) *The Psychology of Attitude Change and Social Influence.* New York: McGraw-Hill.

Zimbardo, P.G., Banks, W.C., Craig, H. and Jaffe, D. (1973, April 8) A Pirandellian prison: the mind is a formidable jailor. *New York Times Magazine*, 38–60.

Zubieta, J.K., Bueller, J.A., Jackson, L.R., Scott, D.J., Xu, Y., Keppe, R.A., Nichols, T.E. and Stohler, C.S. (2005) Placebo effects mediated by endogenous opioid activity on μ-opioid receptors. *The Journal Neuroscience, 25*(34), 7754–7762.

Zubieta, J.K., Smith, Y.R., Bueller, J.A., Xu, Y., Kilbourn, M.R., Jewett, D.M., Meyer, C.R., Koeppe, R.A. and Stohler, C.S. (2002) μ-Opioid receptor-mediated antinociceptive responses differ in men and women. *The Journal of Neuroscience, 22*, 5100–5107.

Index

··